# Advances in Respiratory Management

*Editor*

MANUEL SÁNCHEZ-LUNA

# CLINICS IN PERINATOLOGY

www.perinatology.theclinics.com

*Consulting Editor*
LUCKY JAIN

December 2021 • Volume 48 • Number 4

**ELSEVIER**

1600 John F. Kennedy Boulevard • Suite 1800 • Philadelphia, Pennsylvania, 19103-2899

http://www.theclinics.com

CLINICS IN PERINATOLOGY Volume 48, Number 4
December 2021 ISSN 0095-5108, ISBN-13: 978-0-323-89728-0

Editor: Kerry Holland
Developmental Editor: Karen Solomon

*Clinics in Perinatology* (ISSN 0095-5108) is published quarterly by Elsevier Inc., 360 Park Avenue South, New York, NY 10010-1710. Months of issue are March, June, September, and December. Business and Editorial Offices: 1600 John F. Kennedy Blvd., Ste. 1800, Philadelphia, PA 19103-2899. Customer Service Office: 3251 Riverport Lane, Maryland Heights, MO 63043. Periodicals postage paid at New York, NY and additional mailing offices. Subscription prices are $321.00 per year (US individuals), $788.00 per year (US institutions), $365.00 per year (Canadian individuals), $835.00 per year (Canadian institutions), $435.00 per year (international individuals), $835.00 per year (international institutions), $100.00 per year (US and Canadian students), and $195.00 per year (International students). International air speed delivery is included in all Clinics subscription prices. All prices are subject to change without notice. **POSTMASTER:** Send address changes to *Clinics in Perinatology*, Elsevier Health Sciences Division, Subscription Customer Service, 3251 Riverport Lane, Maryland Heights, MO 63043. **Customer Service: Telephone: 1-800-654-2452** (U.S. and Canada); **1-314-447-8871** (outside U.S. and Canada). **Fax: 1-314-447-8029. E-mail: journalscustomerservice-usa@elsevier.com** (for print support); **journalsonlinesupport-usa@elsevier.com** (for online support).

*Reprints.* For copies of 100 or more, of articles in this publication, please contact the Commercial Reprints Department, Elsevier Inc., 360 Park Avenue South, New York, NY 10010-1710. Tel. 212-633-3874; Fax: 212-633-3820; E-mail: reprints@elsevier.com.

*Clinics in Perinatology* is also published in Spanish by McGraw-Hill Interamericana Editores S.A., P.O. Box 5-237, 06500 Mexico D.F., Mexico.

*Clinics in Perinatology* is covered in *MEDLINE/PubMed (Index Medicus) Current Contents, Excepta Medica, BIOSIS and ISI/BIOMED.*

# Contributors

## CONSULTING EDITOR

**LUCKY JAIN, MD, MBA**
George W. Brumley Jr Professor and Chairman, Emory University School of
Medicine, Department of Pediatrics, Chief Academic Officer, Children's Healthcare of
Atlanta, Executive Director, Emory + Children's Pediatric Institute, Atlanta, Georgia,
USA

## EDITOR

**MANUEL SÁNCHEZ-LUNA, MD, PhD**
Neonatology Division, Instituto de Investigación Sanitaria Hospital General Universitario
Gregorio Marañón, Complutense University of Madrid, Madrid, Spain

## AUTHORS

**MASSIMO AGOSTI, MD**
Division of Neonatology, "F. Del Ponte" Hospital, Woman and Child Department,
University of Insubria, Varese, Italy

**CLAUDIA AURILIA, MD**
Dipartimento Universitario Scienze della Vita e Sanità Pubblica, Unità Operativa
Complessa di Neonatologia, Fondazione Policlinico Universitario Agostino Gemelli
IRCCS, Rome, Italy

**CHRISTOPHER D. BAKER, MD**
Associate Professor, Section of Pulmonary and Sleep Medicine, Department of Pediatrics,
University of Colorado School of Medicine, Aurora, Colorado, USA

**EDUARDO BANCALARI, MD**
Professor of Pediatrics and OB/GYN, Director, Division of Neonatology, Department of
Pediatrics, University of Miami Miller School of Medicine, Miami, Florida, USA

**JENNIFER BECK, PhD**
Department of Critical Care, St. Michael's Hospital, Keenan Research Centre for
Biomedical Science of St. Michael's Hospital, Department of Pediatrics, University
of Toronto, Member, Institute for Biomedical Engineering and Science
Technology (iBEST) at Ryerson University and St-Michael's Hospital, Toronto,
Ontario, Canada

**GUSZTAV BELTEKI, MD, PhD, FRCPCH**
Neonatal Intensive Care Unit, The Rosie Hospital, Cambridge University Hospitals NHS
Foundation Trust, Cambridge, United Kingdom

**ILIA BRESESTI, MD**
Division of Neonatology, "V.Buzzi" Children's Hospital, ASST-FBF-Sacco, Milan, Italy

**MARLIES BRUCKNER, MD**
Centre for the Studies of Asphyxia and Resuscitation, Royal Alexandra Hospital, Department of Pediatrics, University of Alberta, Edmonton, Alberta, Canada; Division of Neonatology, Department of Pediatrics and Adolescent Medicine, Medical University of Graz, Graz, Austria

**ROBERTA CENTORRINO, MD**
Physiopathology and Therapeutic Innovation Unit-INSERM U999, Paris Saclay University, Assistant Professor (non-tenured) and Senior Fellow, Division of Pediatrics and Neonatal Critical Care, "A.Béclère" Medical Centre, Paris Saclay University Hospitals, APHP, Paris, France; Service de Pédiatrie et Réanimation Néonatale, Hôpital "A. Béclère"- GHU Paris Saclay, APHP, Clamart Paris-IDF, France

**NELSON CLAURE, MSc, PhD**
Professor of Pediatrics and Biomedical Engineering, Director, Neonatal Respiratory Physiology Laboratory, Division of Neonatology, Department of Pediatrics, University of Miami Miller School of Medicine, Miami, Florida, USA

**CARLO DANI**
Professor, Division of Neonatology, Careggi University Hospital of Florence, Department of Neurosciences, Psychology, Drug Research and Child Health, University of Florence, Florence, Italy

**PETER G. DAVIS, MD, FRACP**
Newborn Research Centre and Neonatal Services, The Royal Women's Hospital, Department of Obstetrics and Gynaecology, The University of Melbourne, Clinical Sciences, Murdoch Children's Research Institute, Melbourne, Australia

**DANIELE DE LUCA, MD, PhD**
Full Professor of Neonatology, Chief of the Division of Pediatrics and Neonatal Critical Care, "A.Béclère" Medical Centre, Paris Saclay University Hospitals, APHP, Physiopathology and Therapeutic Innovation Unit-INSERM U999, Paris Saclay University, Paris, France; Service de Pédiatrie et Réanimation Néonatale, Hôpital "A. Béclère"- GHU Paris Saclay, APHP, Clamart Paris-IDF, France

**CAMILLA GIZZI, MD, PhD**
Head of Paediatric and Neonatology Unit, 'Sandro Pertini' Hospital, Rome, Italy

**NOELIA GONZÁLEZ-PACHECO, MD, PhD**
Neonatology Division, Instituto de Investigación Sanitaria Hospital General Universitario Gregorio Marañón, Complutense University of Madrid, Madrid, Spain

**ANNE GREENOUGH, MD**
Professor of Neonatology and Clinical Respiratory Physiology, Department of Women and Children's Health, School of Life Course Sciences, Faculty of Life Sciences and Medicine, King's College London, Asthma UK Centre for Allergic Mechanisms in Asthma, NIHR Biomedical Research Centre Based at Guy's and St Thomas' NHS Foundation Trust and King's College London, London, United Kingdom

**SATYAN LAKSHMINRUSIMHA, MD**
Department of Pediatrics, UC Davis Children's Hospital, Sacramento, California, USA

**ALESSANDRA LIO, MD**
Dipartimento Universitario Scienze della Vita e Sanità Pubblica, Unità Operativa Complessa di Neonatologia, Fondazione Policlinico Universitario Agostino Gemelli IRCCS, Rome, Italy

**GIANLUCA LISTA, MD, PhD**
Division of Neonatology, "V.Buzzi" Children's Hospital, ASST-FBF-Sacco, Milan, Italy

**CORRADO MORETTI, MD**
Professor, Emeritus Consultant in Paediatrics, Policlinico Umberto I, Sapienza University of Rome, Rome, Italy; President of Union of European Neonatal and Perinatal Societies (UENPS)

**COLIN J. MORLEY, MD, FRCPCH**
Neonatal Intensive Care Unit, The Rosie Hospital, Cambridge University Hospitals NHS Foundation Trust, Cambridge, United Kingdom

**LOUISE S. OWEN, MD, FRACP**
Newborn Research Centre and Neonatal Services, The Royal Women's Hospital, Department of Obstetrics and Gynaecology, The University of Melbourne, Clinical Sciences, Murdoch Children's Research Institute, Melbourne, Australia

**ANGELA PALADINI, MD**
Dipartimento Universitario Scienze della Vita e Sanità Pubblica, Unità Operativa Complessa di Neonatologia, Fondazione Policlinico Universitario Agostino Gemelli IRCCS, Rome, Italy

**CHRISTOPH M. RÜEGGER, MD**
Newborn Research, Department of Neonatology, University Hospital Zurich, University of Zurich, Zurich, Switzerland

**MANUEL SÁNCHEZ-LUNA, MD, PhD**
Neonatology Division, Instituto de Investigación Sanitaria Hospital General Universitario Gregorio Marañón, Complutense University of Madrid, Madrid, Spain

**MARTÍN SANTOS-GONZÁLEZ, DVM, PhD**
Medical and Surgical Research Unit, Instituto de Investigación Sanitaria Puerta de Hierro–Segovia de Arana, Madrid, Spain

**GEORG M. SCHMÖLZER, MD, PhD**
Centre for the Studies of Asphyxia and Resuscitation, Royal Alexandra Hospital, Department of Pediatrics, University of Alberta, Edmonton, Alberta, Canada

**CHRISTER SINDERBY, PhD**
Department of Critical Care, St. Michael's Hospital, Keenan Research Centre for Biomedical Science of St. Michael's Hospital, Member, Institute for Biomedical Engineering and Science Technology (iBEST) at Ryerson University and St-Michael's Hospital, Department of Medicine and Interdepartmental Division of Critical Care Medicine, University of Toronto, Toronto, Ontario, Canada

**MILENA TANA, MD**
Dipartimento Universitario Scienze della Vita e Sanità Pubblica, Unità Operativa Complessa di Neonatologia, Fondazione Policlinico Universitario Agostino Gemelli IRCCS, Rome, Italy

**FRANCISCO TENDILLO-CORTIJO, DVM, PhD**
Medical and Surgical Research Unit, Instituto de Investigación Sanitaria Puerta de Hierro–Segovia de Arana, Madrid, Spain

**CHIARA TIRONE, MD**
Dipartimento Universitario Scienze della Vita e Sanità Pubblica, Unità Operativa Complessa di Neonatologia, Fondazione Policlinico Universitario Agostino Gemelli IRCCS, Rome, Italy

**GIOVANNI VENTO, PROF**
Dipartimento Universitario Scienze della Vita e Sanità Pubblica, Unità Operativa Complessa di Neonatologia, Fondazione Policlinico Universitario Agostino Gemelli IRCCS, Università Cattolica del Sacro Cuore, Rome, Italy

**EMMA E. WILLIAMS, MBBS**
Clinical Research Fellow, Department of Women and Children's Health, School of Life Course Sciences, Faculty of Life Sciences and Medicine, King's College London, London, United Kingdom

# Contents

Very preterm infants have difficulties establishing effective breathing at birth because their lungs are structurally immature, surfactant-deficient, and not supported by a stiff chest wall. In the past decade, there has been an increased understanding of respiratory physiologic changes during fetal-to-neonatal transition, which could be used to improve respiratory support in the delivery room (DR). This review aims to describe the physiologic changes at birth and how these can be used during respiratory support in the DR.

This study reviews the mechanisms of action and physiologic effects of nasal continuous positive airway pressure (nCPAP) and high-flow nasal cannula (HFNC) in preterm infants with respiratory distress syndrome, discusses the main characteristics of available devices and patients' interfaces, reports on risk of failure and possible adverse effects, and summarizes clinical evidence regarding effectiveness for preventing mechanical ventilation as primary respiratory support or after extubation in the neonatal intensive care unit. nCPAP is preferred to HFNC as primary mode of noninvasive respiratory support in preterm infants with respiratory distress syndrome, whereas HFNC is an effective alternative to nCPAP after extubation.

Nasal or noninvaisve intermittent positive pressure ventilation (NIPPV) refers to well-established noninvasive respiratory support strategies combining a continuous distending pressure with intermittent pressure increases. Uncertainty remains regarding the benefits provided by the various devices and techniques used to generate NIPPV. Our included meta-analyses of trials comparing NIPPV with continuous positive airway pressure (CPAP) in preterm infants demonstrate that both primary and postextubation NIPPV are superior to CPAP to prevent respiratory failure leading to additional ventilatory support. This short-term benefit is associated with a reduction in bronchopulmonary dysplasia, but not with mortality. Benefits are greatest when ventilator-generated, synchronized NIPPV is used.

Avoiding MV is a critical goal in neonatal respiratory care. Different modes of noninvasive respiratory support beyond nasal CPAP, such as nasal intermittent positive pressure ventilation (NIPPV) and synchronized NIPPV (SNIPPV), may further reduce intubation rates. SNIPPV offers consistent benefits over nonsynchronized techniques such as a more efficient positive pressure transmission to the lung, an effective increase in transpulmonary pressure during ventilation, and a better stabilization of the chest wall during inspiration. This review discusses mechanisms of action, benefits and limitations of synchronized noninvasive ventilation, describes the different modes of synchronization, and analyzes properties and clinical results.

Noninvasive high-frequency oscillatory (NHFOV) and percussive (NHFPV) ventilation represent 2 nonconventional techniques that may be useful in selected neonatal patients. We offer here a comprehensive review of physiology, mechanics, and biology for both techniques. As NHFOV is the technique with the wider experience, we also provided a meta-analysis of available clinical trials, suggested ventilatory parameters boundaries, and proposed a physiology-based clinical protocol to use NHFOV.

Patient-ventilator asynchrony is very common in newborns. Achieving synchrony is quite challenging because of small tidal volumes, high respiratory rates, and the presence of leaks. Leaks also cause unreliable monitoring of respiratory metrics. In addition, ventilator adjustment must take into account that infants have strong vagal reflexes, and demonstrate central apnea and periodic breathing, with a high variability in breathing pattern. Neurally adjusted ventilatory assist (NAVA) is a mode of ventilation whereby the timing and amount of ventilatory assist is controlled by the patient's own neural respiratory drive. As NAVA uses the diaphragm electrical activity (Edi) as the controller signal, it is possible to deliver synchronized assist, both invasively and non-invasively (NIV-NAVA), to follow the variability in breathing pattern, and to monitor patient respiratory drive, independent of leaks. This article provides an updated review of the physiology and the scientific literature pertaining to the use of (NAVA) in children (neonatal and pediatric age groups). Both the invasive NAVA and NIV -NAVA publications since 2016 are summarized, as well as the use of Edi monitoring. Overall, the use of NAVA and Edi monitoring is feasible and safe. Compared with conventional ventilation, NAVA improves patient-ventilator interaction, provides lower peak inspiratory pressure, and lowers oxygen requirements.

Evidence from several studies suggests improved comfort, less sedation requirements, less apnea, and some trends towards reduced length of stay, and more successful extubation.

Respiratory care of premature neonates has witnessed substantial advances in the last two decades and has played a crucial role in decreasing early mortality in this population. The use of synchronized ventilation in the neonatal population was delayed as compared to adults, mainly because of technical reasons. Coordinating the infant's respiratory effort and the onset of mechanical ventilation in the neonatal population has requested high sensitivity instruments, but to date there are several modalities available, This review outlines advances in techniques of synchronization and provides an overview of the modes of synchronized mechanical ventilation currently in use in neonatal units.

Volume-targeted ventilation (VTV) has been increasingly used in neonatology. In systemic reviews, VTV has been shown to reduce the risk of neonatal morbidities and improve long-term outcomes. It is adaptive ventilation using complex computer algorithms to deliver ventilator inflations with expired tidal volumes close to a target set by clinicians. Significant endotracheal tube leak and patient–ventilator interactions may complicate VTV and make ventilator parameters and waveforms difficult to interpret. In this article, we review the rationale for using VTV and the evidence supporting its use and provide practical advice for clinicians ventilating newborn infants.

Most extremely premature infants have respiratory instability that can manifest as frequent episodes of intermittent hypoxemia. Although caregivers target clinically recommended ranges of arterial oxygen saturation (oxygen saturation as measured by pulse oximetry [$Spo_2$]), consistent maintenance of these ranges is not always achieved. Excessive administration of supplemental oxygen combined with limited staff resources increases exposure to extreme $Spo_2$ levels. In this population, exposure to hyperoxemia and prolonged episodes of intermittent hypoxemia have been associated with damage to the eye and lung and impaired neurodevelopment. To improve $Spo_2$ targeting, various systems for automated control of inspired oxygen have been developed recently.

High-frequency ventilation (HFV) is an alternative to conventional mechanical ventilation, with theoretic benefits of less risk of ventilator lung injury and more effectivity in washout $CO_2$. Previous clinical studies have not demonstrated advantages of HFV in preterm infants compared with conventional ventilation, so rescue HFV has been used when severe respiratory insufficiency needs aggressive ventilator settings in immature infants. Today it is possible to measure, set directly, and fix tidal volume, which can protect the immature lung from large volumes and fluctuations of the tidal volume. This strategy can be used in preterm infants with respiratory failure needing invasive ventilation.

Mechanical ventilation can be life-saving for the premature infant, but is often injurious to immature and underdeveloped lungs. Lung injury is caused by atelectrauma, oxygen toxicity, and volutrauma. Lung protection must include appropriate lung recruitment starting in the delivery suite and throughout mechanical ventilation. Strategies include open lung ventilation, positive end-expiratory pressure, and volume-targeted ventilation. Respiratory function monitoring, such as capnography and ventilator graphics, provides clinicians with continuous real-time information and an adjunct to optimize lung-protective ventilatory strategies. Further research is needed to assess which lung-protective strategies result in a decrease in long-term respiratory morbidity.

For infants with the most severe forms of chronic lung disease, regardless of etiology, chronic mechanical ventilation can provide stability, reduce acute respiratory events, and alleviate increased work of breathing. This approach prioritizes the baby's growth and development during early life. Once breathing comfortably, these infants can tolerate developmental therapies with the goal of achieving the best neurocognitive outcomes possible.

For the newborns needing respiratory support at 36 weeks postmenstrual age, regardless of the type of ventilation used, it is critical to take into account the mechanics properties of both airways and lungs affected by severe bronchopulmonary dysplasia (sBPD). Ventilator strategies, settings, and weaning must change dramatically after sBPD is established, but to date there is almost no high-quality evidence base supporting a specific approach to guide the optimal ventilator management and weaning in patients with sBPD. Weaning from invasive mechanical ventilation, management of the immediately postextubation period, and weaning from noninvasive ventilation in patients with sBPD are the topics covered in this chapter.

## PROGRAM OBJECTIVE

The goal of *Clinics in Perinatology* is to keep practicing perinatologists, neonatologists, obstetricians, practicing physicians and residents up to date with current clinical practice in perinatology by providing timely articles reviewing the state of the art in patient care.

## TARGET AUDIENCE

Perinatologists, neonatologists, obstetricians, practicing physicians, residents and healthcare professionals who provide patient care utilizing findings from *Clinics in Perinatology*.

## LEARNING OBJECTIVES

Upon completion of this activity, participants will be able to:
1. Review respiratory changes that occur during the transition from the in-utero to postnatal life.
2. Discuss invasive and noninvasive methods of respiratory support.
3. Recognize the challenges and risks of chronic mechanical ventilation.

## ACCREDITATION

The Elsevier Office of Continuing Medical Education (EOCME) is accredited by the Accreditation Council for Continuing Medical Education (ACCME) to provide continuing medical education for physicians.

The EOCME designates this journal-based CME activity for a maximum of 13 *AMA PRA Category 1 Credit*(s)™. Physicians should claim only the credit commensurate with the extent of their participation in the activity.

All other health care professionals requesting continuing education credit for this enduring material will be issued a certificate of participation.

## DISCLOSURE OF CONFLICTS OF INTEREST

The EOCME assesses conflict of interest with its instructors, faculty, planners, and other individuals who are in a position to control the content of CME activities. All relevant conflicts of interest that are identified are thoroughly vetted by EOCME for fair balance, scientific objectivity, and patient care recommendations. EOCME is committed to providing its learners with CME activities that promote improvements or quality in healthcare and not a specific proprietary business or a commercial interest.

**The planning committee, staff, authors and editors listed below have identified no financial relationships or relationships to products or devices they or their spouse/life partner have with commercial interest related to the content of this CME activity:**

Massimo Agosti, MD; Claudia Aurilia, MD; Christopher D. Baker, MD; Ilia Bresesti, MD; Marlies Bruckner, MD; Roberta Centorrino, MD; Regina Chavous-Gibson, MSN, RN; Carlo Dani, MD; Peter G. Davis, MD, FRACP; Camilla Gizzi, MD, PhD; Noelia González-Pacheco, MD, PhD; Satyan Lakshminrusimha, MD; Alessandra Lio, MD; Gianluca Lista, MD, PhD; Louise S. Owen, MD, FRACP; Angela Paladini, MD; Christoph M. Rüegger, MD; Martín Santos-González, DVM, PhD; Georg M. Schmölzer, MD, PhD; Jeyanthi Surendrakumar; Milena Tana, MD; Francisco Tendillo-Cortijo, DVM, PhD; Reni Thomas; Chiara Tirone, MD; Giovanni Vento, MD; Emma E. Williams, MBBS

**The planning committee, staff, authors and editors listed below have identified financial relationships or relationships to products or devices they or their spouse/life partner have with commercial interest related to the content of this CME activity:**

Eduardo Bancalari, MD: Royalties/Patent Beneficiary: Vyaire Medical

Jennifer Beck, PhD: Royalties/Patent Beneficiary and Consultant: Maquet Critical Care; Ownership Interest: Neurovent Research, Inc.

Gusztav Belteki, MD, PhD, FRCPCH: Consultant: Vyaire Medical, Dräger Medical

Nelson Claure, MSc, PhD: Royalties/Patent Beneficiary: Vyaire Medical

Daniele De Luca, MD, PhD: Researcher: Vyaire Medical

Anne Greenough, MD: Researcher/Independent Contractor/Speaker: Abbott Laboratories, SLE

Corrado Moretti, MD: Consultant: GINEVRI srl

Colin J. Morley, MD, FRCPCH: Consultant: Fisher & Paykel Healthcare

Manuel Sánchez-Luna, MD, PhD: Consultant/advisor: Dräger Medical

Christer Sinderby, PhD: Royalties/Patent Beneficiary and Consultant: Maquet Critical Care; Ownership Interest: Neurovent Research, Inc.

## UNAPPROVED/OFF-LABEL USE DISCLOSURE
The EOCME requires CME faculty to disclose to the participants:
1. When products or procedures being discussed are off-label, unlabelled, experimental, and/or investigational (not US Food and Drug Administration [FDA] approved); and
2. Any limitations on the information presented, such as data that are preliminary or that represent ongoing research, interim analyses, and/or unsupported opinions. Faculty may discuss information about pharmaceutical agents that is outside of FDA-approved labelling. This information is intended solely for CME and is not intended to promote off-label use of these medications. If you have any questions, contact the medical affairs department of the manufacturer for the most recent prescribing information.

## TO ENROLL
To enroll in the *Clinics in Perinatology* Continuing Medical Education program, call customer service at 1-800-654-2452 or sign up online at http://www.theclinics.com/home/cme. The CME program is available to subscribers for an additional annual fee of USD 265.00.

## METHOD OF PARTICIPATION
In order to claim credit, participants must complete the following:
1. Complete enrolment as indicated above.
2. Read the activity.
3. Complete the CME Test and Evaluation. Participants must achieve a score of 70% on the test. All CME Tests and Evaluations must be completed online.

## CME INQUIRIES/SPECIAL NEEDS
For all CME inquiries or special needs, please contact elsevierCME@elsevier.com.

# CLINICS IN PERINATOLOGY

---

**SERIES OF RELATED INTEREST**

*Pediatric Clinics of North America*
https://www.pediatric.theclinics.com/
*Obstetrics and Gynecology Clinics of North America*
https://www.obgyn.theclinics.com/

---

**THE CLINICS ARE AVAILABLE ONLINE!**
Access your subscription at:
www.theclinics.com

# Foreword

# The Evolving Respiratory Management of Neonates

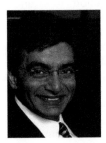

Lucky Jain, MD, MBA
*Consulting Editor*

It is hard to deny the extraordinary influence respiratory ailments and their management have had on the entire discipline of neonatology. The quest to save premature babies and reduce the limit of viability has relied squarely on advances in respiratory management. As we approach the biologic limits at which extrauterine existence appears unlikely, a new quest has begun: achieving handicap-free survival with minimal lung injury.

The journey to better respiratory support accelerated nearly 60 years ago when it became clear that surfactant had a role in preventing hyaline membrane disease.[1] There was also an emerging understanding of the origin of fetal lung fluid and the mechanism(s) involved in its clearance after birth around the same time.[2,3] Simultaneously, assisted ventilation and oxygen supplementation ushered in a new era in respiratory management with dramatically improved survival. However, as survival improved, complications began to tarnish the success and dampen enthusiasm around survival of premature infants. Two of these complications were particularly prominent, the occurrence of chronic lung disease and blindness.[4,5] Much has been written about the checkered history of retinopathy of prematurity, and the reader is referred to many excellent reviews on the topic.[4] The first clear documentation of a new type of lung disease in babies who survived hyaline membrane disease came from Dr Northway and colleagues[5] in 1967 with a classification of the disease severity and its connection to mechanical ventilation used early in life.

It is now clear that some degree of lung function impairment can be seen in up to 10,000 premature infants in the United States and many more worldwide.[6] These infants struggle with secondary complications throughout their infancy, childhood, and adult years. In recent years, the search for identifying underlying predisposition to bronchopulmonary dysplasia has intensified, just as the quest for modes of respiratory support that reduce risk of permanent lung injury has also intensified. It has become

Clin Perinatol 48 (2021) xv–xviii
https://doi.org/10.1016/j.clp.2021.09.001

clear that individual responses are modulated by genetic, epigenetic, and environmental factors. This multifactorial origin and complexity of the disease may also explain the dismal track record of numerous randomized controlled trials of pharmacologic agents, ventilation strategies, nutritional interventions, and more. That is why the focus has shifted to primary prevention (**Fig. 1**).[6] Such an approach would require refinement of endotypes and outcome measures; it would also require precision medicine approaches targeting specific molecular pathways underlying lung injury.

Parallel to these approaches, there is also the hope that efforts to extend gestation using extracorporeal systems will get sophisticated enough to support extrauterine life, allowing the lungs to develop normally. Partridge and colleagues[7] reported the development of an innovative system that closely reproduces the environment of the womb by incorporating a pumpless oxygenator circuit connected to the fetus of a lamb via an umbilical cord interface that is maintained within a closed "amniotic fluid" circuit (**Fig. 2**).[7] In this study published a few years ago, investigators showed that immature fetal lambs that are developmentally equivalent to extremely premature human infants can be physiologically supported in this extrauterine environment for up to 4 weeks, and they demonstrate normal somatic growth, lung maturation, and brain growth.[7]

In this issue of the *Clinics in Perinatology*, Dr Manuel Sanchez-Luna has brought together clinicians and scientists from all over the world to share their expertise and knowledge about advances in the respiratory management of the newborn. As always,

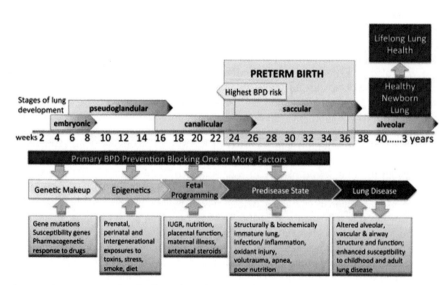

**Fig. 1.** Primary prevention for bronchopulmonary dysplasia (BPD): windows of opportunity. A host of antenatal and postnatal factors can predispose the structurally and biochemically immature lung to the development of BPD. BPD most commonly occurs in extremely premature infants born during the canalicular or early saccular phases of lung development. However, not all extremely premature infants develop BPD, suggesting BPD can be prevented. Shown here are potential windows of opportunity for the primary prevention of BPD. IUGR, intrauterine growth retardation. Reprinted with permission of the American Thoracic Society. Copyright © 2021 American Thoracic Society. All rights reserved.

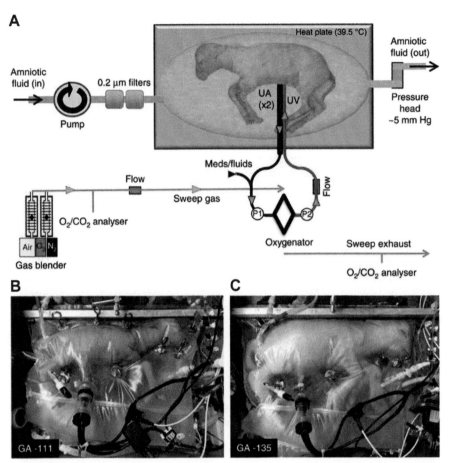

**Fig. 2.** Umbilical artery-umbilical vein biobag system design: an extrauterine system to phys-iologically support the extremely premature lamb. (*A*) Circuit and system components consisting of a pumpless, low-resistance oxygenator circuit, a closed fluid environment with continuous fluid exchange, and an umbilical vascular interface. (*B*) Representative lamb cannulated at 107 days of gestation and on day 4 of support. (*C*) The same lamb on day 28 of support illustrating somatic growth and maturation. UA, Umbilical artery; UV, Umbilical vein. With permission from Partridge EA, Davey MG, Hornick MA, McGovern PE, Mejaddam AY, Vrecenak JD, Mesas-Burgos C, Olive A, Caskey RC, Weiland TR, Han J, Schupper AJ, Connelly JT, Dysart KC, Rychik J, Hedrick HL, Peranteau WH, Flake AW. An extra-uterine system to physiologically support the extreme premature lamb. Nat Commun. 2017;8:15112. https://doi.org/10.1038/ncomms15112. (Page 4).

I am grateful to the publishing staff at Elsevier, including Kerry Holland and Karen Justine Solomon, for their support in bringing this important publication to you.

Lucky Jain, MD, MBA
Emory University School of Medicine, and
Children's Healthcare of Atlanta
1760 Haygood Drive, W409
Atlanta, GA 30322, USA

*E-mail address:*
ljain@emory.edu

## REFERENCES

1. Avery ME, Mead J. Surface properties in relation to atelectasis and hyaline membrane disease. Am J Dis Child 1959;97:517–23.
2. Adams FH, Fujiwara T, Rowshan G. The nature and origin of the fluid in the fetal lamb lung. J Pediatr 1963;63:881–8.
3. Jain L. 50 years ago in the Journal of Pediatrics: the nature and origin of fluid in the fetal lamb lung. J Pediatr 2013;163:1277.
4. Terry TL. Ocular maldevelopment in extremely premature infants: retrolental fibroplasia, VI, general consideration. JAMA 1945;128:582–5.
5. Northway WH, Rosan RC, Porter DY. Pulmonary disease following respirator therapy of hyaline-membrane disease. Bronchopulmonary dysplasia. N Engl J Med 1967;276:357–68.
6. McEvoy CT, Jain L, Schmidt B, et al. Bronchopulmonary dysplasia: NHLBI Workshop on the Primary Prevention of Chronic Lung Diseases. Ann Am Thorac Soc 2014;11:S146–53.
7. Partridge EA, Davey MG, Hornick MA, et al. An extra-uterine system to physiologically support the extreme premature lamb. Nat Commun 2017;25(8):15112.

# Preface

# A New Era in the Respiratory Support of the Sick and Immature Neonate

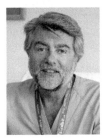

Manuel Sánchez-Luna, MD, PhD
*Editor*

We are living today in a new era in respiratory support of the sick and immature neonate. From the knowledge that ventilator-induced lung injury can be prevented or reduced due to a better understanding of the respiratory physiology, therapies, and more friendly medical devices, a "new respiratory distress syndrome (RDS) of the prematurity" is the leading respiratory problem and represents, instead of the old hyaline membrane disease, a new disease due to the multiple mechanisms involved in the respiratory insufficiency of the immaturity.

This new respiratory support philosophy starts at the very first moments after delivery. The combination of a friendly establishment of the lung volume, minimal invasive support, and early and less invasive rescue surfactant replacement defines this new era. Also, the technology is helping to prevent lung injury due to a better understanding of the respiratory failure, mostly in the more immature infants, but in some cases in the term infant as well. In this issue, we want to update how respiratory support should be focus today based on new physiology and clinical studies.

The issue starts with a review of the transition from the in utero to postnatal life, and most of the information about how this transition occurs is very recent and changing our routine practice. Noninvasive ventilation is the most frequently used respiratory support today. Even so, some of this support is based on weak scientific data and on the availability of adequate equipment to apply it. Nasal continuous positive airway pressure support is probably the best option to prevent invasive mechanical ventilation after delivery, and together with early surfactant administration, can reduce the risk of bronchopulmonary dysplasia. Also, noninvasive nasal ventilation can be an alternative to invasive mechanical ventilation and to decrease lung injury. In a separate article, synchronized nasal ventilation and high-frequency nasal ventilation are discussed,

perinatology.theclinics.com

with new practical information. New data from clinical trials will support the use of Neurally adjusted ventilatory assist (NAVA) synchronization in certain situations. An evidence-based and physiology-based approach to NAVA, invasive and noninvasive, is the goal of this article. Volume target ventilation is also discussed in this issue, as this modality today represents the most friendly and beneficial modality of invasive conventional ventilation. A specific article reviews high-frequency oscillatory ventilation, used most of the time as a rescue therapy. This modality is new alternative to invasive conventional ventilation due to the possibility of combining it with volume guarantee to control the tidal volume and protect the immature lung. Finally, chronic mechanical ventilation in sick neonates, an infrequent but still challenging situation, is discussed as well as the weaning of this in this risky population.

I hope that in this issue we cover most of the recent knowledge, to better understand this new philosophy of respiratory support from early lung stabilization and protective support to prevention of ventilator-induced lung injury. A better understanding of respiratory failure will improve the efficacy of the support to the breath of the immature and sick neonate.

Manuel Sánchez-Luna, MD, PhD
Director of the Neonatology Division
University Hospital Gregorio Marañon
Professor of Pediatrics
Complutense University of Madrid
O'Donnell 48
Madrid 28009, Spain

*E-mail address:*
msluna@salud.madrid.org

# Physiologic Changes during Neonatal Transition and the Influence of Respiratory Support

Marlies Bruckner, MD[a,b,c], Georg M. Schmölzer, MD, PhD[a,b,c],*

## KEYWORDS

- Neonate • Immediate transition • Respiratory support • Resuscitation • Physiology

## KEY POINTS

- To successfully complete fetal-to-neonatal transition newborn infants have to undergo physiologic changes including lung liquid clearance, generation of functional residual capacity, and start of breathing to enable gas exchange and tissue oxygenation.
- Failed or incomplete immediate transition indicates provision of medical support including stimulation, positive pressure ventilation, oxygen supplementation, and/or in very few cases chest compression.
- As medical intervention triggers physiologic reactions health care providers must understand and consider the newborn infants' physiology when performing neonatal resuscitation.
- Health care providers should be aware of physiologic changes including different breathing patterns, the activation of the trigeminocardiac reflex, and glottis closure especially in preterm infants when performing neonatal resuscitation.

No preprints requested.

Conflict of Interest: None.

Author's Contributions: Conception and design, G.M.S. and M.B.; drafting of the manuscript, G.M.S. and M.B.; critical revision of the manuscript, G.M.S. and M.B.; final approval of the manuscript, G.M.S. and M.B.

Very preterm infants have difficulties establishing effective breathing at birth because their lungs are structurally immature, surfactant-deficient, and not supported by a stiff chest wall. In the past decade, there has been an increased understanding of respiratory physiologic changes during fetal-to-neonatal transition, which could be used to improve respiratory support in the delivery room (DR). This review aims to describe the physiologic changes at birth and how these can be used during respiratory support in the DR.

[a] Centre for the Studies of Asphyxia and Resuscitation, Royal Alexandra Hospital, 10240 Kingsway Avenue, Edmonton, Alberta, T5H 3V9, Canada; [b] Department of Pediatrics, University of Alberta, Edmonton, Alberta, Canada; [c] Division of Neonatology, Department of Pediatrics and Adolescent Medicine, Medical University of Graz, Auenbruggerplatz 30, Graz, Austria

* Corresponding author.

E-mail address: georg.schmoelzer@me.com

Clin Perinatol 48 (2021) 697–709

https://doi.org/10.1016/j.clp.2021.07.001

0095-5108/21/© 2021 Elsevier Inc. All rights reserved.

perinatology.theclinics.com

## INTRODUCTION

Very preterm infants have difficulties establishing effective breathing at birth because their lungs are structurally immature, surfactant-deficient, and not supported by a stiff chest wall.[1] Indeed, 10% of newborn infants require respiratory support at birth, which is increasing with decreasing gestational age.[2] The International Liaison Committee on Resuscitation recommends to provide positive pressure ventilation (PPV) for newborns who are apneic, bradycardic, or demonstrate inadequate respiratory effort immediately after birth.[3,4] The purpose of PPV is to create a functional residual capacity (FRC), deliver an adequate tidal volume to facilitate gas exchange, and stimulate breathing while minimizing lung injury.[1] In the past decade, there has been an increased understanding of respiratory physiologic changes during fetal-to-neonatal transition, which could be used to improve respiratory support in the delivery room (DR). This review aims to describe the physiologic changes at birth and how these can be used during respiratory support in the DR.

## PHYSIOLOGIC CHANGES AFTER BIRTH: BACKGROUND
### Clearance of Lung Liquid

Before birth, the airways are liquid-filled and the lungs take no part in gas exchange, which occurs across the placenta. Clearance of lung liquid occurs during a 3-phase process (1) airway liquid clearance, (2) liquid accumulation within the lung's interstitial tissue compartment, and (3) respiratory gas exchange and metabolic homeostasis.[5-7] During the first phase, no gas exchange occurs because the distal airways are liquid-filled airway, with a focus on liquid clearance and movement of liquid through the airways and across the distal airway wall. The focus during this phase is moving liquid through the airways with the goal of uniformly aerating gas exchange regions (**Fig. 1**).[5-7] In rabbit pups, movement of lung liquid was ~9 mL/kg/s resulting in near-complete airway liquid clearance within the first 3 to 5 breaths (or 15–30

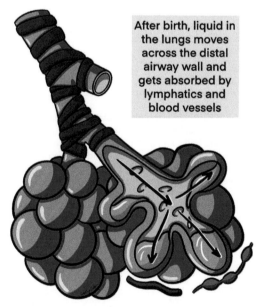

After birth, liquid in the lungs moves across the distal airway wall and gets absorbed by lymphatics and blood vessels

**Fig. 1.** Clearance of Lung Liquid.

seconds).[7] Once the liquid is absorbed, FRC is established with $\sim 3$ mL/kg per breath to a total FRC of 15 mL/kg.[6] During the second phase, liquid, which is leaving the airways, accumulates within the interstitial tissue compartment and results in a transient increase in interstitial tissue pressures and the probability of liquid reentry into the airways, thereby compromising gas exchange.[5-8] Interstitial tissue pressures gradually decrease over 4 to 6 hours due to liquid clearance from the tissue via the lymphatic and blood vessels.[6,8] The third phase occurs after immediate transition, when the liquid has been cleared from the tissue; respiratory support should primarily focus on gas exchange, uniform ventilation, and maintaining respiratory homeostasis.[5-7]

### Gas Exchange

Immediately after birth, the main objective is to clear the airways of liquid because gas exchange can only occur once the liquid in the distal airways is absorbed.[6,9-11] The exchange of carbon dioxide ($CO_2$) and oxygen ($O_2$) should reach a steady state after aeration of the lungs. $CO_2$ produced in the tissue is transported to the lung and exhaled from the lung due to a $P_{CO_2}$ gradient between alveolar capillaries and alveoli, which can only be detected once the lung is aerated.[9-11] In healthy term infants, immediately after birth no $CO_2$ can be detected, which occurs within the next 5 to 10 breaths (or 5–21 seconds).[10,11] Similarly, in preterm infants, the initial $CO_2$ is low and increases over several minutes.[12] However, spontaneously breathing preterm infants achieve lung aeration using different breathing patterns, and levels of expired $CO_2$ vary with different breathing patterns, gestational ages, and over time.[13]

### Crying and Breathing

Most preterm infants cry and breathe at birth,[14,15] leading to establishment of FRC and initiation of spontaneous breathing. To establish FRC, preterm infants use different breathing patterns including normal breathing, crying, grunting, expiratory breaking, and panting.[16,17] Preterm infants frequently brake their expiration by using crying and/or grunting in the first minutes of life. Indeed, crying is the predominant breathing pattern in up to 62 (36–77)%.[16,17] Immediately after birth, most very preterm infants treated with continuous positive airway pressure frequently prolong their expiration by braking the expiratory flow and/or use expiratory breath holds to defend their lung volume.[16,17] As newborns have a very compliant chest wall, it is likely that expiratory braking mechanisms help maintain FRC.[16,17]

There are 2 mechanisms for stopping or slowing expiratory flow and maintaining an elevated lung volume during expiration. Diaphragmatic postinspiratory activity slows the rate of lung deflation by counteracting its passive recoil, and closure or narrowing of the larynx increases the resistance to expiration.[16,17] During braked expiration, the closed or narrowed glottis, with increased intrapulmonary pressure from abdominal muscle contraction, causes the airway pressure to be maintained above atmospheric pressure; this helps clear fluid from the lung, facilitate distribution of gas within the lung, and splint the alveoli and airways open.[5,6,16,17]

### Closure of Glottis/Epiglottis

In utero, glottic adduction maintains elevated airway pressures and thus a high degree of fetal lung expansion, which is an important factor for lung growth development.[18] However, during fetal breathing movements the glottis opens caused by increasing dilator activity with diaphragmatic contractions.[19] Glottic function after birth follows a similar pattern as before birth.[20] Because hypoxia suppresses fetal breathing movements in utero it is suspected that hypoxia in newborn infants results in apnea and glottic adduction after birth.[21] Crawshaw and colleagues[21] used phase contrast X-ray imaging to demonstrate that glottis adduction occurs in preterm rabbit pups with unaerated lungs and unstable breathing patterns immediately after birth. However, once the lungs were aerated and a stable breathing pattern was established, the larynx and epiglottis remained mostly open irrespective of the time after birth. Most concerning, during PPV of preterm rabbit pups that were either apneic or had unstable breathing patterns ventilation was unsuccessful due to glottis closure(**Fig. 2**).[21]

### Trigeminocardiac Reflex

The trigeminocardiac reflex is a brainstem reflex that manifests as sudden cardiac perturbations including bradycardia, arterial hypotension, asystole, apnea, and gastric hypermobility.[22,23] In newborn infants, respiratory depression or apnea during peripheral stimulation of any of the sensory branches of the trigeminal nerve have been described.[24] This depression or apnea might be caused by the cutaneous and mucocutaneous stimulation of the area innervated by the afferent trigeminal nerve, which seems to affect ventilation, the ventilatory pattern, and the cardiovascular system.[25] Reflex stimulation of the face, nose, or nasopharynx due to placement of face mask or insertion of nasal prongs can cause changes in respiration and circulation in newborn infants.[26] Indeed, several studies reported a decrease in breathing rates and an increase in tidal volume when a face mask was placed on newborn infants' face compared with no face mask (see **Fig. 2**).[27–29] Gaertner and colleagues[30] demonstrated that ∼11% of newborn infants born at 34 weeks' gestation or more became apneic with a significant decrease in heart rate (HR) after applying a facemask. In adult animals, cerebral blood flow doubled when the trigeminocardiac reflex was activated; however, this was not confirmed in human studies.[31] The trigeminocardiac reflex is potentially more prominent in pediatric compared with adult patients.[23] However, there are limited data and further research is needed.

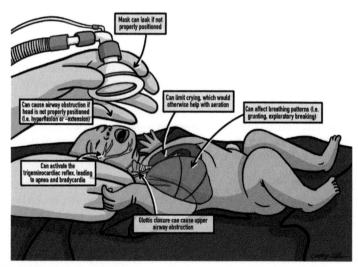

**Fig. 2.** Pitfalls of Mask Ventilation.

## SUPPORT AFTER BIRTH AND ITS IMPACT ON THE NEWBORN INFANT
### Stimulation

Tactile maneuvers including drying and/or rubbing the back or the soles of the feet are recommended to stimulate breathing at birth.[3,4] Many newborn infants receive at least one episode of stimulation within the first minute after birth.[32–34] However, no direct relation between timing to first breath and stimulation was observed because almost half of the infants received stimulation after the first breath.[32–34] In addition, stimulation was less commonly provided to infants born before 30 weeks' gestation; however, it was associated with a significant increase in oxygen saturation as measured by pulse oximetry ($SpO_2$) after stimulation, whereas HR did not increase.[34,35]

The most common response to stimulation was limb movement followed by infant cry and facial grimace. Truncal stimulation (drying, chest rub, back rub) was associated with more crying and movement than foot flicks frequently compared with more mature infants, and many very preterm infants do not receive any stimulation.[35] Most infants were stimulated within the first minute as recommended in resuscitation guidelines.[35] Rubbing the trunk or repetitive tactile stimulation may be most effective, but this needs to be confirmed in prospective studies.[35]

### Oxygen and Oxygen Saturation as Measured by Pulse Oximetry During Fetal-to-Neonatal Transition

The current neonatal resuscitation guidelines state that pulse oximetry should be used to titrate the amount of oxygen needed.[3,4] In the current guidelines, an initial fraction of inspired oxygen ($FiO_2$) of 0.30 for newborn infants born before 28 weeks' gestation, 0.21 to 0.30 for those born before 35 weeks' gestation, and 0.21 for those born at 35 weeks' gestation or more during resuscitation is recommended.[3,4] A meta-analysis of 768 preterm infants born before 32 weeks' gestation reported that $SpO_2$ less than 80% at 5 minutes after birth was associated with a higher risk of intraventricular hemorrhage and risk of death was almost five times.[36] In addition, there was a decreased likelihood of reaching $SpO_2$ 80% at 5 minutes if resuscitation was initiated with $FiO_2$ less than 0.3 (odds ratio [OR], 2.63; 95% confidence interval [CI], 1.21–5.74, $P<.05$).[36] Therefore, an $SpO_2$ of 80% or more should be achieved in preterm infants born before 32 weeks' gestation within 5 minutes.

### Mask Ventilation

The current neonatal resuscitation guidelines recommend a face mask during PPV in the DR.[3,4] Most commonly silicone face masks that cover the infant's mouth and nose are used. Alternatively, a nasal prong could be inserted a short distance into 1 or 2 nostrils.[37–40] During PPV, correct positioning of the infant's head and neck is crucial[3,4] because several factors can interfere with effective ventilation including spontaneous movements of the baby, movements by or distraction of the resuscitator, and procedures such as changing the wraps or fitting a hat.[41–45] Furthermore, during mask PPV, poor face mask technique results in leak or airway obstruction, whereas with a single nasal prong the contralateral nostril and the mouth must be closed to reduce leak (see **Fig. 2**).[37–40]

### Changes in Heart Rate During Mask Ventilation

The current neonatal resuscitation guidelines state that respiratory support must be initiated once the HR is less than 100/min.[3,4] Although an HR of less than 100/min immediately after birth in healthy term and preterm infants born at 32 weeks' gestation or more have been reported,[46] HR less than 100/min is used as a threshold to start PPV. Furthermore, the seventh edition of the neonatal resuscitation program textbook from the American Academy of Pediatrics states that "if PPV was started because the baby had a low HR, the baby's HR should begin to increase within the first 15sec of PPV."[47] However, experimental and clinical data contradict this statement. In asphyxiated term piglets with bradycardia, an increase in HR greater than 100/min was observed in 20%; however, increase in HR in the time epochs 0 to 10 seconds, 5 to 15 seconds, or 10 to 20 seconds of PPV was not observed in any piglet.[48] Similarly, observational studies in the DR reported no increase in HR after 15 seconds of PPV in bradycardic preterm infant.[9,49,50] HR can only increase once gas exchange has occurred; indeed, in preterm infants it took a median (interquartile range) of 126 (96–160) seconds from birth for HR to exceed 100 beats/min.[9] Furthermore, the HR increase only followed 28 (21–36) seconds after gas exchange occurred.[9] During PPV, HR might only increase after gas exchange has occurred, which is followed by either a rapid increase in HR within seconds or gradual increase in HR over at least 60 seconds.

### Peak Inflation Pressure

The viscosity of liquid is considerably higher than that of air, and the airway resistance is about 100 times higher when the lung is liquid-filled versus when it is air-filled.[6] During the first breaths aeration of the lung does not occur uniformly, because the resistance is higher in some parts resulting in irregular pressure distribution during ventilation. During PPV, a peak inflating pressure is chosen with the assumption that this will deliver an appropriate tidal volume. However, lung compliance and therefore the peak inflating pressure required to deliver an appropriate tidal volume vary in the minutes after birth.[43] It is likely that there are even greater differences between infants because the mechanical properties of the lung vary with gestational age and disease states. In addition, many infants breathe during PPV adding to the inconsistency of tidal volume delivered with a set peak inflating pressure.[43] Therefore, relying on a fixed peak inflating pressure might result in either underventilation or overventilation.

### Mask Leak

Mask leak is typically caused by a poor-fitting mask or poor mask position or hold.[41,43,51] Mask leak occurs in about half of the newborn infants who received PPV in the DR during the first 2 minutes after birth, whereby it occurs in most cases at the start of PPV.[45] Mask leak during PPV might delay lung aeration hence effective gas exchange and increase in $SpO_2$ and HR. During mask PPV, simulation studies suggest the 2-point top hold might minimize mask leak during PPV.[52] However, teaching improves technique and significantly reduces mask leak during PPV (see **Fig. 2**).[52]

### Airway Obstruction

During mask ventilation, airway obstruction might occur due to manual compression of the soft tissues of the neck, tongue, and thus the trachea; due to hyperextension or flexion of the head; or due to the face mask being held onto the face to tightly that it obstructs the mouth and nose.[3,4] Using a colorimetric $CO_2$ detector, the airway of preterm infants were obstructed in up to 75% of infants during mask ventilation.[44] An observational study in the DR reported that severe airway obstruction, defined as a reduction in tidal volume of greater than 75%, occurs in 25% of infants receiving mask ventilation.[45] The current neonatal resuscitation guidelines recommend the sniffing position to reduce airway obstruction.[3,4] However, there is lack of data to suggest that the sniffing position reduced airway obstruction.[53] To overcome airway

**Table 1**
**The effects of physiologic changes on the newborn infant and how medical support can improve the newborn infants' condition immediately after birth**

| Physiologic Conditions Immediately After Birth | Effect on the Newborn Infant | Medical Measures to Improve Transition |
|---|---|---|
| Lung liquid clearance | Failed lung liquid clearance results in lung edema and impaired gas exchange | PPV in apneic and/or bradycardic (<100 beats/min) infants forces lung liquid clearance and generates functional residual capacity[3,4] |
| Gas exchange | Failed gas exchange leads to imbalance of $CO_2$ and $O_2$ and results in respiratory acidosis and impaired tissue oxygenation | Using PPV with a peak inspiratory pressure of 20–25 cm $H_2O$ to deliver an appropriate tidal volume and aerate parts in the lung with high resistance[3,4] |
| Glottis closure | Leading to obstruction and resulting in impaired heart rate increase, further medical interventions, hypoxia, and inhibiting breathing efforts | An initial high oxygen boost to open the glottis in preterm infants might be an option to open the glottis[65] |
| Crying and breathing patterns | Failing to cry at birth leads to impaired establishment of functional residual capacity | Tactile maneuvers (drying, rubbing the back or the soles of the feet) to stimulate breathing at birth[3,4] |
| Oxygen saturation ($Spo_2$) | $Spo_2$ <80% at 5 min after birth was associated with a higher risk of intraventricular hemorrhage and risk of death was almost 5 times[36] | Use pulse oximetry to titrate the amount of oxygen needed. Initial $Fio_2$ of 0.30 for newborn infants <28 wk' gestation, 0.21–0.30 for infants <35 wk' gestation, and 0.21 for infants ≥35 wk' gestation.[3,4] |
| End-tidal $CO_2$ | Failed gas exchange due to, eg, obstruction, missing breathing efforts, or failed ventilation results in no detection of end-tidal $CO_2$ within 5–21s after birth resulting in respiratory acidosis | $CO_2$ monitoring might be used to assess lung aeration and guide respiratory support during resuscitation. It is not recommended in the current resuscitation guidelines because there are numerous pitfalls when using different techniques[3,4] |

(continued on next page)

| Table 1 (continued) | | |
| --- | --- | --- |
| **Physiologic Conditions Immediately After Birth** | **Effect on the Newborn Infant** | **Medical Measures to Improve Transition** |
| Activation of the trigeminocardiac reflex | Placing a face mask or nasal prongs on the infants face may lead to apnea and bradycardia | Health care providers should be aware that positioning a face mask could activate the trigeminocardiac reflex causing apnea and bradycardia |
| Activation of the vagus nerve | Endotracheal suctioning may lead to apnea and bradycardia | Current neonatal resuscitation guidelines recommended against routine suction for both vigorous and nonvigorous infants born with meconium-stained amniotic fluid.[3,4] Suctioning may be considered for suspected airway obstruction[3,4] |

obstruction, resuscitation guidelines recommend various airway maneuvers to maintain upper airway patency as well as oropharyngeal airway devices. Indeed, the European Resuscitation guidelines recommend placing an oropharyngeal airway to overcome airway obstruction.[54] However, a recent randomized trial including 137 preterm infants born before 32 weeks' gestation compared mask ventilation with and without oropharyngeal airway and reported a higher frequency of obstructed inflations as well as partial obstruction with an oropharyngeal airway (81% vs 64%; $P = .03$ and 70% vs 54%; $P = .04$, respectively).[55] These data suggest that an oropharyngeal airway significantly increases the incidence of airway obstruction and should not be used during mask ventilation in preterm infants.

## RESPIRATORY SUPPORT AT BIRTH: IMPLEMENTING AVAILABLE KNOWLEDGE
### Using Positive Pressure Ventilation to Improve Lung Liquid Clearance

Inspiration generates a pressure gradient across the airway wall by creating subatmospheric pressures within perialveolar tissue leading to lung liquid clearance.[6] If the newborn does not initiate breathing, lung liquid remains in the airways and impedes gas exchange and oxygenation. The object of PPV is to establish an FRC and deliver an appropriate tidal volume to achieve effective gas exchange. The current neonatal resuscitation guidelines suggest a peak inflation pressure of 20 to 25 cm $H_2O$ with an inspiratory time of 0.3 to 0.5 seconds.[3,4] However, it remains unclear what inflation pressure or inflation times should be used. Animal studies suggest that a prolonged inflation pressure (or sustained inflation) with a peak inflation pressure of ~20 to 30 mm Hg might overcome the high initial resistance, support lung liquid movement, and help expand uniformly.[56] However, a recent systematic review including preterm infants (n = 1502) compared intermittent PPV with sustained inflations (>1 second) reported no improvement in mortality, mechanical ventilation, or key morbidities (eg, bronchopulmonary dysplasia, intraventricular hemorrhage, or retinopathy of prematurity), and long-term neurodevelopmental outcome.[56] More concerning, in a subgroup analysis of infants born at or before 28 weeks' gestation sustained inflation might increase death before discharge (risk ratio, 1.38; 95% CI, 1.00–1.91; $I^2 = 0\%$, $P = .05$).[56] Current neonatal resuscitation guidelines state that in preterm newborn infants, the routine use of sustained inflations to initiate resuscitation is potentially harmful and should not be performed and that it is reasonable to initiate PPV with an inspiratory time of 1 second or less.[3]

### Using $CO_2$ Monitoring to Assess Lung Aeration

$CO_2$ monitoring might be used to assess adequate lung aeration, the degree of pulmonary gas exchange, and ventilation efficiency during mask ventilation.[9–12,44,57–60] Hooper and colleagues[9] reported that during PPV end-tidal $CO_2$ ($ETCO_2$) levels increase to greater than 10 mm Hg at a median 28 (21–36) seconds before the HR increased more than 100/min during resuscitation in preterm infants. $ETCO_2$ levels can indicate the relative degree of lung aeration after birth.[9] However, $ETCO_2$ can only be present when the lung is aerated and gas exchange occurs, and in newborn infants the small tidal volume and high respiratory rate resulting in shorter inspiratory and expiratory time may cause inaccuracy of the measurements.[61] Furthermore, $CO_2$ detectors are useful devices to assess effective ventilation; they cannot differentiate between an inadequate tidal volume, airway obstruction, circulatory failure, or no lung aeration.[60] Alternatively, a respiratory function monitor, which displays flow and tidal volume signals, allows to distinguish between mask leak and airway obstruction.[62]

In addition, $ETCO_2$ could be used to guide respiratory effort in the DR. Ngan and colleagues[63] used $ETCO_2$ to guide the number and duration of sustained inflations at birth, whereas Kong and colleagues[57] and Hawkes and colleagues[64] used exhaled $CO_2$ monitoring to increase the number of infants with normocarbia admitted to the neonatal intensive care unit (NICU). However, neither study increased the number of normocarbic infants at NICU admission. Although $ETCO_2$ monitor might be useful to assess the degree of gas exchange during respiratory support in the DR, the data are limited and randomized trials are needed. In addition, knowledge about the displayed waveforms and their interpretation is required to prevent misdiagnosis or inadequate treatments.

### Using Physiologic Background Knowledge to Improve Neonatal Resuscitation

In utero, glottic adduction helps to maintain elevated airway pressures and thus a high degree of fetal lung expansion, which is important for lung growth development.[18] However, especially in apneic preterm infants, glottis closure might still be present immediately after birth, and noninvasive PPV ventilation is likely to be ineffective in these infants. It is suggested that tactile stimulation immediately after birth might support opening the glottis in apneic infants. In term infants no effect on $SpO_2$ and HR after tactile stimulation was observed,[34] whereas in preterm infants it resulted in a significant increase in $SpO_2$.[34,35]

During PPV glottis closure, which could be unrecognized, could lead to either no change or a decrease in HR and thereby to further interventions and/or more hypoxia inhibiting breathing efforts.[21] Therefore, glottic closure should be considered during PPV in particular when there is no clinical improvement immediately after birth. Dekker and colleagues[65] reported that an initial boost of 100% oxygen (for up to 3 minutes) in infants born before 30 weeks' gestation results in higher minute volumes and tidal volume compared with using 30% oxygen. In addition, no difference in oxidative stress markers or duration of hyperoxemia was observed between the groups.[65] Although further studies are needed, an initial high oxygen boost to open the glottis is preterm infants might be an option to open the glottis.

Another reason for apneic events and bradycardia during PPV is the activation of the trigeminocardiac reflex when a face mask/nasal prongs are placed on an infants' face; however the exact mechanism of trigeminocardiac reflex activation is not fully understood.[26-30] Health care providers should be aware that positioning a face mask could activate the trigeminocardiac reflex causing apnea and bradycardia.[30]

## SUMMARY

The newborn infants' physiologic adaption from intrauterine to extrauterine life includes complex physiologic changes. Biochemical, physical, cardiocirculatory, and respiratory processes are interacting with each other, and every action and intervention during this vulnerable period triggers a chain reaction in the newborn infants' body. Thus, physiologic changes during fetal-to-neonatal transition must be understood and considered when investigating and performing neonatal resuscitation. Although we gained substantial knowledge about this topic over the last decade, further research is strongly needed to improve the outcome of the smallest and most vulnerable ones (**Table 1**).

## BEST PRACTICE BOX

1. Positive pressure ventilation is the cornerstone of respiratory support if infants fail to initiate spontaneous breathing at birth.
2. Healthcare providers should be aware that of a mask or nasal prong onto a newborn infants face can trigger the trigeminocardiac reflex causing apnea and/or bradycardia.
3. Ineffective positive pressure ventilation at birth could be due to glottis closure, mask leak or airway obstruction.

## ACKNOWLEDGMENT

We would like to thank Dr. Cathy Cichon, @DocScribbles for the drawing of the figures.

## REFERENCES

1. Schmölzer GM, te Pas AB, Davis PG, et al. Reducing lung injury during neonatal resuscitation of preterm infants. J Pediatr 2008;153(6):741–5.
2. Aziz K, Chadwick M, Baker M, et al. Ante- and intra-partum factors that predict increased need for neonatal resuscitation. Resuscitation 2008;79(3):444–52.
3. Aziz K, Lee HC, Escobedo MB, et al. Part 5: neonatal resuscitation: 2020 American heart association guidelines for cardiopulmonary resuscitation and emergency cardiovascular care. Circulation 2020;142(16_suppl_2):S524–50.
4. Wyckoff MH, Wyllie J, Aziz K, et al. Neonatal life support 2020 international consensus on cardiopulmonary resuscitation and emergency cardiovascular care Science with treatment recommendations. Resuscitation 2020;156(16 SUPPL. 2):A156–87.
5. te Pas AB, Davis PG, Hooper SB, et al. From liquid to air: breathing after birth. J Pediatr 2008;152(5):607–11.
6. Hooper SB, Te Pas AB, Kitchen MJ. Respiratory transition in the newborn: a three-phase process. Arch Dis Child Fetal Neonatal Ed 2016;101(3):F266–71.
7. Hooper SB, Kitchen MJ, Wallace MJ, et al. Imaging lung aeration and lung liquid clearance at birth. FASEB J 2007;21(12):3329–37.

8.  Miserocchi G, Poskurica BH, Del Fabbro M. Pulmonary interstitial pressure in anesthetized paralyzed newborn rabbits. J Appl Physiol 1994;77(5):2260–8.

9.  Hooper SB, Fouras A, Siew ML, et al. Expired CO2 levels indicate degree of lung aeration at birth. PLoS One 2013;8(8):e70895.

10. Schmölzer GM, Hooper SB, Wong C, et al. Exhaled carbon dioxide in healthy term infants immediately after birth. J Pediatr 2015;166(4):844–9.e3.

11. Blank DA, Gaertner VD, Kamlin COF, et al. Respiratory changes in term infants immediately after birth. Resuscitation 2018;130:105–10.

12. Kang LJ, Cheung P, Pichler G, et al. Monitoring lung aeration during respiratory support in preterm infants at birth. PLoS One 2014;9(7):e102729.

13. Nicoll J, Cheung PY, Aziz K, et al. Exhaled carbon dioxide and neonatal breathing patterns in preterm infants after birth. J Pediatr 2015;167(4):829–33.e1.

14. O'Donnell CPF, Kamlin COF, Davis PG, et al. Crying and breathing by extremely preterm infants immediately after birth. J Pediatr 2010;156(5):846–7.

15. Murphy MC, McCarthy LK, O'Donnell CPF. Crying and breathing by new-born preterm infants after early or delayed cord clamping. Arch Dis Child Fetal Neonatal Ed 2020;105(3):F331–3.

16. Te Pas AB, Davis PG, Kamlin COF, et al. Spontaneous breathing patterns of very preterm infants treated with continuous positive airway pressure at birth. Pediatr Res 2008;64(3):281–5.

17. te Pas AB, Wong C, Kamlin COF, et al. Breathing patterns in preterm and term infants immediately after birth. Pediatr Res 2009;65(3):352–6.

18. Harding R, Hooper SB. Regulation of lung expansion and lung growth before birth. J Appl Physiol 1996;81(1):209–24.

19. Harding R, Bocking AD, Sigger JN. Upper airway resistances in fetal sheep: the influence of breathing activity. J Appl Physiol 1986;60(1):160–5.

20. Hooper SB, Kitchen MJ, Polglase GR, et al. The physiology of neonatal resuscitation. Curr Opin Pediatr 2018;30(2):187–91.

21. Crawshaw JR, Kitchen MJ, Binder-Heschl C, et al. Laryngeal closure impedes non-invasive ventilation at birth. Arch Dis Child Fetal Neonatal Ed 2018;103(2):F112–9.

22. Schaller B, Cornelius JF, Prabhakar H, et al. The trigemino-cardiac reflex. J Neurosurg Anesthesiol 2009;21(3):187–95.

23. Chowdhury T, Mendelowith D, Golanov E, et al. Trigeminocardiac Reflex: the current clinical and physiological knowledge. J Neurosurg Anesthesiol 2015;27(2):136–47.

24. Tesoriere H. A trigeminal-respiratory reflex in depressed newborn infants. Anesth Analg 1960;39(4):352–4.

25. White S, McRitchie R. Nasopharyngeal reflexes: integrative analysis of evoked respiratory and cardiovascular effects. Aust J Exp Biol Med Sci 1973;51(1):17–31.

26. Haddad GG, Mellins RB. The role of airway receptors in the control of respiration in infants: a review. J Pediatr 1977;91(2):281–6.

27. Fleming PJ, Levine MR, Goncalves A. Changes in respiratory pattern resulting from the use of a facemask to record respiration in newborn infants. Pediatr Res 1982;16(12):1031–4.

28. Dolfin T, Duffty P, Wilkes D, et al. Effects of a face mask and pneumotachograph on breathing in sleeping infants. Am Rev Respir Dis 1983;128(6):977–9.

29. Søvik S, Eriksen M, Lossius K, et al. A method of assessing ventilatory responses to chemoreceptor stimulation in infants. Acta Paediatr Int J Paediatr 1999;88(5):563–70.

30. Gaertner VD, Ruëgger CM, O'Currain E, et al. Physiological responses to face-mask application in newborns immediately after birth. Arch Dis Child Fetal Neonatal Ed 2020;106(4):381–5.

31. Schaller B, Cornelius JF, Prabhakar H, et al. The trigemino-cardiac reflex: an update of the current knowledge. J Neurosurg Anesthesiol 2009;21(3):187–95.

32. van Henten TMA, Dekker J, te Pas AB, et al. Tactile stimulation in the delivery room: do we practice what we preach? Arch Dis Child - Fetal Neonatal Ed 2019;104(6):F661–2.

33. Gaertner VD, Flemmer SA, Lorenz L, et al. Physical stimulation of newborn infants in the delivery room. Arch Dis Child Fetal Neonatal Ed 2018;103(2):F132–6.

34. Baik-Schneditz N, Urlesberger B, Schwaberger B, et al. Tactile stimulation during neonatal transition and its effect on vital parameters in neonates during neonatal transition. Acta Paediatr Int J Paediatr 2018;107(6):952–7.

35. Dekker J, Martherus T, Cramer SJE, et al. Tactile stimulation to stimulate spontaneous breathing during stabilization of preterm infants at birth: a retrospective analysis. Front Pediatr 2017;5:61.

36. Oei JL, Vento M, Rabi Y, et al. Higher or lower oxygen for delivery room resuscitation of preterm infants below 28 completed weeks gestation: a meta-analysis. Arch Dis Child Fetal Neonatal Ed 2017;102(1):F24–30.

37. Machumpurath S, O'Currain E, Dawson JA, et al. Interfaces for non-invasive neonatal resuscitation in the delivery room: a systematic review and meta-analysis. Resuscitation 2020;156:244–50.

38. Kamlin COF, Schilleman K, Dawson JA, et al. Mask versus nasal tube for stabilization of preterm infants at birth: a randomized controlled trial. Pediatrics 2013; 132(2):e381–8.

39. Lindner W, Högel J, Pohlandt F. Sustained pressure—controlled inflation or intermittent mandatory ventilation in preterm infants in the delivery room? A randomized, controlled trial on initial respiratory support via nasopharyngeal tube. Acta Paediatr 2005;94(3):303–9.

40. McCarthy LK, Twomey AR, Molloy EJ, et al. A randomized trial of nasal prong or face mask for respiratory support for preterm newborns. Pediatrics 2013;132(2): e389–95.

41. Kaufman J, Schmölzer GM, Kamlin COF, et al. Mask ventilation of preterm infants in the delivery room. Arch Dis Child Fetal Neonatal Ed 2013;98(5):405–10.

42. Poulton DA, Schmölzer GM, Morley CJ, et al. Assessment of chest rise during mask ventilation of preterm infants in the delivery room. Resuscitation 2011; 82(2):175–9.

43. Schmölzer GM, Kamlin OCOF, O'Donnell CPF, et al. Assessment of tidal volume and gas leak during mask ventilation of preterm infants in the delivery room. Arch Dis Child Fetal Neonatal Ed 2010;95(6):393–7.

44. Finer NN, Rich W, Wang C, et al. Airway obstruction during mask ventilation of very low birth weight infants during neonatal resuscitation. Pediatrics 2009; 123(3):865–9.

45. Schmölzer GM, Dawson JA, Kamlin COF, et al. Airway obstruction and gas leak during mask ventilation of preterm infants in the delivery room. Arch Dis Child Fetal Neonatal Ed 2011;96(4):254–7.

46. Dawson JA, Kamlin COF, Wong C, et al. Changes in heart rate in the first minutes after birth. Arch Dis Child Fetal Neonatal Ed 2010;95(3):F177–81.

47. Weiner GM, Zaichkin J. Textbook of neonatal resuscitation. 7th edition. Chicago (US): American Academy of Pediatrics; 2016.

48. Espinoza ML, Cheung P-Y, Lee T-F, et al. Heart rate changes during positive pressure ventilation after asphyxia-induced bradycardia in a porcine model of neonatal resuscitation. Arch Dis Child - Fetal Neonatal Ed 2019;104(1):F98–101.
49. Yam CH, Dawson JA, Schmolzer GM, et al. Heart rate changes during resuscitation of newly born infants <30 weeks gestation: an observational study. Arch Dis Child - Fetal Neonatal Ed 2011;96(2):F102–7.
50. Palme-Kilander C, Tunell R. Pulmonary gas exchange during facemask ventilation immediately after birth. Arch Dis Child 1993;68(1 Spec No):11–6.
51. O'Shea JE, Thio M, Owen LS, et al. Measurements from preterm infants to guide face mask size. Arch Dis Child Fetal Neonatal Ed 2016;101(4):F294–8.
52. Wood FE, Morley CJ, Dawson JA, et al. Improved techniques reduce face mask leak during simulated neonatal resuscitation: study 2. Arch Dis Child Fetal Neonatal Ed 2008;93(3):F230–4.
53. Chua C, Schmölzer GM, Davis PG. Airway manoeuvres to achieve upper airway patency during mask ventilation in newborn infants - an historical perspective. Resuscitation 2012;83(4):411–6.
54. Wyllie J, Bruinenberg J, Roehr CC, et al. European resuscitation council guidelines for resuscitation 2015. Section 7. Resuscitation and support of transition of babies at birth. Resuscitation 2015;95:249–63.
55. Kamlin COF, Schmölzer GM, Dawson JA, et al. A randomized trial of oropharyngeal airways to assist stabilization of preterm infants in the delivery room. Resuscitation 2019;144:106–14.
56. Kapadia VS, Urlesberger B, Soraisham A, et al. Sustained lung inflations during neonatal resuscitation at birth: a meta-analysis. Pediatrics 2021;147(1). e2020021204.
57. Kong JY, Rich W, Finer NN, et al. Quantitative end-tidal carbon dioxide monitoring in the delivery room: a randomized controlled trial. J Pediatr 2013;163(1):104–8.e1.
58. Blank D, Rich W, Leone T, et al. Pedi-cap color change precedes a significant increase in heart rate during neonatal resuscitation. Resuscitation 2014;85(11):1568–72.
59. Murthy V, O'Rourke-Potocki A, Dattani N, et al. End tidal carbon dioxide levels during the resuscitation of prematurely born infants. Early Hum Dev 2012;88(10):783–7.
60. van Os S, Cheung P-Y, Pichler G, et al. Exhaled carbon dioxide can be used to guide respiratory support in the delivery room. Acta Paediatr 2014;103(8):796–806.
61. Humberg A, Herting E, Göpel W, et al. Beatmung in Pädiatrie und Neonatologie. Germany: Georg Thieme Verlag; 2017. p. 41–53.
62. Schmolzer GM, Kamlin OCOF, Dawson JA, et al. Respiratory monitoring of neonatal resuscitation. Arch Dis Child Fetal Neonatal Ed 2010;95(4):F295–303.
63. Ngan AY, Cheung PY, Hudson-Mason A, et al. Using exhaled CO 2 to guide initial respiratory support at birth: a randomised controlled trial. Arch Dis Child Fetal Neonatal Ed 2017;102(6):F525–31.
64. Hawkes GA, O'Connell BJ, Livingstone V, et al. Efficacy and user preference of two CO2 detectors in an infant mannequin randomized crossover trial. Eur J Pediatr 2013;172(10):1393–9.
65. Dekker J, Martherus T, Lopriore E, et al. The effect of initial high vs. low FiO2 on breathing effort in preterm infants at birth: a randomized controlled trial. Front Pediatr 2019;7:1–11.

# Nasal Continuous Positive Airway Pressure and High-Flow Nasal Cannula Today

Carlo Dani[a,b]

## KEYWORDS

- Noninvasive respiratory support • Continuous positive airway pressure
- High-flow nasal cannula • Respiratory distress syndrome • Premature infants

## KEY POINTS

- Nasal continuous positive airway pressure (nCPAP) and high-flow nasal cannula (HFNC) are widely diffused as primary and postextubation noninvasive respiratory support in preterm infants with respiratory distress syndrome (RDS).
- Physiologic effects of nCPAP and to a lesser extent of HFNC are well known, as are the risk factors for failure and adverse effects.
- Available evidences suggests that nCPAP should be preferred to HFNC as primary mode of noninvasive respiratory support in preterm infants with RDS, whereas HFNC is an effective alternative to nCPAP after extubation.

## INTRODUCTION

Although the respiratory support of preterm infants with respiratory distress syndrome (RDS) has improved and new modes of mechanical ventilation (MV) have been developed, the incidence of bronchopulmonary dysplasia (BPD) has remained high.[1] It has been reported that BPD increased in infants born at 22 to 28 weeks of gestation from 32% to 47% between 1993 and 2012.[1] The cause of BPD is multifactorial and, although its most important risk factor is extreme prematurity, the role of MV in favoring its development has been clearly demonstrated.[2,3] MV often causes secondary lung damage, the so-called ventilator-induced lung injury, especially by inducing volutrauma, atelectrauma, and oxygen toxicity.[4–6] Moreover, there is a strong association between the need for MV and the development of severe neurologic complications, such as intraventricular hemorrhage, periventricular leukomalacia, and neurodevelopmental impairment.[7,8] Therefore, interventions aimed at limiting the need for MV, such

[a] Division of Neonatology, Careggi University Hospital of Florence, Florence, Italy;
[b] Department of Neurosciences, Psychology, Drug Research and Child Health, University of Florence, Florence, Italy
E-mail address: carlo.dani@unifi.it

Clin Perinatol 48 (2021) 711–724
https://doi.org/10.1016/j.clp.2021.07.002          perinatology.theclinics.com

as noninvasive respiratory support and surfactant treatment, have been advocated to improve the outcome of extremely preterm infants.

Among noninvasive respiratory support, nasal continuous positive airway pressure (nCPAP) and high-flow nasal cannula (HFNC) are widely diffused, although it seems that in the last 15 years the use of nCPAP has remained stable over time, whereas that of HFNC has rapidly increased.[1,9,10] In this regard, it has recently been reported that all Italian neonatal intensive care units (NICUs) use nCPAP, whereas HFNC is used in 60% of clinical settings.[11]

Although nCPAP, and to a lesser extent HFNC, is used for the treatment of different neonatal respiratory disorders (eg, transient tachypnea of the newborn, meconium aspiration syndrome, and so forth), preterm infants with RDS represent the most widely studied patient population for these modes of noninvasive support. Thus, the focus of this article is the use of nCPAP and HFNC in preterm infants with RDS. We review their mechanisms of action and physiologic effects, discuss the main characteristics of available devices and patients' interfaces, report on their risk of failure and possible adverse effects, and summarize the clinical evidence about their effectiveness for preventing MV as primary respiratory support or after extubation in the setting of NICU.

## CONTINUOUS POSITIVE AIRWAY PRESSURE

The first report on the use of CPAP in preterm infants with RDS was published by Gregory and coworkers in 1971.[12] They found a 55% increase in expected survival by providing CPAP through an endotracheal tube or a head box. These important results favored a quick diffusion of nCPAP for the treatment of infant RDS.

### Physiologic Effects of Nasal Continuous Positive Airway Pressure

nCPAP is used to assist infants with respiratory failure who spontaneously breathe. In preterm infants narrow flow-resistive airway and high chest wall/lung compliance ratio may contribute to lower the development of an adequate end-expiratory lung volume.[13,14] Moreover, high chest wall compliance, which can allow the paradoxic inward movement of rib cage during the inspiratory phase of respiration, and a low concentration of alveolar surfactant can contribute to lower the functional residual capacity (FRC) and this, in turn, can result in airway occlusion, parenchymal atelectasis, and ventilation-perfusion mismatch. These pathophysiologic disadvantages are overcome in preterm infants with RDS through the application of nCPAP, which generates a distending pressure that stents the airways, helps patients increase and maintain FRC, increases end-expiratory lung volume, and stabilizes the highly compliant chest wall, thereby improving lung compliance, ventilation-perfusion mismatch, and thoracoabdominal synchrony.[15] Thus, all these different effects allow nCPAP to improve patients' oxygenation, promote conservation of surfactant on the alveolar surface, and reduce the dynamic and resistive work of breathing (WOB) (**Table 1**).

### Methods of Generating Continuous Airway Pressure

nCPAP is delivered from either a continuous flow or a variable flow source. In ventilator-derived continuous-flow CPAP, the pressure is generated by a gas flow directed against a valve-adjusted resistance of the expiratory limb of the circuit. In bubble CPAP, the pressure is generated by a gas flow directed against resistance of the expiratory limb of the circuit, which is adjusted by the depth of its immersion under water.[13] It has been reported that during bubble CPAP pressure oscillations occur able to generate volumes similar to those generated by high-frequency oscillatory

**Table 1**
**Physiologic effects of nCPAP and HFNC**

| nCPAP | HFNC |
|---|---|
| Provides a continuous distending pressure | Provides a continuous distending pressure |
| Increases and maintains FRC | Increases average airway pressure by 0.8 cm $H_2O$ for each 1 L/min increase in flow, but is characterized by a considerable variability |
| Increases the end-expiratory lung volume | |
| Stabilizes the highly compliant chest wall | |
| Improves lung compliance | |
| Stents the airways | Washouts upper airways, which leads to a reduction of the physiologic dead space as suggested by the decrease of patient's respiratory rate and $Paco_2$ and by the improvement of oxygenation |
| Decreases the inspiratory resistance | |
| Improves ventilation-perfusion mismatch | |
| Improves thoracoabdominal synchrony | |
| Improves patient's oxygenation and to lesser extent $Paco_2$ (washout effect) | |
| Promotes conservation of surfactant | Decreases the inspiratory resistance |
| Reduces the dynamic and resistive WOB | Decreases the dynamic and resistive WOB to a lesser extent than nCPAP |
| | Improves airway conductance by reducing the effect of cold air |
| | Reduces the metabolic cost of gas conditions by providing air with 100% relative humidity |

ventilation and this might enhance gas exchange by delivering a low amplitude.[16,17] However, the main limitation of this mode of CPAP is the lack of pressure monitoring and alarms.

In variable-flow CPAP (ie, Arabella System [US-MED EQUIP, Houston, Tx], Infant Flow System [Vyaire Medical, Hirzel, Switzerland]) there is a dedicated flow driver and gas generator: in the inspiratory phase the Bernoulli effect directs gas flow toward nares, but when infants expire the Coanda effect induces the inspiratory flow to flip and exit the generator chamber via the expiratory limb.[13]

Comparison of physiologic and clinical effects of continuous- and variable-flow CPAP has been undertaken in several studies. Klausner and colleagues[18] demonstrated in a simulated airway model that variable-flow CPAP decreases the WOB to a quarter and the pressure generated shows less variability in comparison with continuous-flow CPAP (generated by infant ventilator). Pandit and colleagues[19] confirmed these results in very preterm infants: variable-flow CPAP lowered the WOB from 13% to 29% maintaining a more stable pressure level and increasing more significantly lung compliance in comparison with continuous-flow CPAP (generated by infant ventilator). Consistently with these findings, variable-flow CPAP was found to allow a greater lung recruitment than continuous-flow CPAP (generated by infant ventilator).[20]

The WOB was found to be lower in preterm infants treated with variable-flow than with bubble CPAP in very preterm infants.[21] Lipstein and colleagues[22] reported in a similar population that inspiratory WOB and pressure fluctuations were similar with bubble CPAP ventilator-derived CPAP during the inspiratory phase but were higher during the expiration phase. These results were partially confirmed by Kahn and colleagues who found a similar inspiratory WOB with bubble CPAP and ventilator-derived CPAP.[23]

### Nasal Continuous Positive Airway Pressure Interfaces

Variable-flow CPAP is generally delivered through short nasal prongs or a nasal mask specifically designed for the device (ie, ArabellaSystem, Infant FlowSystem).

Conversely, different interfaces are used to delivery continuous-flow CPAP, such as short (6–15 mm) and long (40–90 mm) binasal prongs or a shortened endotracheal tube used as nasopharyngeal single prong.[13] However, long binasal prongs are not recommended because they are prone to obstruction and increase the WOB. Moreover, the use of an endotracheal tube is declining after the advent of binasal prongs and the publication of data suggesting it is less effective in improving respiratory parameters and preventing extubation failure.[23]

There are different types of nasal prongs and their effectiveness can vary. Sharma and colleagues[24] compared the level of CPAP delivered by three different CPAP delivery interfaces (RAM cannula system, Hudson prongs, and nasal mask) in preterm neonates with RDS and reported that maximum drop in oropharyngeal pressure was observed with RAM cannula (1 and 1.2 cm $H_2O$ less than set CPAP of 5 and 6 cm $H_2O$, respectively). Pharyngeal pressure best correlated to set CPAP level with the use of nasal mask.[24] These results were confirmed by Singh and colleagues[25] who found that for a given set CPAP pressure level in preterm infants, the RAM cannula system delivers lower pharyngeal pressure levels than Hudson prongs. Consistently, Green and colleagues[26] demonstrated in an in vitro setting that there is considerable variation in measured resistance of available CPAP interfaces (Hudson prong, RAM Cannula, Fisher & Paykel prong, Infant Flow prong, Fisher & Paykel mask, Infant Flow mask) at gas flows (6, 8, and 10 L/min) commonly applied in clinical neonatal care. They found that RAM Cannula had the highest resistance and nasal mask had the lowest resistance at all assessed sizes and gas flows.[26]

Kieran and colleagues[27] demonstrated that in preterm infants nCPAP was more effective in preventing intubation and MV within 72 hours of starting therapy when given via nasal masks compared with nasal prongs. Goel and colleagues[28] confirmed these results because they found that nasal mask decreased the need for MV within 72 hours of starting therapy (8% vs 25%) in comparison with nasal prongs, but the difference was not statistically significant. However, a recent meta-analysis demonstrated that nasal mask significantly decreases the risk of CPAP failure (number needed to treat = 9) and the incidence of moderate to severe nasal trauma (number needed to treat = 6).[29]

### Continuous Positive Airway Pressure Failure

It has been reported that nCPAP, used as primary respiratory support in extremely preterm infants with RDS, failed to prevent MV in about 50% of cases.[30] This failure occurs most frequently within 8 hours of starting therapy in association with increasing oxygen requirement.[30] Among the risk factors male sex, fraction of inspired oxygen ($F_{IO_2}$) greater than 0.40 in the first hours of life, and increased CPAP requirement (>6 cm $H_2O$) have been reported.[31,32] Other authors found risk factors for CPAP failure to be birth weight less than 1000 g and $F_{IO_2}$ requirement greater than 30%[33]; or gestational age, hypertensive disorders of pregnancy, and severe RDS requiring surfactant more than twice, and $F_{IO_2}$ greater than 0.30.[34] It is worth noting that Gulczyńska and colleagues[35] detailed that each gestational week can reduce the odds of CPAP failure by 19%, and each 100 g of birth weight can reduce the odds by 16%. Moreover, they found that a prognostic threshold of $F_{IO_2}$ of 0.29 in the second hour of life predicts CPAP failure with a sensitivity of 73% and a specificity of 57% (**Table 2**).[35]

### Continuous Positive Airway Pressure Adverse Effects

Despite its several beneficial effects, nCPAP can cause adverse side effects and complications. The most severe is air leak, namely pneumothorax, pneumomediastinum, and pulmonary interstitial emphysema. Physiopathologic mechanisms leading to

| Table 2 Risk factors for failure of nCPAP and HFNC | |
| --- | --- |
| **nCPAP** | **HFNC** |
| Low gestational age | Low gestational age ($\leq$30 wk) |
| Birth weight <1000 g | $F_{IO_2}$ >0.30 |
| Male sex | Birth weight $\leq$1200 g |
| $F_{IO_2}$ >0.30–0.40 in the first hours of life | |
| Increased CPAP requirement (>6 cm $H_2O$) | |
| Hypertensive disorders of pregnancy | |
| Severe RDS requiring surfactant more than twice | |

complications are the development of air trapping and/or lung overdistention. The former is induced by the inadvertent positive end-expiratory pressure caused by the patient's high respiratory rate and too short expiratory time; the latter is elicited by the uneven distribution of tidal volume, which causes the overdistention of the more compliant areas of the lung.[36,37] Consistently, it has been demonstrated that CPAP, as primary therapy for RDS, is associated with an increased risk of pneumothorax (number needed to treat for an additional harmful outcome = 11).[38]

Another frequent adverse effect is the so-called CPAP belly syndrome.[39] Pressurized gases can easily pass into the esophagus and cause bowel distention. Although nCPAP might contribute to the development of feeding intolerance, a correlation between noninvasive respiratory supports and the occurrence of necrotizing enterocolitis (NEC) has never been demonstrated.[40] Answers to these issues might come from the ENTARES study, which is currently evaluating the impact of nCPAP versus HFNC on enteral feeding to identify the most suitable technique for preterm infants with RDS.[40]

Binasal and single prongs for nCPAP are commonly reported to induce nasal traumas of different severity. The following staging has been suggested for nasal injuries: mild (stage I), persistent hyperemia on intact septal skin; moderate (stage II), with superficial ulcer or erosion; and severe (stage III), with necrosis and complete loss of skin thickness.[41] To protect nares, the use of material barriers, such as hydrocolloid gel or soft silicon, has been proposed but scarce data are available on their effectiveness. However, Guimarães and colleagues[41] reported that nasal traumas were found in 65% of 135 very low birth weight infants at stage I, II, and III in 49%, 16%, and 1% of patients, respectively. These findings are important because without proper care these lesions may progress to permanent deformity (ie, nares or columella asymmetry, nasal tip deviation, or collapse).[42]

## HIGH-FLOW NASAL CANNULA

HFNC allows the delivery of heated, humidified gas flow at rates greater than 1 L/min through a specialized nasal prong. This has become increasingly popular as an option for noninvasive respiratory support for preterm infants in the last two decades thanks to easy application, which facilitates nursing and greater patient comfort, which improves parental interaction.[14]

### Physiologic Effects of Nasal Continuous Positive Airway Pressure

One of the most relevant working mechanisms of HFNC is the provision of a distending pressure, which contributes to developing and maintaining FRC and lung recruitment and airway patency. Wilkinson and colleagues[43] demonstrated that HFNC increases average airway pressure by 0.8 cm $H_2O$ for each 1 L/min increase in flow. Liew and colleagues[44] substantially confirmed this finding but also found that the increase of pressure correlated to the increase of flow is characterized by considerable variability significantly higher with mouth closed and in infants with smaller weight (<1000 g), while unaffected by prong-to-nares ratio. Lavizzari and colleagues[45] confirmed the fluctuations of airway pressure (although not clinically relevant) and observed that during HFNC (for 6 L/min of flow) only 75% of infants reached a pressure of 4 cm $H_2O$ and values greater than 5 cm $H_2O$ were rarely achieved.

Another major mechanism of action of HFNC is its ability to wash out upper airways, which leads to a reduction of the physiologic dead space. This effect has never been demonstrated in preterm infants but its existence is supported by the associated decrease of patients' respiratory rate and $Paco_2$, and by the improvement of oxygenation.[46]

It has been reported that HFNC can decrease the inspiratory resistance associated with the nasopharynx by providing nasopharyngeal gas flows that match or exceed the patient's peak inspiratory flow.[46] This might contribute to decrease the resistive WOB but to a lesser extent than nCPAP (see **Table 1**).[45]

Other suggested mechanisms of action of HFNC are improvement of airway conductance and pulmonary compliance by reducing the effect of cold air, and reduction of the metabolic cost of gas conditions by providing air with 100% relative humidity.[47]

### Methods of Generating High-Flow Nasal Cannula

The basic functional theories behind HFNC devices are the same. They are respiratory support systems that deliver gas to near body temperature and near 100% relative humidity at a flow of 2.0 to 8.0 L/min. Two devices are most widely used for HFNC: Optiflow (Fisher & Paykel Healthcare, Auckland, New Zealand) and Vapotherm (Exeter, NH). Studies comparing the clinical effectiveness of these devices are scarce. In a randomized pilot study of extubation in 40 very preterm infants, Miller and Dowd[48] found that they were similarly effective in preventing reintubation within 7 days. Fernandez-Alvarez and colleagues[49] performed a retrospective study evaluating the effectiveness of Optiflow and Vapotherm in weaning preterm infants from nCPAP. They found them equally effective and safe for weaning from nCPAP. However, infants weaned to Vapotherm spent less time on noninvasive respiratory support.[49]

### High-Flow Nasal Cannula Failure

Knowledge about the risk factors for HFNC failure is useful to guide decisions regarding the most appropriate initial respiratory support in the most appropriate patients. Manley and colleagues[50] performed a secondary analysis of the HIPSTER trial and found that in infants born from 28 to 36 weeks of gestation lower gestational age (<30 weeks) and higher $Fio_2$ (>0.30) before randomization predicted HFNC treatment failure. Similar results were found by McKimmie-Doherty and colleagues,[51] who performed a secondary analysis of the HUNTER trial and found that HFNC failed less frequently in infants born greater than or equal to 31 weeks of gestation and with a birth weight greater than 1200 g. They detailed that lower gestational age (odds ratio, 1.13 per week) and higher $Fio_2$ (>0.30) before randomization predicted HFNC treatment failure.[51] Data on risk factors for HFNC failure in extremely preterm infants are lacking (see **Table 2**).

### High-Flow Nasal Cannula Adverse Effects

Most studies have reported no adverse events for preterm infants on HFNC and have concluded that the use of HFNC is safe. However, a nationwide survey in Germany reported that 4.5% of clinics experienced greater than three cases of pneumothorax in NICU or pediatric intensive care unit.[52] However, clinicians are unable to continuously measure the pressures delivered by HFNC and high pressures have been reported among infants treated with this support.[53] Thus, to avoid an unpredictable sudden increase of pressure, it is important to ensure a large leak around the nasal prongs when HFNC is used.

However, Jasin and colleagues[54] reported a case of subcutaneous scalp emphysema/pneumocephalus in a preterm infant, and a similar case of pneumocephalus was reported more recently by Iglesias-Deus and colleagues.[55]

The Vapotherm was temporarily removed from the market because of recovery of a bacterium (*Ralstonia mannitolilytica*) in infants who were treated with the device. It has since been marketed again with new guidelines on cleaning and no further infectious complications have been reported.

## NASAL CONTINUOUS POSITIVE AIRWAY PRESSURE VERSUS HIGH-FLOW NASAL CANNULA: COMPARATIVE STUDIES

### Nasal Continuous Positive Airway Pressure Versus High-Flow Nasal Cannula for Primary Respiratory Support

Ramaswamy and colleagues[56] performed a network meta-analysis of 10 randomized controlled studies (RCTs) including 1504 neonates comparing the outcome of infants treated with nCPAP or HFNC for primary respiratory support of preterm infants with RDS. They found similar effects on the risk of MV, treatment failure (ie, need for other forms of respiratory support because of respiratory acidosis, repeated apnea, high oxygen-dependence), air leak, mortality, and BPD or mortality.[56] The risk of nasal trauma was higher with nCPAP than with HFNC (relative risk [RR], 6.75%; 95% confidence interval [CI], 1.67–72.94).[56] More recently Bruet and colleagues[57] conducted a further meta-analysis of 10 RCTs including 1803 neonates. They found that nCPAP decreases the risk of treatment failure (RR, 1.34; 95% CI, 1.01–1.68) in comparison with HFNC, but it did not affect the risk of MV.[57] Moreover, they showed that HFNC decreases the risk of nasal injuries (RR, 0.48; 95% CI, 0.31–0.65) in comparison with nCPAP. In these studies, meta-regression analysis excluded any influence of gestational age,[56,57] birth weight, HFNC flow rate, type of CPAP generator, and use of surfactant.

### Nasal Continuous Positive Airway Pressure Versus High-Flow Nasal Cannula for Preventing Extubation Failure

Wilkinson and colleagues[58] meta-analyzed six RCTs including 934 infants to compare the effect of nCPAP and HFNC after extubation. They did not find differences with regard to the risk of mortality, BPD, treatment failure, or reintubation.[58] In addition, they showed that HFNC reduced nasal trauma (RR, 0.64; 95% CI, 0.51–0.79) and the risk of pneumothorax (RR, 0.35; 95% CI, 0.11–1.06) compared with nCPAP.[58] These findings were substantially confirmed by Ramaswamy and colleagues[59] who performed the network meta-analysis of 11 RCTs including 1631 neonates. Continuous- and variable-flow CPAP had the same effect of HFNC on the risk of reintubation, mortality, and BPD or mortality.[59] However, HFNC decreased the risk of air leaks (RR, 0.35%; 95% CI, 0.07–0.98) and nasal injuries (RR, 0.37%; 95% CI, 0.15–0.65) in comparison with continuous-flow nCPAP.[59] Regression analysis showed a trend of decreasing efficacy at lower gestational ages for HFNC when compared with continuous-flow CPAP.[59]

Recently, Uchiyama and colleagues[60] carried out an RCT in 372 preterm infants to compare the postextubation outcome of preterm infants treated with HFNC or with nCPAP/nasal intermittent positive pressure ventilation (NIPPV). They found that

HFNC treatment failed more frequently than nCPAP/NIPPV (31% vs 16%; $P = .001$), but the reintubation rate was similar (6% vs 9%; $P = .290$). These results are partially explained by the fact that 24% of infants in the nCPAP/NIPPV group received NIPPV, which is well known to be more effective in preventing reintubation than HFNC and nCPAP.[60]

## DISCUSSION

It has been reported that during nCPAP pressure is generated within the device and is dependent on the flow in the expiratory line, whereas resistance is provided by the expiratory valve. Conversely, during HFNC pressure is developed within the nasal cavity and results from the flow through the cannula in combination with the infant's breathing, whereas resistance is determined by the nasal leak around the cannula.[45] These different mechanisms of action can support different effects and possible clinical application of nCPAP and HFNC.

The most recent meta-analyses comparing the effectiveness of nCPAP and HFNC as primary care of RDS demonstrated that nCPAP reduced the risk of treatment failure,[57] but not that of MV.[56,57] However, these findings are not generalizable with regard to extreme preterm infants because most of the studies enrolled infants with gestational age of more than 28 weeks.[56,57] In fact, it has been demonstrated that the more immature and small babies have the greatest probability of HFNC failure.[50,51]

However, to correctly interpret the results of these meta-analyses it is important to consider that in about half of the evaluated studies infants who failed HFNC treatment were successfully rescued with nCPAP.[56,57] This fact introduced a high risk of bias because this deviation of initial intended mode of respiratory support masks the fact that many of the reported successes of HFNC were actually caused by the effect of nCPAP.

Thus, in agreement with previous considerations, the American Academy of Pediatrics did not recommend HFNC as primary respiratory support for preterm infants with RDS,[61] which is in line with a European Consensus of experts who suggest that "At present, CPAP remains the preferred initial method of non-invasive support."[62]

When the effect of nCPAP and HFNC was compared after extubation, there were not differences in term of risk of reintubation, mortality, and BPD or mortality, whereas HFNC decreased the risk of air leak in treated preterm infants.[58,59] Thus, the American Academy of Pediatrics concluded that HFNC "may be an effective alternative to nCPAP for postextubation failure,"[61] in agreement with the European Consensus of experts, which reports that "During weaning, HFNC can be used as an alternative to CPAP for some babies."[62]

With regard to adverse effects, it has been reported that the risk of air leaks is increased by nCPAP,[38] and to a lesser extent by HFNC[52] for which fewer data are available. However, it is right to remember that some concerns remain for the lack of pressure monitoring during HFNC. Many studies demonstrated that HFNC decreases the risk of nasal trauma in comparison with nCPAP, as primary respiratory support[56,57] and in the postextubation phase.[58,59] This point, although less important for the risk of treatment failure and reintubation, nevertheless deserves due consideration in choosing nCPAP or HFNC as noninvasive respiratory support in preterm infants with RDS.

## SUMMARY

Despite different mechanisms of action and that physiologic effects are not always superimposable, in many NICUs nCPAP and HFNC are considered interchangeable.

However, today nCPAP should remain the first choice as primary mode of noninvasive respiratory support in preterm infants with RDS,[61–63] especially in very preterm infants. Some centers have a great deal of experience with HFNC and use it as primary support even in the most immature infants, but this approach is not generalizable. Conversely, in the postextubation phase, HFNC was found as effective as nCPAP. Thus, because it also decreases the risk of air leak and nasal trauma,[58,59] this mode of noninvasive support can represent an effective alternative in the weaning phase of RDS.[61–63]

## BEST PRACTICE BOX

- Interventions aimed at limiting the need for mechanical ventilation, such as noninvasive respiratory support and surfactant treatment have been advocated to improve the outcome of extremely preterm infants with respiratory distress syndrome (RDS).
- Among noninvasive respiratory support, nasal continuous positive airway pressure (nCPAP) and high flow nasal cannula (HFNC) are widely diffused.
- On the basis of current literature, nCPAP should remain the first-choice as primary mode of noninvasive respiratory support in preterm infants with RDS, especially in very preterm infants.
- Conversely, in the post-extubation phase HFNC is as effective as nCPAP and can represent an effective alternative in the weaning phase of RDS.

## CLINICS CARE POINTS

- the main limitation of this mode of CPAP is the lack of pressure monitoring and alarms.
- variable-flow CPAP lowered the WOB from 13% to 29% maintaining a more stable pressure level and increasing more significantly lung compliance in comparison with continuous-flow CPAP.
- The WOB was found to be lower in preterm infants treated with variable-flow than with bubble CPAP in very preterm infants.
- RAM Cannula had the highest resistance and nasal mask had the lowest resistance at all assessed sizes and gas flows.
- recent meta-analysis demonstrated that nasal mask significantly decreases the risk of CPAP failure (number needed to treat 5 9) and the incidence of moderate to severe nasal trauma (number needed to treat 5 6).
- nCPAP, used as primary respiratory support in extremely preterm infants with RDS, failed to prevent MV in about 50% of cases.
- Gulczynska and colleagues[35] detailed that each gestational week can reduce the odds of CPAP failure by 19%, and each 100 g of birth weight can reduce the odds by 16%.
- nCPAP can cause adverse side effects and complications. The most severe is air leak, namely pneumothorax.
- HFNC increases average airway pressure by 0.8 cm H2O for each 1 L/min increase in flow.
- lower gestational age (odds ratio, 1.13 per week) and higher FIO2 (>0.30) before randomization predicted HFNC treatment failure.
- nCPAP decreases the risk of treatment failure (RR, 1.34; 95% CI, 1.01–1.68) in comparison with HFNC, but it did not affect the risk of MV.[57] Moreover, they showed that HFNC decreases the risk of nasal injuries (RR, 0.48; 95% CI, 0.31–0.65) in comparison with nCPAP.

- They did not find differences with regard to the risk of mortality, BPD, treatment failure, or reintubation.[58] In addition, they showed that HFNC reduced nasal trauma (RR, 0.64; 95% CI, 0.51–0.79) and the risk of pneumothorax (RR, 0.35; 95% CI, 0.11–1.06) compared with nCPAP.

- to correctly interpret the results of these meta-analyses it is important to consider that in about half of the evaluated studies infants who failed HFNC treatment were successfully rescued with nCPAP.[56,57] This fact introduced a high risk of bias because this deviation of initial intended mode of respiratory support masks the fact that many of the reported successes of HFNC were actually caused by the effect of nCPAP.

- the American Academy of Pediatrics did not recommend HFNC as primary respiratory support for preterm infants with RDS,[61] which is in line with a European Consensus of experts who suggest that "At present, CPAP remains the preferred initial method of non-invasive support."

- the American Academy of Pediatrics concluded that HFNC "may be an effective alternative to nCPAP for postextubation failure,"[61] in agreement with the European Consensus of experts, which reports that "During weaning, HFNC can be used as an alternative to CPAP for some babies.

## DISCLOSURE

The author has nothing to disclose.

## REFERENCES

1. Stoll BJ, Hansen NI, Bell EF, et al. Trends in care practices, morbidity, and mortality of extremely preterm neonates, 1993-2012. JAMA 2015;314:1039–51.
2. Jensen A, Schmidt B. Epidemiology of bronchopulmonary dysplasia. Birth Defects Res A Clin Mol Teratol 2014;100(3):145–57.
3. Lapcharoensap W, Gage SC, Kan P, et al. Hospital variation and risk factors for bronchopulmonary dysplasia in a population-based cohort. JAMA Pediatr 2015;169(2):e143676.
4. Dreyfuss D, Saumon G. Role of tidal volume, FRC, and end-inspiratory volume in the development of pulmonary edema following mechanical ventilation. Am Rev Respir Dis 1993;148(5):1194–203.
5. Tsuchida S, Engelberts D, Peltekova V, et al. Atelectasis causes alveolar injury in nonatelectatic lung regions. Am J Respir Crit Care Med 2006;174(3):279–89.
6. Davis JM, Dickerson B, Metlay L, et al. Differential effects of oxygen and barotrauma on lung injury in the neonatal piglet. Pediatr Pulmonol 1991;10(3):157–63.
7. Walsh MC, Morris BH, Wrage LA, et al. Extremely low birth weight neonates with protracted ventilation: mortality and 18-month neurodevelopmental outcomes. J Pediatr 2005;146(6):798–804.
8. Zhang H, Dysart K, Kendrick DE, et al. Prolonged respiratory support of any type impacts outcomes of extremely low birth weight infants. Pediatr Pulmonol 2018; 53(10):1447–55.
9. D'Apremont I, Marshall G, Musalem C, et al. Trends in perinatal practices and neonatal outcomes of very low birth weight infants during a 16-year period at NEOCOSUR centers. J Pediatr 2020;225:44–50.e1.
10. Habas F, Durand S, Milesi C, et al. 15-year trends in respiratory care of extremely preterm infants: contributing factors and consequences on health and growth during hospitalization. Pediatr Pulmonol 2020;55(8):1946–54.

11. Petrillo F, Gizzi C, Maffei G, et al. Neonatal respiratory support strategies for the management of extremely low gestational age infants: an Italian survey. Ital J Pediatr 2019;45(1):44.

12. Gregory GA, Kitterman JA, Phibbs RH, et al. Treatment of the idiopathic respiratory-distress syndrome with continuous positive airway pressure. N Engl J Med 1971;284(24):1333–40.

13. Gupta S, Donn SM. Continuous positive airway pressure: physiology and comparison of devices. Semin Fetal Neonatal Med 2016;21(3):204–11.

14. Ekhaguere O, Patel S, Kirpalani H. Nasal intermittent mandatory ventilation versus nasal continuous positive airway pressure before and after invasive ventilatory support. Clin Perinatol 2019;46(3):517–36.

15. Hammer J. Nasal CPAP in preterm infants: does it work and how? Intensive Care Med 2001;27(11):1689–91.

16. Lee KS, Dunn FM. A comparison of underwater bubble continuous positive airway pressure with ventilator-derived continuous positive airway pressure in premature neonates ready for extubation. Biol Neonate 1998;73(2):69–75.

17. Pillow JJ, Hillman N, Moss TJ, et al. Bubble continuous positive airway pressure enhances lung volume and gas exchange in preterm lambs. Am J Respir Crit Care Med 2007;176(1):63–9.

18. Klausner JF, Lee Ay, Hutchinson AA. Decreased imposed work with a new nasal continuous positive airway pressure device. Pediatr Pulmonol 1996;22(3):188–94.

19. Pandit PB, Courtney SE, Pyon KH, et al. Work of breathing during constant- and variable-flow nasal continuous positive airway pressure in preterm neonates. Pediatrics 2001;108(3):682–5.

20. Courtney SE, Pyon KH, Saslow JG, et al. Lung recruitment and breathing pattern during variable versus continuous flow nasal continuous positive airway pressure in premature infants: an evaluation of three devices. Pediatrics 2001;107(2):304–8.

21. Courtney SE, Aghai ZH, et al. Work of breathing (WOB) during nasal continuous positive airway pressure (NCPAP): a pilot study of bubble vs. variable-flow (VF) NCPAP. J Perinatol 2003;53:2039.

22. Liptsen E, Aghai ZH, Pyon KH, et al. Work of breathing during nasal continuous positive airway pressure in preterm infants: a comparison of bubble vs variable-flow devices. J Perinatol 2005;25(7):453–8.

23. Kahn DJ, Courtney SE, Steele AM, et al. Unpredictability of delivered bubble nasal continuous positive airway pressure role of bias flow magnitude and nares-prong air leaks. Pediatr Res 2007;62(3):343–7.

24. De Paoli AG, Davis PG, Faber B. Devices and pressure sources for administration of nasal continuous positive airway pressure in preterm neonates. Cochrane Database Syst Rev 2008;23(1):CD002977.

25. Sharma D, Murki S, Maram S, et al. Comparison of delivered distending pressures in the oropharynx in preterm infant on bubble CPAP and on three different nasal interfaces. Pediatr Pulmonol 2020;55(7):1631–9.

26. Singh N, McNally MJ, Darnall RA. Does the RAM cannula provide continuous positive airway pressure as effectively as the Hudson prongs in preterm neonates? Am J Perinatol 2019;36(8):849–54.

27. Green EA, Dawson JA, Davis PG, et al. Assessment of resistance of nasal continuous positive airway pressure interfaces. Arch Dis Child Fetal Neonatal Ed 2019;104(5):F535–9.

28. Kieran EA, Twomey AR, Molloy EJ, et al. Randomized trial of prongs or mask for nasal continuous positive airway pressure in preterm infants. Pediatrics 2012; 130(5):e1170–6.
29. Goel S, Mondkar J, Panchal H, et al. Nasal mask versus nasal prongs for delivering nasal continuous positive airway pressure in preterm infants with respiratory distress: a randomized controlled trial. Indian Pediatr 2015;52(12):1035–40.
30. Jasani B, Ismail A, Rao S, et al. Effectiveness and safety of nasal mask versus binasal prongs for providing continuous positive airway pressure in preterm infants: a systematic review and meta-analysis. Pediatr Pulmonol 2018;53(7): 987–92.
31. Wright CJ, Polin RA, Kirpalani H. Continuous positive airway pressure to prevent neonatal lung injury: how did we get here, and how do we improve? J Pediatr 2016;173:17–24.e2.
32. Rocha G, Flor-de-Lima F, Proenca E, et al. Failure of early nasal continuous positive airway pressure in preterm infants of 26 to 30 weeks gestation. J Perinatol 2013;33(4):297–301.
33. De Jaegere AP, van der Lee JH, Cante C, et al. Early prediction of nasal continuous positive airway pressure failure in preterm infants less than 30 weeks gestation. Acta Paediatr 2012;101(4):374–9.
34. Permatahati WI, Setyati A, Haksari EL. Predictor factors of continuous positive airway pressure failure in preterm infants with respiratory distress. Glob Pediatr Health 2021;8. 2333794X211007464.
35. Multicenter Study Collaborative Group for Evaluation of Outcomes in Very Low Birth Weight Infants. Failure of non-invasive continuous positive airway pressure as the initial respiratory support in very preterm infants: a multicenter prospective cohort study. Zhonghua Er Ke Za Zhi 2021;59(4):273–9.
36. Gulczyńska E, Szczapa T, Hożejowski R, et al. Fraction of inspired oxygen as a predictor of CPAP failure in preterm infants with respiratory distress syndrome: a prospective multicenter study. Neonatology 2019;116(2):171–8.
37. Hall RT, Rhodes PG. Pneumothorax and pneumomediastinum in infants with idiopathic respiratory distress syndrome receiving continuous positive airway pressure. Pediatrics 1975;55(4):493–6.
38. Morley C. Continuous distending pressure. Arch Dis Child Fetal Neonatal Ed 1999;81(2):F152–6.
39. Ho JJ, Subramaniam P, Davis PG. Continuous positive airway pressure (CPAP) for respiratory distress in preterm infants. Cochrane Database Syst Rev 2020; 10(10):CD002271.
40. Jaile JC, Levin T, Wung JT, et al. Benign gaseous distension of the bowel in premature infants treated with nasal continuous airway pressure: a study of contributing factors. AJR Am J Roentgenol 1992;158(1):125–7.
41. Cresi F, Maggiora E, Borgione SM, et al. Enteral nutrition tolerance and respiratory support (entares) study in preterm infants: study protocol for a randomized controlled trial. Trials 2019;20(1):67.
42. Guimarães AR, Rocha G, Rodrigues M, et al. Nasal CPAP complications in very low birth weight preterm infants. J Neonatal Perinatal Med 2020;13(2):197–206.
43. Fischer C, Bertelle V, Hohlfeld J, et al. Nasal trauma due to continuous positive airway pressure in neonates. Arch Dis Child Fetal Neonatal Ed 2010;95(6): F447–51.
44. Wilkinson DJ, Andersen CC, Smith K, et al. Pharyngeal pressure with high-flow nasal cannulae in premature infants. J Perinatol 2008;28(1):42–7.

45. Liew Z, Fenton AC, Harigopal S, et al. Physiological effects of high-flow nasal cannula therapy in preterm infants. Arch Dis Child Fetal Neonatal Ed 2020; 105(1):87–93.
46. Lavizzari A, Veneroni C, Colnaghi M, et al. Respiratory mechanics during NCPAP and HHHFNC at equal distending pressures. Arch Dis Child Fetal Neonatal Ed 2014;99(4):F315–20.
47. Dysart K, Miller TL, Wolfson MR, et al. Research in high flow therapy: mechanisms of action. Respir Med 2009;103(10):1400–5.
48. Mikalsen IB, Davis P, Oymar K. High flow nasal cannula in children: a literature review. Scand J Trauma Resusc Emerg Med 2016;24:93.
49. Miller SM, Dowd SA. High-flow nasal cannula and extubation success in the premature infant: a comparison of two modalities. J Perinatol 2010;30(12):805–8.
50. Fernandez-Alvarez JR, Mahoney L, Gandhi R, et al. Optiflow vs Vapotherm as extended weaning mode from nasal continuous positive airway pressure in preterm infants 28 weeks gestational age. Pediatr Pulmonol 2020;55(10):2624–9.
51. Manley BJ, Roberts CT, Frøisland DH, et al. Refining the use of nasal high-flow therapy as primary respiratory support for preterm infants. J Pediatr 2018;196: 65–70.e1.
52. McKimmie-Doherty M, Arnolda GRB, Buckmaster AG, et al. Predicting nasal high-flow treatment success in newborn infants with respiratory distress cared for in nontertiary hospitals. J Pediatr 2020;227:135–41.e1.
53. Schmid F, Olbertz DM, Ballmann M. The use of high-flow nasal cannula (HFNC) as respiratory support in neonatal and pediatric intensive care units in Germany: a nationwide survey. Respir Med 2017;131:210–4.
54. Locke RG, Wolfson MR, Shaffer TH. Inadvertent administration of positive end-distending pressure during nasal cannula flow. Pediatrics 1993;91(1):135–8.
55. Jasin LR, Kern S, Thompson S, et al. Subcutaneous scalp emphysema, pneumo-orbitis and pneumocephalus in a neonate on high humidity high flow nasal cannula. J Perinatol 2008;28(11):779–81.
56. Iglesias-Deus A, Pérez-Muñuzuri A, López-Suárez O, et al. Tension pneumocephalus induced by high-flow nasal cannula ventilation in a neonate. Arch Dis Child Fetal Neonatal Ed 2017;102(2):F173–5.
57. Ramaswamy VV, More K, Roehr CC, et al. Efficacy of noninvasive respiratory support modes for primary respiratory support in preterm neonates with respiratory distress syndrome: systematic review and network meta-analysis. Pediatr Pulmonol 2020;55(11):2940–63.
58. Bruet S, Butin M, Dutheil F. Systematic review of high-flow nasal cannula versus continuous positive airway pressure for primary support in preterm infants. Arch Dis Child Fetal Neonatal Ed 2021.
59. Wilkinson D, Andersen C, O'Donnell CPF, et al. High flow nasal cannula for respiratory support in preterm infants. Cochrane Database Syst Rev 2016;2: CD006405.
60. Ramaswamy VV, Bandyopadhyay T, Nanda D, et al. Efficacy of noninvasive respiratory support modes as postextubation respiratory support in preterm neonates: a systematic review and network meta-analysis. Pediatr Pulmonol 2020; 55(11):2924–39.
61. Uchiyama A, Okazaki K, Kondo M, et al. Randomized controlled trial of high-flow nasal cannula in preterm infants after extubation. Pediatrics 2020;146(6): e20201101.

62. Cummings JJ, Polin RA. Committee on Fetus and Newborn, American Academy of Pediatrics. Noninvasive respiratory support. Pediatrics 2016;137(1): e20153758.
63. Sweet DG, Carnielli V, Greisen G, et al. European Consensus guidelines on the management of respiratory distress syndrome: 2019 update. Neonatology 2019;115(4):432–50.

# Nasal Intermittent Positive Pressure Ventilation for Neonatal Respiratory Distress Syndrome

Christoph M. Rüegger, MD[a],*, Louise S. Owen, MD, FRACP[b,c,d],
Peter G. Davis, MD, FRACP[b,c,d]

## KEYWORDS

- Infant • Premature • Respiratory distress syndrome • Noninvasive ventilation
- Nasal positive pressure ventilation

## KEY POINTS

- Two device types have typically been used to deliver NIPPV: ventilators and flow-drivers, both devices can incorporate the option to synchronize pressure changes with spontaneous breathing.
- Ventilator-generated NIPPV is traditionally set up to deliver NIPPV with settings mimicking settings used during endotracheal ventilation.
- Flow-driver-generated NIPPV may also be set up in this manner, albeit with lower peak pressures, but it is more typically used with settings reflective of bilevel CPAP.
- Overall, NIPPV is superior to CPAP as primary and postextubation support for the prevention of respiratory failure in preterm infants, especially when ventilator-generated, synchronized NIPPV is used.
- Ventilator-generated, synchronized NIPPV as either primary or postextubation support in preterm infants may reduce the risk of bronchopulmonary dysplasia, but is not associated with a decrease in mortality.

## INTRODUCTION

In the past, preterm infants with signs of moderate or severe respiratory distress were intubated and mechanically ventilated. This invasive approach resulted in inflammation of the lungs in the short-term and impaired development and scarring known as bronchopulmonary dysplasia (BPD) in the long-term.[1] Efforts to decrease rates

[a] Newborn Research, Department of Neonatology, University Hospital Zurich, University of Zurich, Frauenklinikstrasse 10, Zurich 8091, Switzerland; [b] Newborn Research Centre and Neonatal Services, The Royal Women's Hospital, Melbourne, Australia; [c] Department of Obstetrics and Gynaecology, The University of Melbourne, Melbourne, Australia; [d] Clinical Sciences, Murdoch Children's Research Institute, Melbourne, Australia
* Corresponding author.
*E-mail address:* christoph.rueegger@usz.ch

Clin Perinatol 48 (2021) 725–744
https://doi.org/10.1016/j.clp.2021.07.004
perinatology.theclinics.com
0095-5108/21/© 2021 The Authors. Published by Elsevier Inc. This is an open access article under
the CC BY license (http://creativecommons.org/licenses/by/4.0/).

of BPD in the surfactant/antenatal steroid era have led to an increased use of noninvasive respiratory support for even the most immature infants.[2]

Prophylactic nasal continuous positive airway pressure (CPAP), started soon after birth, is now recommended for spontaneously breathing very preterm or very low-birth-weight infants with respiratory distress syndrome (RDS).[3] Prophylactic CPAP reduces the need for mechanical ventilation and surfactant administration, and lowers the rates of both BPD alone and the combined outcome of death or BPD when compared with immediate endotracheal ventilation.[3]

Despite the physiologic and clinical benefits, CPAP failure rates remain at approximately 50% in the first week of life in extremely preterm newborns at highest risk for developing BPD.[4-7] CPAP failure is associated with a substantial increase in important adverse outcomes including air leak, BPD, intraventricular hemorrhage, and death.[8]

As a result, methods to augment the effectiveness of CPAP have gained interest.[9] Noninvasive intermittent positive pressure ventilation (NIPPV) applied at the nose has become a well-established therapy for preterm infants.[10] Despite its frequent use, uncertainty remains regarding the precise terminology, the appropriate clinical indications, the different devices and techniques used to generate NIPPV, and the level of benefit they provide. These differences complicate the interpretation of the available evidence.[11,12] In this review, we address these uncertainties, with a particular focus on NIPPV as primary and postextubation respiratory support for preterm infants with RDS. For both indications, we summarize the current evidence from randomized controlled trials (RCTs) comparing NIPPV with CPAP.

## NASAL INTERMITTENT POSITIVE PRESSURE VENTILATION
### Terminology

NIPPV is a form of noninvasive respiratory support that combines a continuous positive end-expiratory airway pressure (PEEP) with intermittent higher pressures delivered by a nasal mask or nasal prongs. The terminology surrounding NIPPV is confusing. There are many alternative pressure generating devices, interfaces, and settings available. In addition, some devices allow synchronization with the infant's own breathing efforts. The most common abbreviations include nsNIPPV (nonsynchronized NIPPV), sNIPPV (synchronized NIPPV), BiPAP (biphasic CPAP), bilevel CPAP, and bilevel NIPPV.

Although all these modes are considered forms of NIPPV, 2 main NIPPV modalities must be distinguished: traditional NIPPV, with settings designed to mimic ventilator settings, typically generated using a ventilator, or alternatively settings that are more reflective of bilevel CPAP, typically generated using flow-drivers. There are devices of both types which have the capacity to synchronize pressure changes with spontaneous breathing (**Table 1**).

### Pressure and Volume Delivery

The lower pressure level (PEEP) during NIPPV offers the same physiologic benefits as CPAP, that is, stabilization of the upper airways and the compliant preterm chest wall and prevention of end-expiratory alveolar collapse. This maintains functional residual capacity and reduces ventilation-perfusion mismatch, which improves oxygenation and work of breathing. The intermittent pressure peaks increase the mean airway pressure (MAP) above the PEEP level, potentially further recruiting the lung, which may improve functional residual capacity more efficiently than CPAP alone.[13]

**Table 1**
Characteristics of 'traditional' NIPPV and bilevel CPAP[18,22,33]

| | 'Traditional' NIPPV | Bilevel CPAP |
|---|---|---|
| Device | Mostly ventilator, can be flow-driver with lower peak pressure settings | Flow-driver |
| Principle | Mimics timings and settings used during endotracheal ventilation | Independent breathing on two PEEP levels |
| Interface | Short binasal prongs, nasal masks, nasopharyngeal tubes | Short binasal prongs, nasal masks |
| Maximum pressure | Similar to endotracheal ventilation, usually $\leq 25$ cm $H_2O$ | 11–15 cm $H_2O$, depending on operating mode[a] |
| Peak and PEEP pressure difference | $\geq 5$ cm $H_2O$ | $\leq 4$ cm $H_2O$ |
| High pressure delivery rate | Variable (10–60 per min) | Low (10–30 per min) |
| High pressure duration | Short (<0.5 s) | Long (0.5–1 s) |
| Synchronization | Possible, available with some ventilators | Possible, usually not intended, available with some devices |
| Method of synchronization | Pneumatic capsule (eg, Graseby), flow sensor, pressure sensor, neurally adjusted ventilator assist (NAVA) | Pneumatic capsule (eg, Graseby)[34] |
| Pressure curves | | |

[a] Infant Flow SiPAP (Vyaire Medical, Mettawa, Il, USA): theoretic maximum at 11 cm $H_2O$ if nonsynchronized and at 15 cm $H_2O$ if synchronized, although delivered pressures are often well below these maximums.[9,19]

Because of large and variable leaks around the nose and mouth, the transmission of applied NIPPV pressures to the lung is substantially attenuated.[14,15] Moreover, observational studies demonstrate that the majority of nonsynchronized pressure peaks occur during spontaneous expiration and do not contribute to tidal volume.[16] When the pressure rises coincided with spontaneous inspiration, only a 15% increase in relative tidal volume was noted. During apneic episodes, pressure peaks resulted in measurable tidal volumes only 5% of the time, and produced tidal volumes a quarter of those seen during spontaneous breathing. Higher peak inspiratory pressures did not increase the likelihood of a visible chest inflation, suggesting that higher set pressures may not provide additional respiratory assistance during apnoea.[16]

Whether nonsynchronized NIPPV confers any benefit over CPAP when the PEEP during CPAP is matched to the generated MAP during NIPPV is still a matter of debate. A small crossover study including 10 infants on nonsynchronized NIPPV and CPAP delivered at the same MAP found minimal differences in short-term outcomes, suggesting that any advantage of nonsynchronized NIPPV may arise from a higher MAP rather than from the effect of the intermittent pressure peaks themselves.[13]

### Synchronization

Observations of low pressure and volume delivery during nonsynchronized NIPPV suggest support may be more effective if inflations are synchronized with the infant's own inspiratory efforts. Synchronization may be achieved by airway flow detection, which ensures that the glottis is open before pressure is applied.[17] However, this is challenging because of air leakage around the prongs and masks and from the open mouth. Graseby capsules are unaffected by air leak, but may be affected by movement artifact; however, they are the most commonly used method for NIPPV synchronization.[18] These cheap, lightweight, and disposable capsules are noninvasively attached to the anterior abdominal wall below the xiphoid process; they consist of a small, flat balloon filled with air, which is sensitive to pressure variations. The balloon connects to a pressure transducer capable of detecting the beginning of the diaphragmatic contraction, which enables the synchronization of the pressure peak. Although the accuracy of the Graseby capsule is affected by its position, method of fixation, and movement artifacts, it produces reliable signals that rapidly trigger the set pressure peak with most spontaneous breaths.[19–21] Other potential synchronization methods include neurally adjusted ventilatory assist, currently available with the Servo-n ventilator (Maquet, Solna, Sweden) and respiratory inductance plethysmography.[22]

### Safety

Although there were initial concerns regarding an increased risk of gastrointestinal side effects with NIPPV, recent evidence suggests that NIPPV is a safe therapy in preterm infants.[23] This has been confirmed by 2 systematic reviews of the Cochrane Collaboration on NIPPV for initial support of neonatal RDS and for preterm infants after extubation.[11,12] Both reviews reported no significant differences between the NIPPV and CPAP groups in rates of feeding intolerance, gastrointestinal perforation, necrotizing enterocolitis, or air leak. The incidence of nasal injury through tight-fitting binasal prongs has not been assessed systematically for infants receiving NIPPV. Since the risk of nasal injury, and the strategies to prevent it are considered the same for NIPPV and CPAP, use of nasal masks, rotating nasal interfaces, and nasal barrier dressings may be equally effective in reducing nasal injury during NIPPV.[24]

## CLINICAL EVIDENCE

The majority of clinical trials in preterm infants have compared NIPPV with CPAP as either the primary mode of treatment for neonatal RDS, or after extubation. Of these trials, Kirpalani's *NIPPV Trial* dominates the literature.[25] This large, pragmatic trial differs from the smaller studies in that it recruited a heterogeneous study population and permitted a variety of devices to deliver NIPPV, including some that delivered synchronized pressure changes. Although pragmatic, the considerable degree of methodological and clinical heterogeneity makes interpretation of pooled trial results difficult. To evaluate the impact of these variations, we begin with a review of Kirpalani's *NIPPV Trial* and its substudies, and provide updated meta-analyses of trials comparing NIPPV with CPAP as primary or postextubation support for neonatal RDS.

### Kirpalani's Nasal Intermittent Positive Pressure Ventilation Trial

This large randomized, controlled, multicenter trial conducted between 2007 and 2011 hypothesized that NIPPV would reduce the risk of BPD in extremely low-birth-weight infants by minimizing the duration of endotracheal intubation.[25] Infants with a birth weight of less than 1000 g and a gestational age of less than 30 weeks, eligible for noninvasive support within the first 28 days of life, were randomly assigned to 1 of 2 forms of noninvasive respiratory support, NIPPV or CPAP. Initial settings for respiratory support were provided, but not mandated and clinicians could individualize care. No NIPPV delivery devices were specified, NIPPV synchronization was permitted but not mandated. The primary outcome was a composite of death or moderate/severe BPD according to National Institutes of Health criteria.[26] Three preplanned subgroup analyses were performed according to birth weight, prior intubation status (intubated or nonintubated before randomization), and the form of the intervention used in the NIPPV group (synchronized or nonsynchronized).

A total of 1009 infants with a mean gestational age of 26 weeks and a mean birth weight of 800 g were enrolled. The primary outcome, death or BPD occurred in 38.4% (191 of 497 infants) randomized to NIPPV and in 36.7% (180 of 490) randomized to CPAP (adjusted odds ratio, 1.09; 95% confidence interval [CI], 0.83–1.43; $P = .56$). There were no significant differences between NIPPV and CPAP in the individual components of death or BPD, in other prespecified secondary outcomes including potential adverse effects of treatment, or in the subgroup analyses according to birth weight, prior intubation status, or synchronization.

In the years following the publication of Kirpalani's *NIPPV Trial* results, 2 secondary analyses have been published with the following aims: (1) to examine whether important outcomes differed in infants who received ventilator-generated or flow-driver-generated NIPPV, and (2) to compare noninvasive ventilation failure rates in intubation-naïve extremely low-birth-weight infants randomized to NIPPV or CPAP.[27,28]

### Substudy 1: ventilator-generated versus flow-driver-generated nasal intermittent positive pressure ventilation

This nonrandomized comparison from Kirpalani's *NIPPV Trial* provides outcome data on the 497 infants in the NIPPV group.[27] NIPPV could be delivered by a ventilator or a flow-driver device based on unit preference, practice, and device availability. Irrespective of the device, traditional NIPPV settings or bilevel CPAP settings could be used. In the NIPPV group, 215 infants received ventilator-generated NIPPV and 241 received flow-driver-generated NIPPV. Forty-one infants, in whom both devices had been used, were excluded. The composite outcome, death or BPD at 36 weeks was 39% in the ventilator-generated NIPPV group and 37% in the flow-driver-generated NIPPV group (adjusted odds ratio, 0.88; 95% CI, 0.57–1.35; $P = .56$). Although rates of BPD were not significantly different between groups (adjusted odds ratio, 0.64; 95% CI, 0.41–1.02; $P = .061$), more deaths occurred before 36 weeks gestational age in the flow-driver-generated NIPPV group (2.3% vs 9.4%; adjusted odds ratio, 5.01; 95% CI, 1.74–14.4; $P = .003$).

### Substudy 2: nasal intermittent positive pressure ventilation versus continuous positive airway pressure in intubation-naïve infants

The second substudy compared the rate of 'failure of noninvasive support' in infants who were never intubated before enrollment and randomization.[28] As opposed to the original trial and substudy 1, the primary outcome was defined as failure of noninvasive respiratory support requiring endotracheal intubation at any time in the first 7 days after randomization. Of the 1009 extremely low-birth-weight infants initially enrolled in the NIPPV trial, 142 had not been intubated before randomization. Of those, 27.5% in the NIPPV group and 30.1% in the CPAP group were subsequently intubated (relative risk, 0.91; 95% CI, 0.54–1.53). The combined outcome of death or BPD at 36 weeks postmenstrual age was not different between groups (19.7% vs 16.7%; risk ratio, 1.18; 95% CI, 0.58–2.40). There was no significant difference in rates of air leak.

### What do the results of Kirpalani's nasal intermittent positive pressure ventilation trial and its substudies mean?

In contrast with the results obtained from the pooled analysis of smaller trials that favored the use of NIPPV in preterm infants, Kirpalani's *NIPPV trial* and its substudies found no significant benefit of NIPPV with respect to the risk of death or survival without BPD.[11,12,29–31] There may be several reasons for the differences in findings. First, more immature infants were included in Kirpalani's *NIPPV trial* (**Tables 2** and **3**); failure of noninvasive support is more prevalent in extremely preterm infants and is associated with a marked increase in the rate of adverse outcomes, including death and BPD.[4,8] In such a high-risk population with RDS due to surfactant-deficient lungs, collapsing airways and poor muscle strength, a number of infants may still be inadequately supported with NIPPV despite the modest increase in MAP provided by additional positive pressure breaths. Second, the pragmatic trial design did not specify the ventilator device, settings, or use of synchronization. In the NIPPV group, approximately half of infants received flow-driver-generated NIPPV, typically set to deliver modest peak pressures, lower than pressures set during ventilator-generated NIPPV. Indeed, mortality was higher in infants who mostly received flow-driver-generated NIPPV, possibly due to a higher reintubation rate compared with infants receiving ventilator-generated NIPPV (adjusted rate ratio for number of reintubations, 1.23; 95% CI, 1.02–1.49).[27] Moreover, a subgroup analysis by synchronization rather than by device revealed that ventilator-generated NIPPV was mostly applied in a nonsynchronized manner, and synchronization was more often used during flow-driver-generated NIPPV (suggesting that traditional NIPPV settings with short high-pressure durations were still commonly used during flow-driver-generated NIPPV, cf. **Table 1**). Both combinations of device and technique may be associated with a lack of effective pressure transmission to the lungs, and may contribute to the finding of no significant benefit of NIPPV.

### Meta-Analyses of Trials Comparing Nasal Intermittent Positive Pressure Ventilation with Continuous Positive Airway Pressure

The updated meta-analyses were performed using RevMan, version 5.4.[32] Relevant studies were identified by searching PubMed, The Cochrane Library, and the reference lists of included articles. Studies were included if they were RCTs that enrolled

**Table 2**
Trials comparing NIPPV with CPAP for primary respiratory support (by device and synchronization)

| | Mean GA[a] at Birth [wk] | Surfactant | Device[f] | NIPPV Set Peak Pressure [cm H₂O] | NIPPV High Pressure Duration [s] | NIPPV High Pressure Delivery Rate [per minute] | NIPPV PEEP[b] [cm H₂O] | CPAP PEEP[b] [cm H₂O] |
|---|---|---|---|---|---|---|---|---|
| **1.1.1 Ventilator-generated, nonsynchronized NIPPV** | | | | | | | | |
| Bisceglia et al,[35] 2007 | NDA[c] | No | 1 | 14–20 | NDA[c] | 40 | 4–6 | 4–6 |
| Sai Sunil Kishore et al,[36] 2009 | 30.8 | Mixed | 2, 3 | 15–26 | 0.30–0.35 | 50–60 | 5–6 | 5–7 |
| Meneses et al,[37] 2011 | 29.6 | No | 4 | 15–20 | 0.40–0.50 | 20–30 | 4–6 | 5–6 |
| Armanian et al,[38] 2014 | 30.0 | No | 4 | 16–20 | 0.40 | 40–50 | 5–6 | 5–6 |
| Oncel et al,[39] 2015[e] | 29.2 | No | 5 | 15–20 | NDA[c] | 20–30 | 5–6 | 5–6 |
| Sabzehei et al,[40] 2018[e] | 30.1 | Yes | 4 | 14–20 | 0.30–0.35 | 30–50 | 5–6 | 5–6 |
| Skariah & Lewis,[41] 2019[e] | 31.8 | No | 2 | 11–18 | 0.36–0.40 | 18–30 | 3–5 | 3–5 |
| **1.1.2 Ventilator-generated, synchronized NIPPV** | | | | | | | | |
| Kugelman et al,[42] 2007 | 30.9 | No | 5 | 14–22 | 0.30 | 12–30 | 6–7 | 6–7 |
| Salama et al,[43] 2015 | 31.2 | Mixed | 6 | 5–12 | 0.30–0.50 | 15–18 | 4–6 | 6 |
| Dursun et al,[44] 2019[e] | 29.3 | No | 5 | 16–24 | 0.40 | 30–40 | 6–8 | 6–8 |
| Gharehbaghi et al,[45] 2019[e] | 30.1 | No | 7 | 18–20 | 0.35–0.40 | 30–40 | 5–6 | 5–6 |
| **1.1.3 Flow-driver-generated, nonsynchronized NIPPV** | | | | | | | | |
| Kong et al,[46] 2012[e] | 32.9 | No | 8 | 12–15 | 0.35–0.50 | 20–30 | 4–6 | 4–6 |
| Aguiar et al,[47] 2015[e] | 31.0 | No | 9 | 8 | 2 | 10 | 6 | 6–8 |
| Sadeghnia et al,[48] 2016[e] | 29.9 | No | 10 | 8 | 0.50 | 30 | 4 | 6 |
| **1.1.4 Flow-driver-generated, synchronized NIPPV** | | | | | | | | |
| Lista et al,[49] 2010 | 30.3 | Yes | 9 | 8 | 0.50–0.70 | 30 | 4.5 | 6 |
| Wood et al,[50] 2013 | 29.8 | No | 9 | 6–9 | 0.3 | 10 | 4–6 | 4–6 |

(continued on next page)

**Table 2**
*(continued)*

| | Mean GA[a] at Birth [wk] | Surfactant | Device[f] | NIPPV Set Peak Pressure [cm H₂O] | High Pressure Duration [s] | High Pressure Delivery Rate [per minute] | PEEP[b] [cm H₂O] | CPAP PEEP[b] [cm H₂O] |
|---|---|---|---|---|---|---|---|---|
| **1.1.5 Mixed methods** | | | | | | | | |
| Ramanathan et al,[51] 2012 | 27.8 | Yes | 9, 11 | 15–20 | 0.50 | 30–40 | 5 | 5–8 |
| Kirpalani et al,[25] 2013 | 26.2 | No | 2, 3, 9 | ≤18[d] | 0.30–0.50[d] | 10–40[d] | 5–8[d] | 5–8[d] |

[a] GA, gestational age.
[b] PEEP, positive end expiratory pressure.
[c] NDA, no data available.
[d] Suggested initiating and maximal settings.
[e] Trials not yet included in the corresponding meta-analysis of the Cochrane Collaboration.
[f] 1: Bear Infant Ventilator CUB 750 (Ackrad Laboratories, Cranford, NJ, USA). 2: Drager Babylog 8000 (Drager Medical Inc, Lubeck, Germany). 3: VIP Bird-R Sterling (Vyaire Medical, II, USA). 4: Continuous flow ventilator, not specified. 5: SLE 2000 (Specialised Laboratory Equipment, Croydon, UK). 6. Neoport E100 M (DRE Medical, Louisville, KY, USA). 7: Inspiration 5i ventilator (eVent Medical Ltd, Ireland). 8: BiPAP device, not specified. 9: Infant Flow SiPAP System (Vyaire Medical, II, USA). 10: Fabian (Acutronic Medical Systems AG, Hirzel, Switzerland). 11: Avea CVS Ventilator (Vyaire Medical, II, USA).

**Table 3**
Trials comparing NIPPV with CPAP for postextubation support (by device and synchronization)

| | Mean GA[a] at Birth [wk] | Device[g] | NIPPV Set Peak Pressure [cm H2O] | NIPPV High Pressure Duration [s] | NIPPV High Pressure Delivery Rate [per minute] | NIPPV PEEP[b] [cm H2O] | CPAP PEEP[b] [cm H2O] |
|---|---|---|---|---|---|---|---|
| **1.2.1 Ventilator-generated, nonsynchronized NIPPV** | | | | | | | |
| Khorana et al,[52] 2008 | NDA[c] | 1 | Pre-ext[d] | Pre-ext[d] | Pre-ext[d] | Pre-ext[d] | Pre-ext[d] |
| Kahramaner et al,[53] 2014 | 28.8 | 2 | Pre-ext[d] +2 | NDA[c] | 25 | 6 | 6 |
| Jasani et al,[54] 2016 | 30.7 | 1 | Pre-ext[d] +4 | NDA[c] | Pre-ext[d] | ≤5 | 5-6 |
| Komatsu et al,[55] 2016[f] | 30.8 | 3 | 16 | NDA[c] | 12 | 6 | 6 |
| Ribeiro et al,[56] 2017[f] | 29.6 | 4 | 14-16 | 0.30-0.35 | 12-18 | 4-6 | 4-5 |
| Estay et al,[57] 2020[f] | 27.9 | 5 | 12-18 | 0.45-0.60 | 20 | 5-6 | 5-6 |
| **1.2.2 Ventilator-generated, synchronized NIPPV** | | | | | | | |
| Friedlich et al,[58] 1999 | 27.8 | 6 | Pre-ext[d] | 0.60 | 10 | 4-6 | 4-6 |
| Barrington et al,[59] 2001 | 26.1 | 6 | 16 | NDA[c] | 12 | 6 | 6 |
| Khalaf et al,[60] 2001 | 28.0 | 6 | Pre-ext[d] +2 – +4 | NDA[c] | Pre-ext[d] | ≤5 | 4-6 |
| Moretti et al,[61] 2008 | 27.0 | 7 | 10-20 | NDA[c] | Pre-ext[d] | 3-5 | 3-5 |
| Gao et al,[62] 2010 | 32.5 | 5 | 20 | NDA[c] | 40 | 5 | 4-8 |
| Ding et al,[63] 2020[f] | 29.8 | 8 | 15-25 | NDA[c] | 15-50 | 4-6 | 6 |
| **1.2.3 Flow-driver-generated, nonsynchronized NIPPV** | | | | | | | |
| O'Brien et al,[64] 2012 | 27.4 | 9 | 8-10 | 1 | 20 | 5-7 | 5-7 |
| Victor et al,[65] 2016[f] | 27.3 | 9 | 8 | 1 | 30 | 4 | 6 |
| **1.2.4 Mixed methods** | | | | | | | |
| Kirpalani et al,[25] 2013 | 26.2 | 2, 9, 10 | ≤18[e] | 0.30-0.50[e] | 10-40[e] | 5-8[e] | 5-8[e] |

[a] GA, gestational age.
[b] PEEP, positive end expiratory pressure.
[c] NDA, no data available.
[d] pre-ext, pre-extubation settings.
[e] Suggested initiating and maximal settings.
[f] Trials not yet included in the corresponding meta-analysis of the Cochrane Collaboration.
[g] 1: Bear Infant Ventilator CUB 750 (Ackrad Laboratories, Cranford, NJ, USA). 2: Drager Babylog 8000 (Drager Medical Inc, Lubeck, Germany). 3. Neoport E100 M (DRE medical, Louisville, KY, USA). 4. Inter 3/5plus (Intermed, Sao Paulo, Brazil). 5: Continuous flow ventilator, not specified. 6. Infantstar 500/950 (Infrasonics, San Diego, CA, USA). 7. Giulia (Ginevri, Rome, Italy). 8. Comen nv8 (Comen Medical, Shenzen, China). 9: Infant Flow SiPAP System (Vyaire Medical, II, USA). 10: VIP Bird-R Sterling (Vyaire Medical, II, USA).

preterm infants (born <37 weeks' gestation), compared any form of NIPPV with CPAP, and reported the primary outcome. Four subgroup analyses included whether NIPPV was delivered by a ventilator or by a flow-driver-device and whether pressure changes were synchronized with spontaneous breathing or not. No differentiation was made between the type of settings (traditional NIPPV vs bilevel CPAP) applied in each trial. A fixed-effect model was used to pool data of included trials.

### Primary respiratory support

This meta-analysis aimed to compare the efficacy of NIPPV versus CPAP when used as primary respiratory support in preterm infants with RDS who were less than 6 hours old. We defined the primary outcome as respiratory failure leading to additional ventilatory support during the first week of life. An early and brief period of endotracheal ventilation for an INSURE (intubate—surfactant administration—extubate) procedure was not considered as respiratory failure.

We pooled data from 18 trials and 1900 infants (see **Table 2**). We added data from 8 newly published trials comprising 850 infants to the existing meta-analysis of the Cochrane Collaboration.[11] In 11 trials, ventilator-generated NIPPV with variable peak pressures of 12 to 26 cm $H_2O$ were used. Five trials used flow-driver-generated support with peak pressures of 8 to 15 cm $H_2O$. Two trials, including Kirpalani's *NIPPV trial* used mixed methods: both ventilator-generated and flow-driver-generated NIPPV, with or without synchronization, and with variable pressure settings. None of the included studies attempted to match the PEEP in the CPAP group with the generated MAP in the NIPPV group.

Six individual trials reported a significant reduction in rates of respiratory failure during the first week of life in infants managed with NIPPV. Twelve showed no significant difference, and none showed a significant benefit for CPAP. Pooled data from all 18 trials demonstrated a clinically important, 37% relative reduction in the risk of respiratory failure with NIPPV (**Fig. 1**). This beneficial effect was most obvious in the trials using ventilator-generated NIPPV (combined subgroups 1.1.1 and 1.1.2: RR 0.60; 95% CI, 0.48–0.76), and was greatest when synchronization was used (subgroup 1.1.2), with 7 infants needing to be treated with ventilator-generated, synchronized NIPPV to prevent one respiratory failure. Flow-driver devices provided a smaller (subgroup 1.1.3) and nonsignificant effect (subgroup 1.1.4) on the risk of respiratory failure (combined subgroups 1.1.3 and 1.1.4: RR 0.70; 95% CI, 0.49–1.01). These findings are consistent with those of the corresponding 2016 Cochrane Review.[11]

### Postextubation respiratory support

This meta-analysis evaluated the efficacy of NIPPV versus CPAP when used as post-extubation respiratory support for preterm infants. We defined the primary outcome as respiratory failure leading to additional ventilatory support during the week postextubation.

Fifteen trials enrolling 2444 infants were included (see **Table 3**). Data from 5 trials published between 2016 and 2020 enrolling 1013 infants were added to the existing meta-analysis of the Cochrane Collaboration.[12] Twelve trials used ventilator-generated NIPPV, 2 trials delivered flow-driver-generated NIPPV, the final study being the Kirpalani mixed methods study.

Overall, infants extubated to NIPPV had a 22% relative risk reduction for respiratory failure within the first week postextubation compared with those managed with CPAP (**Fig. 2**). Extubation of 12 infants to NIPPV would prevent one case of extubation failure. Again, this benefit was greatest in trials using ventilator-generated NIPPV (combined subgroups 1.2.1 and 1.2.2: RR 0.51; 95% CI, 0.40–0.65) and was strongest

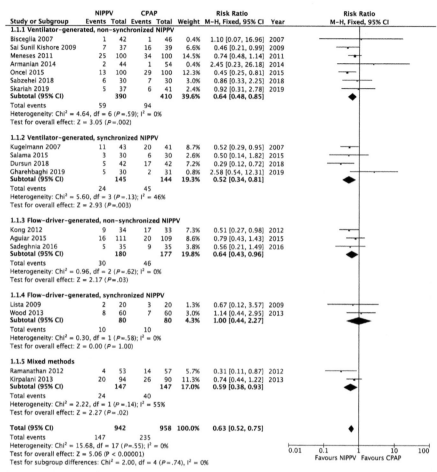

**Fig. 1.** Forest plot of trials comparing NIPPV versus CPAP for primary respiratory support (by device and synchronization).

when ventilator-generated, synchronized NIPPV was used (subgroup 1.2.2). On average, only 3 infants would need to be extubated to ventilator-generated, synchronized NIPPV to prevent one case of postextubation failure. No beneficial effect was found for flow-driver devices (subgroup 1.2.3).

### Mortality

Results from 17 trials enrolling 1834 infants could be pooled for this analysis. Overall and within subgroups, no difference in mortality was noted when NIPPV was compared with CPAP as primary respiratory support for preterm infants with neonatal RDS (**Table 4**). After extubation, no significant reduction in mortality was found in the meta-analysis of 10 trials and 2178 infants, and no significant difference was detected when mortality was examined by device or synchronization for either primary or post-extubation support.

These findings contrast the results of the respective meta-analysis of the Cochrane Collaboration on NIPPV versus CPAP for preterm neonates after extubation, where a

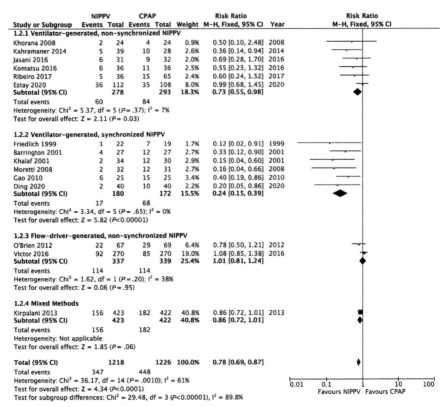

**Fig. 2.** Forest plot of trials comparing NIPPV versus CPAP for postextubation support (by device and synchronization).

small difference in mortality between treatment groups was reported, favoring NIPPV (RR 0.69; 95% CI, 0.48–0.99).[12]

### Bronchopulmonary dysplasia
Fourteen of the 18 trials (1534 infants) evaluating NIPPV versus CPAP as primary respiratory support reported BPD at 36 weeks' corrected gestational age. We noted a 28% relative reduction in the risk of BPD with NIPPV (**Table 5**). However, this overall difference was fully attributable to the reduction in BPD seen in studies using ventilator-generated, synchronized NIPPV. None of the other subanalyses showed a significant difference in the rate of BPD between groups. In the meta-analysis of the Cochrane Collaboration on NIPPV as primary respiratory support for preterm infants, no reduction in BPD was observed in any of the subgroups.[11]

After extubation, meta-analysis of 11 studies enrolling 2128 infants revealed a borderline lower rate of BPD when infants were randomized to NIPPV compared with infants randomized to CPAP (see **Table 5**). Once again, within subgroups, only ventilator-generated, synchronized NIPPV was associated with a reduction in BPD. In the corresponding meta-analysis of the Cochrane Collaboration, both ventilator-generated (RR 0.69; 95% CI, 0.50–0.95) and synchronized NIPPV (RR 0.64; 95% CI, 0.44–0.95) were associated with a reduction in BPD.

**Table 4**
**Meta-analysis of trials comparing NIPPV with CPAP for primary and postextubation support**

| | Number of Trials | NIPPV | | CPAP | | Risk Ratio (95% CI) |
|---|---|---|---|---|---|---|
| | | Deaths | Total | Deaths | Total | |
| Primary respiratory support | | | | | | |
| Ventilator-generated, nonsynchronized NIPPV | 7 | 40 | 390 | 49 | 410 | 0.83 (0.57–1.20) |
| Ventilator-generated, synchronized NIPPV | 4 | 2 | 145 | 3 | 144 | 0.76 (0.17–3.30) |
| Flow-driver-generated, nonsynchronized NIPPV | 2 | 6 | 146 | 8 | 144 | 0.75 (0.28–1.99) |
| Flow-driver-generated, synchronized NIPPV | 2 | 0 | 80 | 2 | 80 | 0.20 (0.01–4.08) |
| Mixed methods | 2 | 4 | 148 | 5 | 147 | 0.78 (0.21–2.83) |
| Total | 17 | 52 | 909 | 67 | 925 | 0.79 (0.57–1.09) |
| Postextubation care | | | | | | |
| Ventilator-generated, nonsynchronized NIPPV | 5 | 17 | 238 | 27 | 261 | 0.61 (0.35–1.06) |
| Ventilator-generated, synchronized NIPPV | 2 | 5 | 72 | 7 | 71 | 0.70 (0.23–2.11) |
| Flow-driver-generated, nonsynchronized NIPPV | 2 | 21 | 337 | 22 | 339 | 0.96 (0.54–1.71) |
| Flow-driver-generated, synchronized NIPPV | 0 | — | — | — | — | — |
| Mixed methods | 1 | 35 | 430 | 41 | 430 | 0.85 (0.55–1.31) |
| Total | 10 | 78 | 1077 | 97 | 1101 | 0.80 (0.60–1.06) |

Outcome: Mortality during study period.

**Table 5**
**Meta-analysis of trials comparing NIPPV with CPAP for primary and postextubation support**

| | Number of Trials | NIPPV | | CPAP | | Risk Ratio (95% CI) |
|---|---|---|---|---|---|---|
| | | BPD | Total | BPD | Total | |
| **Primary Respiratory Support** | | | | | | |
| Ventilator-generated, nonsynchronized NIPPV | 4 | 32 | 257 | 43 | 256 | 0.73 (0.48–1.11) |
| Ventilator-generated, synchronized NIPPV | 4 | 9 | 145 | 24 | 144 | 0.37 (0.18–0.78) |
| Flow-driver-generated, nonsynchronized NIPPV | 2 | 9 | 146 | 7 | 144 | 1.27 (0.48–3.32) |
| Flow-driver-generated, synchronized NIPPV | 2 | 5 | 80 | 7 | 80 | 0.71 (0.24–2.13) |
| Mixed methods | 2 | 28 | 140 | 34 | 142 | 0.85 (0.54–2.72) |
| Total | 14 | 83 | 768 | 115 | 766 | 0.72 (0.56–0.93) |
| **Postextubation care** | | | | | | |
| Ventilator-generated, nonsynchronized NIPPV | 4 | 52 | 209 | 58 | 229 | 0.91 (0.66–1.27) |
| Ventilator-generated, synchronized NIPPV | 4 | 30 | 133 | 45 | 128 | 0.63 (0.44–0.91) |
| Flow-driver-generated, nonsynchronized NIPPV | 2 | 153 | 328 | 165 | 327 | 0.92 (0.79–1.08) |
| Flow-driver-generated, synchronized NIPPV | 0 | — | — | — | — | — |
| Mixed methods | 1 | 144 | 394 | 143 | 380 | 0.97 (0.81–1.17) |
| Total | 11 | 379 | 1064 | 411 | 1064 | 0.91 (0.81–1.01) |

Outcome: Bronchopulmonary dysplasia

## SUMMARY

There is clear evidence that NIPPV is superior to CPAP as primary and postextubation respiratory support for the prevention of respiratory failure in preterm infants with RDS. For both indications, ventilator-generated, synchronized NIPPV is most effective to prevent respiratory failure. Results show no reduction in mortality overall or within subgroups, irrespective of whether primary or postextubation NIPPV support is delivered. Longer-term pulmonary benefits include a reduction in BPD, but only with ventilator-generated, synchronized NIPPV. Implementation of this evidence may be hampered by the limited availability of ventilators able to deliver synchronized pressure changes. There is little evidence of harm during NIPPV generated by any device or delivered in any mode, with no reported increase in abdominal adverse events.

In view of the high heterogeneity among trials included in our meta-analyses, results may not be generalizable and must be interpreted with caution. It is important for clinicians to understand that not all modes of noninvasive support are the same, and variations in the applied strategy may not provide the same level of benefit. Superiority of ventilator-generated NIPPV over flow-driver-generated NIPPV is explained by higher peak pressures used during ventilator-generated NIPPV. If MAPs were matched across all devices and all modes, there may be little difference between CPAP, flow-driver-generated NIPPV, and ventilator-generated NIPPV.

Additional data from adequately powered RCTs are warranted to determine the benefits of NIPPV in smaller and more immature infants. A particular focus should be placed on clinically relevant outcomes such as death, BPD, and long-term respiratory function following prolonged NIPPV use. Moreover, the role of synchronized NIPPV as primary respiratory support starting directly after birth in the delivery room deserves further attention.

## BEST PRACTICES

- NIPPV is preferable over CPAP as primary and post-extubation respiratory support in preterm infants with RDS.
- For both indications, ventilator-generated, synchronized NIPPV should be used to prevent respiratory failure.
- Ventilator-generated, synchronized NIPPV may reduce the risk of bronchopulmonary dysplasia when used as either primary or post-extubation support in preterm infants, but is not associated with a decrease in mortality.

## CLINICS CARE POINTS

- Not all modes of NIPPV are the same, and variations in the applied strategy may affect the level of benefit.
- During nonsynchronized NIPPV, most pressure peaks occur during spontaneous expiration and do not contribute to tidal volume.
- Any advantage of nonsynchronized NIPPV may arise from a higher mean airway pressure rather than from the effect of the intermittent pressure peaks themselves.
- Synchronization of the positive pressure peaks with the infant's own breathing efforts results in a more effective pressure and volume delivery.

- Superiority of ventilator-generated NIPPV over flow-driver-generated NIPPV is explained by higher peak pressures used during ventilator-generated NIPPV.
- There is little evidence of harm during NIPPV generated by any device or delivered in any mode.

## DISCLOSURE

The authors have nothing to disclose.

## REFERENCES

1. Baraldi E, Filippone M. Chronic lung disease after premature birth. N Engl J Med 2007;357(19):1946–55.
2. Doyle LW, Carse E, Adams A-M, et al. Ventilation in extremely preterm infants and respiratory function at 8 years. N Engl J Med 2017;377(4):329–37.
3. Subramaniam P, Ho JJ, Davis PG. Prophylactic nasal continuous positive airway pressure for preventing morbidity and mortality in very preterm infants. Cochrane Database Syst Rev 2016;6:CD001243.
4. Dargaville PA, Aiyappan A, Paoli AGD, et al. Continuous positive airway pressure failure in preterm infants: incidence, predictors and consequences. Neonatology 2013;104(1):8–14.
5. SUPPORT Study Group of the Eunice Kennedy Shriver NICHD Neonatal Research Network. Target ranges of oxygen saturation in extremely preterm infants. N Engl J Med 2010;362(21):1959–69.
6. Morley CJ, Davis PG, Doyle LW, et al. Nasal CPAP or intubation at birth for very preterm infants. N Engl J Med 2008;358(7):700–8.
7. Sandri F, Plavka R, Ancora G, et al. Prophylactic or early selective surfactant combined with nCPAP in very preterm infants. Pediatrics 2010;125(6):e1402–9.
8. Dargaville PA, Gerber A, Johansson S, et al. Incidence and outcome of CPAP failure in preterm infants. Pediatrics 2016;138(1):e20153985.
9. Owen LS, Morley CJ, Davis PG. Neonatal nasal intermittent positive pressure ventilation: a survey of practice in England. Arch Dis Child Fetal Neonatal Ed 2008;93(2):F148.
10. Kieran EA, Walsh H, O'Donnell CPF. Survey of nasal continuous positive airways pressure (NCPAP) and nasal intermittent positive pressure ventilation (NIPPV) use in Irish newborn nurseries. Arch Dis Child Fetal Neonatal Ed 2011;96(2):F156.
11. Lemyre B, Laughon M, Bose C, et al. Early nasal intermittent positive pressure ventilation (NIPPV) versus early nasal continuous positive airway pressure (NCPAP) for preterm infants. Cochrane Database Syst Rev 2016;12(12):CD005384.
12. Lemyre B, Davis PG, Paoli AGD, et al. Nasal intermittent positive pressure ventilation (NIPPV) versus nasal continuous positive airway pressure (NCPAP) for preterm neonates after extubation. Cochrane Database Syst Rev 2017;2(2): CD003212.
13. Owen LS, Morley CJ, Davis PG. Do the pressure changes of neonatal non-synchronised NIPPV (NS nasal intermittent positive pressure ventilation) confer advantages over cpap, or are high CPAP pressures as effective? Pediatr Res 2011;70(Suppl 5):16.
14. Schmölzer GM, Dawson JA, Kamlin COF, et al. Airway obstruction and gas leak during mask ventilation of preterm infants in the delivery room. Arch Dis Child Fetal Neonatal Ed 2011;96(4):F254.

15. Owen LS, Morley CJ, Davis PG. Pressure variation during ventilator generated nasal intermittent positive pressure ventilation in preterm infants. Arch Dis Child Fetal Neonatal Ed 2010;95(5):F359.

16. Owen LS, Morley CJ, Dawson JA, et al. Effects of non-synchronised nasal intermittent positive pressure ventilation on spontaneous breathing in preterm infants. Arch Dis Child Fetal Neonatal Ed 2011;96(6):F422.

17. Dimitriou G, Greenough A, Laubscher B, et al. Comparison of airway pressure-triggered and airflow-triggered ventilation in very immature infants. Acta Paediatr 1998;87(12):1256–60.

18. Waitz M, Mense L, Kirpalani H, et al. Nasal intermittent positive pressure ventilation for preterm neonates synchronized or not? Clin Perinatol 2016;43(4): 799–816.

19. Owen LS, Morley CJ, Davis PG. Effects of synchronisation during SiPAP-generated nasal intermittent positive pressure ventilation (NIPPV) in preterm infants. Arch Dis Child Fetal Neonatal Ed 2015;100(1):F24.

20. Stern DJ, Weisner MD, Courtney SE. Synchronized neonatal non-invasive ventilation-a pilot study: the graseby capsule with bi-level NCPAP. Pediatr Pulm 2014; 49(7):659–64.

21. Chang H-Y, Claure N, D'Ugard C, et al. Effects of synchronization during nasal ventilation in clinically stable preterm infants. Pediatr Res 2011;69(1):84–9.

22. Owen LS, Manley BJ. Nasal intermittent positive pressure ventilation in preterm infants: Equipment, evidence, and synchronization. Semin Fetal Neonatal Med 2016;21(3):146–53.

23. Garland JS, Nelson DB, Rice T, et al. Increased risk of gastrointestinal perforations in neonates mechanically ventilated with either face mask or nasal prongs. Pediatrics 1985;76(3):406–10.

24. Imbulana DI, Manley BJ, Dawson JA, et al. Nasal injury in preterm infants receiving non-invasive respiratory support: a systematic review. Arch Dis Child Fetal Neonatal Ed 2018;103(1):F29.

25. Kirpalani H, Millar D, Lemyre B, et al. A trial comparing noninvasive ventilation strategies in preterm infants. N Engl J Med 2013;369(7):611–20.

26. Jobe AH, Bancalari E. Bronchopulmonary dysplasia. Am J Resp Crit Care 2012; 163(7):1723–9.

27. Millar D, Lemyre B, Kirpalani H, et al. A comparison of bilevel and ventilator-delivered non-invasive respiratory support. Arch Dis Child Fetal Neonatal Ed 2016;101(1):21.

28. Bourque SL, Roberts RS, Wright CJ, et al. Nasal intermittent positive pressure ventilation versus nasal continuous positive airway pressure to prevent primary noninvasive ventilation failure in extremely low Birthweight infants. J Pediatr 2019;216:218–21.e1.

29. Meneses J, Bhandari V, Alves JG. Nasal intermittent positive-pressure ventilation vs nasal continuous positive airway pressure for preterm infants with respiratory distress syndrome: a systematic review and meta-analysis. Arch Pediat Adol Med 2012;166(4):372–6.

30. Ramaswamy VV, Bandyopadhyay T, Nanda D, et al. Efficacy of noninvasive respiratory support modes as postextubation respiratory support in preterm neonates: A systematic review and network meta-analysis. Pediatric Pulmonology. 2020;55:2924–39.

31. Ramaswamy VV, More K, Roehr CC, et al. Efficacy of noninvasive respiratory support modes for primary respiratory support in preterm neonates with respiratory

distress syndrome: Systematic review and network meta-analysis. *Pediatric Pulmonology.* 2020;55:2940–63.

32. Centre TCCNC. Nordic Cochrane centre, the Cochrane collaboration. Review Manager (RevMan) [Computer program]. Version 5.3. Copenhagen: The Nordic Cochrane Centre, The Cochrane Collaboration, 2014.

33. Ekhaguere O, Patel S, Kirpalani H. Nasal intermittent mandatory ventilation versus nasal continuous positive airway pressure before and after invasive ventilatory support. Clin Perinatol 2019;46(3):517–36.

34. Miedema M, Burg PS, Beuger S, et al. Effect of nasal continuous and biphasic positive airway pressure on lung volume in preterm infants. J Pediatr 2013; 162(4):691–7.

35. Bisceglia M, Belcastro A, Poerio V, et al. A comparison of nasal intermittent versus continuous positive pressure delivery for the treatment of moderate respiratory syndrome in preterm infants. Minerva Pediatr 2007;59(2):91–5.

36. Kishore MSS, Dutta S, Kumar P. Early nasal intermittent positive pressure ventilation versus continuous positive airway pressure for respiratory distress syndrome. Acta Paediatr 2009;98(9):1412–5.

37. Meneses J, Bhandari V, Alves JG, et al. Noninvasive ventilation for respiratory distress syndrome: a randomized controlled trial. Pediatrics 2011;127(2):300–7.

38. Armanian A-M, Badiee Z, Heidari G, et al. Initial treatment of respiratory distress syndrome with nasal intermittent mandatory ventilation versus nasal continuous positive airway pressure: a randomized controlled trial. Int J Prev Med 2014; 5(12):1543–51.

39. Oncel MY, Arayici S, Uras N, et al. Nasal continuous positive airway pressure versus nasal intermittent positive-pressure ventilation within the minimally invasive surfactant therapy approach in preterm infants: a randomised controlled trial. Arch Dis Child Fetal Neonatal Ed 2015;101(4):F323–8.

40. Sabzehei MK, Basiri B, Shokouhi M, et al. A comparative study of treatment response of respiratory distress syndrome in preterm infants: early nasal intermittent positive pressure ventilation versus early nasal continuous positive airway pressure. Int J Pediatr 2018;6(10):8339–46.

41. Skariah TA, Lewis LE. Early nasal intermittent positive pressure ventilation (NIPPV) versus nasal continuous positive airway pressure (NCPAP) for respiratory distress syndrome (RDS) in infants of 28-36 weeks gestational age: a randomized controlled trial. Iranian J Neonatal 2019;10(2):1–8.

42. Kugelman A, Feferkorn I, Riskin A, et al. Nasal intermittent mandatory ventilation versus nasal continuous positive airway pressure for respiratory distress syndrome: a randomized, controlled, prospective study. J Pediatr 2007;150(5): 521–6.e1.

43. Salama GSA, Ayyash FF, Al-Rabadi AJ, et al. Nasal-imv versus nasal-CPAP as an initial mode of respiratory support for premature infants with RDS: a prospective randomized clinical trial. Rawal Med J 2015;40(2):197–202.

44. Dursun M, Uslu S, Bulbul A, et al. Comparison of early nasal intermittent positive pressure ventilation and nasal continuous positive airway pressure in preterm infants with respiratory distress syndrome. J Trop Pediatr 2018;65(4):352–60.

45. Gharehbaghi MM, Hosseini MB, Eivazi G, et al. Comparing the efficacy of nasal continuous positive airway pressure and nasal intermittent positive pressure ventilation in early management of respiratory distress syndrome in preterm infants. Oman Med J 2019;34(2):99–104.

46. Kong L-K, Kong X-Y, Li L-H, et al. Comparative study on application of duo positive airway pressure and continuous positive airway pressure in preterm

neonates with respiratory distress syndrome. Zhongguo Dang Dai Er Ke Za Zhi 2012;14(12):888–92.

47. Aguiar T, Macedo I, Voutsen O, et al. Nasal bilevel versus continuous positive airway pressure in preterm infants: a randomized controlled trial. J Clin Trials 2015;5(221). 2167–0870.

48. Sadeghnia A, Barekateyn B, Badiei Z, et al. Analysis and comparison of the effects of N-BiPAP and Bubble-CPAP in treatment of preterm newborns with the weight of below 1500 grams affiliated with respiratory distress syndrome: a randomised clinical trial. Adv Biomed Res 2016;5(1):3.

49. Lista G, Castoldi F, Fontana P, et al. Nasal continuous positive airway pressure (CPAP) versus bi-level nasal CPAP in preterm babies with respiratory distress syndrome: a randomised control trial. Arch Dis Child Fetal Neonatal Ed 2010; 95(2):F85.

50. Wood F, Gupta S, Tin W, et al. G170 randomised controlled trial of synchronised intermittent positive airway pressure (SiPAP™) versus continuous positive airway pressure (CPAP) as a primary mode of respiratory support in preterm infants with respiratory distress syndrome. Arch Dis Child 2013;98(Suppl 1):A78.

51. Ramanathan R, Sekar KC, Rasmussen M, et al. Nasal intermittent positive pressure ventilation after surfactant treatment for respiratory distress syndrome in preterm infants <30 weeks' gestation: a randomized, controlled trial. J Perinatol 2012;32(5):336–43.

52. Khorana M, Paradeevisut H, Sangtawesin V, et al. A randomized trial of non-synchronized Nasopharyngeal Intermittent Mandatory Ventilation (nsNIMV) vs. Nasal Continuous Positive Airway Pressure (NCPAP) in the prevention of extubation failure in pre-term < 1,500 grams. J Med Assoc Thai 2008;91(Suppl 3): S136–42.

53. Kahramaner Z, Erdemir A, Turkoglu E, et al. Unsynchronized nasal intermittent positive pressure versus nasal continuous positive airway pressure in preterm infants after extubation. J Matern Fetal Neonatal Med 2013;27(9):926–9.

54. Jasani B, Nanavati R, Kabra N, et al. Comparison of non-synchronized nasal intermittent positive pressure ventilation versus nasal continuous positive airway pressure as post-extubation respiratory support in preterm infants with respiratory distress syndrome: a randomized controlled trial. J Matern Fetal Neonatal Med 2015;29(10):1546–51.

55. Komatsu DFR, Diniz EM, Ferraro AA, et al. Randomized controlled trial comparing nasal intermittent positive pressure ventilation and nasal continuous positive airway pressure in premature infants after tracheal extubation. Rev Assoc Med Bras (1992) 2016;62(6):568–74.

56. Ribeiro S, Fontes M, Bhandari V, et al. Noninvasive ventilation in newborns ≤1,500 g after tracheal extubation: randomized clinical trial. Am J Perinat 2017;34(12):1190–8.

57. Estay AS, Mariani GL, Alvarez CA, et al. Randomized controlled trial of non-synchronized nasal intermittent positive pressure ventilation versus nasal CPAP after extubation of VLBW infants. Neonatology 2020;117(2):193–9.

58. Friedlich P, Lecart C, Posen R, et al. A randomized trial of nasopharyngeal-synchronized intermittent mandatory ventilation versus nasopharyngeal continuous positive airway pressure in very low birth weight infants after extubation. J Perinatol 1999;19(6):413–8.

59. Barrington KJ, Bull D, Finer NN. Randomized trial of nasal synchronized intermittent mandatory ventilation compared with continuous positive airway pressure after extubation of very low birth weight infants. Pediatrics 2001;107(4):638–41.

60. Khalaf MN, Brodsky N, Hurley J, et al. A prospective randomized, controlled trial comparing synchronized nasal intermittent positive pressure ventilation versus nasal continuous positive airway pressure as modes of extubation. Pediatrics 2001;108(1):13–7.
61. Moretti C, Gizzi C, Papoff P, et al. Comparing the effects of nasal synchronized intermittent positive pressure ventilation (nSIPPV) and nasal continuous positive airway pressure (nCPAP) after extubation in very low birth weight infants. Early Hum Dev 1999;56(2–3):167–77.
62. Gao W-W, Tan S-Z, Chen Y-B, et al. Randomized trail of nasal synchronized intermittent mandatory ventilation compared with nasal continuous positive airway pressure in preterm infants with respiratory distress syndrome. Zhongguo Dang Dai Er Ke Za Zhi 2010;12(7):524–6.
63. Ding F, Zhang J, Zhang W, et al. Clinical study of different modes of non-invasive ventilation treatment in preterm infants with respiratory distress syndrome after extubation. Front Pediatr 2020;8:63.
64. O'Brien K, Campbell C, Brown L, et al. Infant flow biphasic nasal continuous positive airway pressure (BP- NCPAP) vs. infant flow NCPAP for the facilitation of extubation in infants' ≤1,250 grams: a randomized controlled trial. BMC Pediatr 2012;12(1):43.
65. Victor S, Roberts SA, Mitchell S, et al. Biphasic positive airway pressure or continuous positive airway pressure: a randomized trial. Pediatrics 2016;138(2): e20154095.

# Synchronized Nasal Intermittent Positive Pressure Ventilation

Corrado Moretti, MD[a], Camilla Gizzi, MD, PhD[b],*

## KEYWORDS

• Synchronized NIPPV • Noninvasive ventilation • Preterm infant • RDS

## KEY POINTS

- Synchronization is needed to improve the efficacy of the noninvasive ventilatory treatment of premature infants.
- The ideal triggering device for noninvasive ventilation must meet the dual challenges of being rapidly activated by a physiologic signal of spontaneous inspiration and being reliable despite working in a circuit with leaks.
- Abdominal capsule, pressure-trigger, flow-trigger, and NAVA are used as triggering devices for noninvasive ventilation.
- The physiologic benefits of synchronized mechanical breaths during noninvasive ventilation depend on various factors such as a more efficient positive pressure transmission to the lung, an effective increase in transpulmonary pressure during ventilation, and a better stabilization of the chest wall during the inspiratory phase.
- Clinical data suggest beneficial effects of synchronized nasal ventilation in preterm infants when compared with nasal CPAP, with regard to early treatment of RDS, extubation failure, and incidence of bronchopulmonary dysplasia.

## INTRODUCTION

Mechanical ventilation (MV) has an important role in neonatal respiratory care, but severe and long-lasting complications may be a consequence of this invasive technique. The best strategy to prevent neonatal morbidity is to avoid or shorten MV in favor of noninvasive respiratory support but, despite early nasal continuous positive airway pressure (NCPAP) and selective surfactant, a high percentage of neonates develop respiratory failure and need to be intubated[1]; in addition, many of them fail extubation and must be reintubated. For this reason, in recent years, research has been oriented toward developing noninvasive techniques that are more effective than NCPAP.

[a] Department of Paediatrics, Policlinico Umberto I, Sapienza University of Rome, Viale Regina Elena 324, Rome 00185, Italy; [b] Paediatric and Neonatology Unit, "Sandro Pertini" Hospital, Via Monti Tiburtini 385, Rome 00157, Italy
* Corresponding author.
*E-mail address:* camillagizzi@tin.it

Clin Perinatol 48 (2021) 745–759
https://doi.org/10.1016/j.clp.2021.07.005
0095-5108/21/© 2021 Elsevier Inc. All rights reserved.
perinatology.theclinics.com

Nonsynchronized nasal intermittent positive pressure ventilation (NIPPV) is a technique extensively used in daily clinical care, which uses a common ventilator to provide intermittent breaths with parameters similar to those for invasive MV. NIPPV is known as nasal intermittent mandatory ventilation (NIMV) when unassisted spontaneous breaths are possible between mandatory inflations. However, infant-ventilator asynchrony is a problem with NIPPV, as already occurred with MV.

Asynchronous cycles delivered late in the spontaneous inspiration or during expiration alter the infant's spontaneous breathing pattern, which probably occurs because the mandatory cycles stimulate the activity of the pulmonary stretch receptors. These elicit active expiratory efforts against the ventilator cycle, delay spontaneous exhalation, and therefore the onset of the next inspiration (**Fig. 1**), and they may also activate laryngeal closure.[2] Moreover, clinical studies conducted on preterm infants treated with NIPPV have demonstrated that the rate of asynchrony is very high and that only a low percentage ($\sim$25–33%) of mechanical inflations are in synchrony with spontaneous inspirations.[3,4] Other clinical trials showed that asynchronous mechanical breaths are not effective, and that ventilation only improves when synchronization occurs.[3,5,6] The beneficial effect of NIPPV in reducing the need for MV, compared with NCPAP,[7–10] is probably for several reasons: the higher mean airway pressure (MAP), a washout of the anatomic dead space in the upper airways, and a stimulatory effect on the respiratory drive. Another important consideration is the quality of the patient's comfort during ventilation. Setting a rate of 20 to 40 cycles/min on the ventilator means that 28,800 to 57,600 pressure waves will be delivered to the infant through the interface every day, and most of them will be asynchronous. Synchronization is therefore needed to improve the efficacy and the care of the noninvasive ventilatory treatment of premature infants, exactly as it was for invasive ventilation.

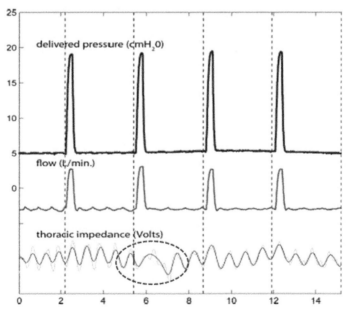

**Fig. 1.** Scalar traces of ventilator pressure, flow and thoracic impedance of a preterm neonate assisted with NIPPV. Mechanical breaths are not synchronized with the infant. The second mechanical breath occurred immediately after the end of a spontaneous inspiration activating a forced expiration and altering the infant's respiratory rhythm.

## TRIGGERING DEVICES TO SYNCHRONIZE NONINVASIVE VENTILATION

The ideal triggering device for synchronized NIPPV (SNIPPV) and NIMV (SNIMV) of the newborn infants must meet the dual challenges of firstly being rapidly activated (<100 ms) by a physiologic signal determined by the start of a spontaneous breath, and secondly being reliable despite working in a circuit with leaks. Characteristics of the currently available trigger devices are summarized in **Table 1**.

The first randomized trial to evaluate SNIMV in preterm infants was performed in 1999 by Friedlich and colleagues,[11] who first used this technique successfully to treat 22 very low birth weight (VLBW) infants after extubation. Synchronization was obtained using the abdominal pneumatic or Graseby capsule, a sensor that should be placed where abdominal expansion is maximal, usually between the sternal xiphoid apophysis and the umbilicus. Although it is a relatively simple device, the abdominal pneumatic capsule has several disadvantages because of which its accuracy is questioned (**Tab.1**); moreover, breath detection based on this technique is relatively slow,[12] and its reliability is less consistent when the patient is breathing faster.[13]

With pressure triggering, the ventilator must detect a pressure drop in the system that is created by the inspiratory effort of the patient (see **Table 1**). Preterm infants have a very weak inspiratory effort, and therefore it is difficult to set trigger sensitivity because of the small drop in pressure.

Flow-trigger ventilation is the most used technique for invasive ventilation of the newborn, but a flow-sensor used with nasal prongs has important drawbacks, such as low reliability and instability of the flow-signal, which are problems caused mainly by the continuous and variable leaks from the open circuit (see **Table 1**). An advanced flow-trigger designed to overcome these problems has been developed[14]: this device, a simple differential pressure transducer pneumotachograph, is connected to a software program that only detects the abrupt flow-signal from the patient's spontaneous inspiration and discards the slow-changing flow-signal of the leaks. The increase in dead space is a theoretic disadvantage of a flow-sensor but, during nasal ventilation, expiratory flow vents mainly from the patient's mouth with no rebreathing, as confirmed by the absence of the expiratory wave during flow monitoring (**Fig. 2**). This means that there is a difference between the inspiratory and expiratory flow through the sensor, making the flow-signal unstable. In the advanced flow-trigger, the software automatically resets the flow-signal to zero after every inspiration to obviate this problem. Bench tests have demonstrated that this device is capable of detecting very small inspiratory flow and volumes, that its performance is not affected by the size of leaks, and that its response time is <100 ms.[14] Several clinical trials have demonstrated the efficacy of flow-SNIPPV in decreasing intubation and MV need within a few hours of birth (primary mode)[15,16] and in reducing extubation failure (secondary mode),[16,17] and for treatment of apnea of prematurity (AOP).[18]

Neurally adjusted ventilatory assist (NAVA) is a more recently developed ventilatory mode that uses the electrical activity of the diaphragm (Edi) to trigger the ventilator (see **Table 1**). The Edi signal detected from the crural portion of the diaphragm is obtained using a dedicated indwelling nasogastric feeding tube with electrodes incorporated in its wall. The ventilator is therefore controlled by the neural respiratory drive of the patient and delivers mechanical breaths that are synchronized with initiation, size and termination of each breath, and proportional to the infant's inspiratory effort.[19] Recent studies suggest that NAVA triggering can be helpful in preterm infants to prevent endotracheal intubation or allow early extubation.[20] However, there is some worry both about their ability to self-regulate breath size and that the neural feedback for protection from lung overinflation seems to be insufficient in preterm infants.[21] At

**Table 1**
Triggering devices to synchronize noninvasive ventilation

| Trigger Device | Signal | Response Time | Advantages | Disadvantages |
|---|---|---|---|---|
| Abdominal capsule (Graseby Capsule) | Pneumatic signal determined by the compression of the capsule and generated by the expansion of the abdomen during spontaneous inspiration | $53 \pm 13$ ms | • No dead space<br>• Not affected by leaks<br>• Simple and inexpensive | • Efficacy depends on its proper placement, which requires practice<br>• If the capsule is stuck too close to the rib margin, asynchrony may be determined by paradoxic breathing movements<br>• Movement may be misinterpreted as breathing<br>• Abdominal distension may decrease sensitivity<br>• No flow monitoring |
| Pressure-trigger | Pressure drop in the ventilator circuit determined by the inspiratory effort | Not reported | • No dead space<br>• Simple and inexpensive | • Low sensitivity with frequent autotriggering or no triggering<br>• Autotriggering from secretions or moisture<br>• Pressure-signal is affected by leaks<br>• No flow monitoring |
| Flow-trigger | Flow signal produced by spontaneous inspiration | $64 \pm 7$ ms | • Good sensitivity<br>• Flow is the specific signal of spontaneous inspiration<br>• Flow monitoring | • Flow-signal is affected by leaks (see text)<br>• Increased dead space (see text)<br>• Autotriggering from secretions or moisture |
| NAVA-trigger | Electrical activity of the diaphragm (Edi) | $35 \pm 8$ ms | • Good sensitivity<br>• No dead space<br>• Not affected by leaks | • Requires practice to place and keep the sensor stable<br>• The catheter is partially invasive<br>• No flow monitoring<br>• Expensive |

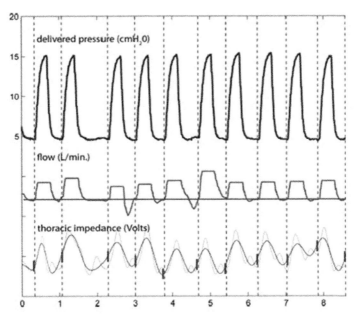

**Fig. 2.** Scalar traces of ventilator pressure, flow and thoracic impedance of a preterm neonate assisted with flow-SNIPPV. Note the good synchronization and the absence of the expiratory flow trace.

the time of writing, there have been no systematic reviews on the use of NIV-NAVA as a mode of respiratory support in preterm infants.[22]

## EFFECTS OF SYNCHRONIZED NASAL INTERMITTENT POSITIVE PRESSURE VENTILATION ON THE RESPIRATORY PHYSIOLOGY OF PRETERM INFANTS

The physiologic benefits of synchronized mechanical breaths during noninvasive ventilation depend on various factors. The first factor is that with synchronization, positive pressure is transmitted efficiently to the lungs because it is delivered when the glottis is opening, with consequent reduced risk of abdominal distension. The mechanisms that determine upper airway patency and modulate its resistance are very complex because they depend on coordination between upper-airway muscles and the activity of the diaphragm. To reduce the resistance, one critical function of the upper-airway abductor muscles (hypoglossal, genioglossus, and posterior cricoarytenoid, the dilator of the vocal cords) is to stiffen and widen the upper-airway when negative pressure is generated by contraction of the diaphragm (**Fig. 3**A). By contrast, closure of the glottis (thyroarytenoid muscle), that is, grunting, is frequently seen during expiration and contributes to maintaining functional residual capacity in infants (**Fig. 3**B). The second factor is that, with synchronization, there is an effective increase in the transpulmonary pressure produced by the sum of the negative pressure from the patient and the positive pressure from the ventilator. The third factor is that synchronized mechanical pressure waves stabilize the chest wall of the premature infant during the inspiratory phase. We must consider that in the mature respiratory system, the diaphragm moves downward during inspiration increasing intra-abdominal pressure, which causes the abdominal wall to move outward. Almost simultaneously, the chest wall is stabilized by the contractile activity of the intercostal muscles, and the

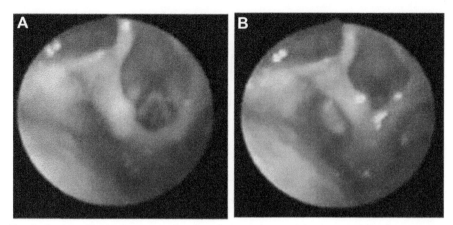

**Fig. 3.** During the respiratory cycle, the glottis opens widely during inspiration (*A*) and closes during expiration (*B*), that is, grunting.

transverse diameter of its lower part is increased by the action of the diaphragm through the area of apposition to the inner rib cage wall, the so-called 'bucket-handle' effect (**Fig. 4**A). By contrast, in premature infants, the transmission of the negative intrapleural pressure to the highly compliant chest wall results in its inward collapse during the inspiratory phase (**Fig. 4**B). Anatomic factors include less ribcage ossification, immature contractile activity of the intercostal muscles, and reduced efficiency of diaphragmatic contraction due to limited excursion. This phenomenon is called thoracoabdominal asynchrony (TAA), and its highest degree occurs when one compartment moves in the opposite direction to the other, commonly referred to as paradoxic breathing movements.[23,24] This condition determines an increase in work of breathing (WOB) because the inward collapse of the rib cage is compensated by augmenting the excursion of the diaphragm and by increasing the respiratory rate (RR) to maintain adequate gas exchange.

A physiologic study on SNIMV by Kiciman and colleagues published in 1998 is essential to understanding the effects of synchronization on the respiratory

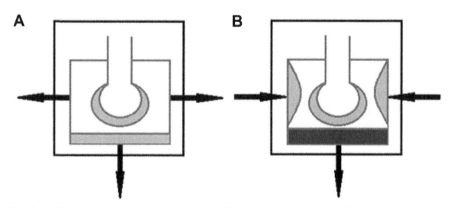

**Fig. 4.** In the mature respiratory system, the diaphragm and chest wall move in unison (*A*). In premature infants, the transmission of negative intrapleural pressure to the highly compliant chest wall results in its inward collapse during the inspiratory phase (*B*).

physiology of preterm infants during noninvasive ventilation.[25] Kiciman and colleagues measured the degree of TAA in a group of 14 premature infants during treatment with CPAP applied by endotracheal tube (ETT-CPAP), NCPAP, and SNIMV. At the time of the study, the infants had a median GA of 30 weeks (range 26–36), a median postnatal age of 6 days (range 1–40), and a median weight of 1413 g (range 730–2825 g). Two strain gauges placed around the chest and around the abdomen were used to record their movements. The phase angle was calculated to measure TAA. The phase angle is the difference in degrees between 2 waves that move at the same frequency (**Fig. 5**). The complete phase of a waveform can be defined as 360°. When 2 waves are in phase, the phase angle is 0°; when 2 waves are in opposite phases, the phase angle is 180°. In full-term infants, the phase angle is significantly smaller than in preterm infants, respectively, 12.5 ± 5.0° versus 60.6 ± 39.8°,[23] probably also because in the latter up to 60% of breaths commence with diaphragmatic contraction in advance of glottic opening.[26] Kiciman and colleagues reported that TAA was significantly diminished during NCPAP compared with ETT-CPAP. This may be secondary to the elimination of airway resistance imposed by the ETT, thereby reducing the requirement for negative pleural pressure and chest wall distortion. Further significant reduction in TAA, with a phase angle close to the physiologic values of premature infants, was obtained during SNIMV due to more effective stabilization of the chest wall throughout the inspiratory phase. One year later in 1999, the physiologic effects of SNIPPV compared to NCPAP were analyzed in 11 VLBW infants (BW: 1141 ± 53g; GA: 28.1 ± 0.5 weeks) immediately after extubation[5]: the 2 techniques were applied in random order; the median age at the time of the study was 6 days; $Fio_2$ was 0.25 ± 0.01; and synchronization was obtained by a flow-sensor (flow-SNIPPV) interposed between the Y-piece and the short binasal prongs (SBP). Recordings of esophageal pressure (Pe) showed a significant difference between the 2 modes of ventilation, with the lowest values consistently observed during SNIPPV as a result of the ventilator unloading WOB. Moreover, during flow-

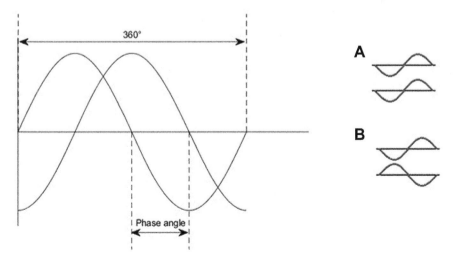

**Fig. 5.** The complete phase of a waveform can be defined as 360°. The phase angle is the difference in degrees between 2 waves that move at the same frequency. When 2 waves are in phase (A), the phase angle is 0°. When 2 waves are in opposite phases (B), the phase angle is 180°. The phase angle in the figure is about 90°.

SNIPPV, transcutaneous (Tc) $Pco_2$ and the infant's mean RR were significantly lower than during NCPAP, whereas Vt and minute volume (Ve) were significantly greater. One of the most important criticisms of this trial is that PEEP and NCPAP were set at a low value (+3 $cmH_2O$) and this factor may have positively influenced the physiologic effects of SNIPPV on lung mechanics. A few years later in 2006, Aghai and colleagues confirmed that compared with NCPAP, SNIPPV was able to reduce the patient's WOB.[27] The 2 techniques were applied in random order in a group of 15 infants with mild RDS (BW: 1367 $\pm$ 325g; GA: 29.5 $\pm$ 2.4 weeks). At the time of the study, the mean age of the patients was 4 $\pm$ 4 days and $Fio_2$ was 0.26 $\pm$ 0.1. In this study, NCPAP and PEEP were set at +5 $cmH_2O$ and no significant difference was found in Vt, Ve, or RR during SNIPPV compared to NCPAP. Aghai and colleagues speculated that the disparity with the previous trial was probably due to the study population or because the lung recruitment was enhanced by a higher PEEP and did not change significantly with the addition of the ventilator's inspiratory pressure wave. In 2011, Chang and colleagues compared the short-term effects of NIMV and SNIMV with NCPAP on ventilation, gas exchange, and infant-ventilator interaction.[28] The 3 techniques were applied in random order in 16 clinically stable preterm infants (BW: 993 $\pm$ 248 g; GA: 27.6 $\pm$ 2.3 weeks; age at the time of the study 15 $\pm$ 14 days, and $Fio_2$ 0.25 $\pm$ 0.4). Chang and colleagues concluded that there were no short-term benefits of NIMV or SNIMV on ventilation or gas exchange compared with NCPAP. However, SNIMV reduced breathing effort and resulted in better infant-ventilator interaction than NIMV. By contrast, Owen and colleagues studied the effects of NIPPV on 10 spontaneously breathing preterm infants (median GA, BW, age, and weight at the time of the study were: 25 + 3 weeks, 797 g, 24 days, and 1076 g) and concluded that this technique increases the Vt of individual breaths by 15% ($P$ = .01) only when the onset of inflation coincides with spontaneous inspiration.[3] In 2015, Huang and colleagues performed a randomized crossover study comparing the short-term effects of NIMV and SNIMV after extubation in 14 VLBW infants recovering from RDS.[6] The characteristics of the infants were: mean GA 26.3 $\pm$ 2.3 weeks; BW 928 g (range 475–1310 g); postnatal age 6.5 days (range 2–43 days); weight at the time of the study 839 g (range 450–1310 g). The 2 techniques were applied with the same MAP: the RR was set to 40 cycles for NIMV, and only 40 breaths were assisted during SNIMV. The infants enrolled were still suffering from residual RDS as indicated by the supplemental oxygen needed immediately before extubation ($Fio_2$ 26.7 $\pm$ 7.6%) and by the spontaneous RR of greater than 60 breaths/min. The results showed that during SNIMV, there was a significant decrease in Pe, spontaneous RR, and $TcPCO_2$, and a significant increase in $TcPO_2$ and synchrony rate. The authors concluded that, compared to NIMV, SNIMV decreases the respiratory effort in VLBW infants recovering from RDS and improves gas exchange. It can therefore be considered to provide more efficient respiratory support. More recently in 2018, Charles and colleagues compared the WOB during flow-SNIPPV and heated humidified high flow nasal cannula (HHHFNC) when used as postextubation support in preterm infants.[29] A randomized crossover study was undertaken of 9 infants with a median GA of 27 weeks (range 24–31 weeks) and postnatal age of 7 days (range 2–50 days). Flow-SNIPPV compared to HHHFNC postextubation reduced WOB and TAA and, owing to the highly significant difference between the 2 modes of support, the study was terminated before reaching the planned number of infants. Another interesting study is an *in-vivo* model of RDS performed in rabbits treated with surfactant immediately followed by noninvasive ventilation. This trial demonstrated that SNIPPV, compared with NCPAP and NIPPV, is associated with a significantly better response in terms of gas exchange, dynamic compliance, and lung injury scores, probably due to a better distribution of surfactant.[30]

## SUGGESTED PARAMETERS AND NASAL INTERFACES

The parameters usually suggested for SNIPPV and SNIMV are very similar to those set for MV: peak inspiratory pressure 10 to 25 cmH$_2$O, PEEP 4 to 8 cmH$_2$O, inspiratory time (Ti) 0.33 to 0.40 sec, and flow usually in the range of 6 to 10 L/min. The less invasive parameters are set after extubation or for AOP, and the more aggressive ones are set as primary mode for infants with RDS. Unfortunately, owing to the leaks, the value of expiratory Vt is currently not easily measurable during nasal ventilation, but technical developments will certainly help overcome this problem. However, no trial on synchronized noninvasive ventilation has reported an increase in air leak syndromes, probably due to the open circuit.

Choice of interface is critical to successful ventilation. Nasal ventilation is currently performed using various different models, of which SBP are the most widespread device. The different shapes and properties of these interfaces lead to varying impacts on the pressure transmission to the lungs, which in turn influences clinical outcomes, and the considerable difference in resistance to gas-flow is a key point.[31] In the last few years, treatment with HHHFNC has become increasingly popular because of reduced incidence of nasal trauma, increased infant comfort, improved mother and child bonding, and high popularity among parents and nursing staff. Initially developed for the delivery of low or high-flow oxygen therapy, the HHHFNC has been adopted into routine clinical practice in many centers for NIPPV delivery. The main characteristic of this device is that both the tubes between the Y-piece and the nasal prongs only conduct inspiratory flow, and for this reason, this device can be defined 'double-inspiratory loop cannula' (DILC). One of the main problems with the DILC is its higher intrinsic resistance compared to SBP, which is likely to compromise flow and pressure delivery to the airway and to reduce the efficacy of nasal support or ventilation treatments.[32,33] Recently, a DILC with low resistance was developed for flow-SNIPPV with a sensor placed at the level of Y piece. Bench tests and preliminary clinical data confirm that this device can be successfully used for flow-SNIPPV, combining the physiologic advantages of synchronized ventilation with the comfort and ease of use of an HHHFNC.[34]

Nasal masks are also increasingly being used to deliver NCPAP in preterm infants. This device was found to have lower resistance and give less risk of nasal trauma,[31] but to date, no data are available on SNIPPV applied with nasal masks.

## SYNCHRONIZED NASAL VENTILATION AS PRIMARY MODE OF VENTILATION

Four observational studies are available in this category. Santin and colleagues[35] prospectively compared early SNIPPV by Graseby Capsule following INSURE versus continued MV and later extubation to SNIPPV. In this study, early SNIPPV was associated with a significantly shorter duration of MV (2.4 ± 0.4 vs 0.3 ± 0.0 days; $P = .001$), supplemental oxygen (15 ± 3.2 vs 8.2 ± 3.3 days; $P = .04$), and hospital stay (37.5 ± 3.0 vs 29.1 ± 3.3 days; $P = .04$). In a retrospective study, NCPAP was compared to flow-SNIPPV following INSURE.[15] Significantly fewer infants were reintubated within the first 72 hours in the flow-SNIPPV group (35.5% vs 6.1%; $P = .004$); the incidence of bronchopulmonary dysplasia (BPD) was lower, and infants needed less surfactant and less methylxanthine compared with the NCPAP group. Ricotti and colleagues[36] performed a retrospective study assessing the use of bilevel NIPPV versus flow-SNIPPV as primary mode with or without INSURE in VLBW infants with clinical signs of RDS. They did not find a significant difference between the groups in the duration or failure of noninvasive respiratory ventilation. Finally, Ramos-Navarro and colleagues[16] performed a prospective observational study on flow-SNIPPV used on 78 preterm infants of less than 32 weeks' GA. In 53 patients, SNIPPV was applied as rescue therapy after NCPAP failure to prevent intubation. In the same study, SNIPPV was electively applied in 25 ventilator-dependent patients to support extubation. MV was avoided over the following 72 hours in 66% of patients of the rescue group and in 92% of the elective group.

Five randomized control trials (RCTs) have assessed the effect of synchronization during NIPPV in preterm neonates as a primary mode of ventilation. Bhandari and colleagues[37] observed that early extubation of 41 preterm infants to SNIPPV by Graseby Capsule resulted in a significantly lower rate of BPD or death when compared with continued MV and later extubation (20% vs 52%; $P = .03$). Kugelman and colleagues[38] randomized 84 infants with RDS to early NCPAP or pressure-triggered SNIPPV without foregoing MV or administration of surfactant. In this study, infants assigned to early SNIPPV were less likely to be intubated (49% vs 25%; $P = .04$) and had a lower incidence of BPD (17% vs 2%; $P = .03$). However, few infants weighing less than 1000 g were included in this trial. Salvo and colleagues[39] compared flow-SNIPPV with bilevel NIPPV in 124 preterm infants (<1500 g and <32 weeks) and found no difference in failure or duration of noninvasive respiratory ventilation between the 2 groups. None of the RCTs using SNIPPV as primary mode reported adverse side effects.

More recently, 2 RCTs have been published on NIV-NAVA. One unblinded RCT[40] compared NCPAP and NIV-NAVA in 123 infants with BW <1500 g and RDS after birth. The study showed no difference in primary outcome (MV at ≤72 hours of life), or secondary outcomes (need for surfactant, duration of noninvasive support, duration of MV, BPD, and death). Similarly, Kallio and colleagues[41] randomized 40 preterm infants (GA 28–36 weeks) requiring NCPAP and supplemental oxygen for respiratory distress at less than 48 h of postnatal age to NIV-NAVA or NCPAP. The primary outcome was oxygen need 12 h after inclusion in the study. Secondary outcomes were the total duration of oxygen treatment, respiratory support and parenteral nutrition, blood gas values, patient comfort, need for MV, and treatment complications. In the trial, NIV-NAVA had no statistically significant effect on primary or secondary outcomes.

## SYNCHRONIZED NASAL VENTILATION AFTER EXTUBATION

Five RCTs, comparing SNIPPV (abdominal or flow -trigger) with NCPAP as a secondary mode of noninvasive ventilation were included in a Cochrane review.[9] A subgroup meta-analysis of the 5 RCTs showed that SNIPPV significantly reduced respiratory failure after extubation (RR 0.25; 95% confidence interval [CI], 0.15–0.41), the need for endotracheal reintubation within the first week after extubation (RR 0.33; 95% CI, 0.19–0.57), and the incidence of BPD (RR 0.64; 95% CI, 0.44–0.95). None of the RCTs using SNIPPV as secondary mode reported adverse side effects. Similar results have been reported in a systematic review and network meta-analysis.[11]

More recently, 3 observational and retrospective studies have become available on NIV-NAVA after extubation. In a retrospective study, Yonehara and colleagues[42] enrolled 34 patients (GA <30 weeks), who received NIPPV or NIV-NAVA after extubation. Treatment failure was defined as a switch between the 2 modes or reintubation ≤7 days after extubation. No significant difference was observed between the 2 groups in treatment failure or adverse events. In a retrospective study, Yagui and colleagues[43] included 49 infants considered at high risk of reintubation (BW <1000 g; MV for ≥7 days or previous failed extubation), who were extubated to NCPAP or NIV-NAVA. The reintubation rate until 72 h after extubation decreased significantly in the NIV-NAVA group compared with NCPAP (50.0 vs 11.7, P<.02) while there was no difference in secondary outcomes. Finally, Lee and colleagues[44] performed a retrospective study that included 32 infants of less than 30 weeks GA who were intubated with MV for longer than 24 h and weaned to NCPAP or NIV-NAVA. Despite similar ventilatory variables before weaning, extubation failure within 72 h was significantly reduced in the NIV-NAVA group (6.3% vs 37.5%; P = .041).

## SYNCHRONIZED NASAL VENTILATION TO TREAT APNOEA OF PREMATURITY

Two RCTs using SNIPPV compared with NCPAP[45,46] reported on reduction in apneic episodes as a secondary outcome. A crossover RCT[18] assessed the effect of different noninvasive ventilation strategies on symptoms of AOP. Nineteen infants were enrolled in this study (median GA 27 weeks; median BW 800 g) and were allocated randomly to flow-SNIPPV, NIPPV, and NCPAP (4 h each period). The median event rates of desaturations and/or bradycardia per hour were as follows: 2.9 (range 0.75–6.8) during flow-SNIPPV; 6.1 (range 3.1–9.4) during NIPPV; and 5.9 (range 2–10.3) during NCPAP (P<.001 for NIPPV vs SNIPPV; P<.009 for NCPAP vs SNIPPV). The median central apnea rates per hour were as follows: 2.4 (range 1–3.6) during SNIPPV; 6.3 (range 2.8–17) during NIPPV; and 5.4 (range 3.1–12) during NCPAP (P<.001 for both NIPPV and NCPAP vs SNIPPV).

Tabacaru and colleagues[47] retrospectively investigated if NIV-NAVA ventilation was better than NIPPV for the treatment of symptomatic apnea in VLBW infants. NIV-NAVA was associated with a significant reduction in the number of isolated bradycardic events/d (0.48 ± 0.14 vs 1.35 ± 0.27; P = .019) and overall bradycardias/d (2.42 ± 0.47 vs 4.02 ± 0.53; P = .042), and there were more periods with no events (23.0% vs 6.8%; P = .004). Finally, Bai and colleagues[48] evaluated the efficacy of SNIPPV in preterm infants with primary AOP. Forty-four preterm infants were divided into SNIPPV or NCPAP groups. The SNIPPV group had a lower incidence of failure of respiratory support (9.1% vs 27.3%; P<.05), a lower incidence of hypercarbia (4.5% vs 18.2%; P<.05), and a lower incidence of gastrointestinal complications (4.5% vs 13.6%; P<.05).

## SUMMARY

Synchronized nasal ventilation is an effective technique that ensures an excellent interaction between the machine and the patient. Physiologic and clinical positive effects are currently widely demonstrated. As happened for MV, synchronization is becoming the basic method for noninvasive ventilation of the neonate, as reported by many papers in the literature. Finally, further studies are needed to confirm the effects of this mode on long-term outcomes of preterm infants.

---

**Best practices**

**What is the current practice?**

Continuous positive airway pressure (CPAP), heated humidified high-flow nasal cannula (HHHFNC) and noninvasive intermittent positive pressure ventilation (NIPPV) are the mainstays of primary and postextubation respiratory support in preterm infants.

Available evidence suggests that NIPPV is superior to CPAP for primary and postextubation respiratory support in preterm infants, and that HHHFNC is slightly inferior.

Synchronization of NIPPV improves the efficacy of noninvasive respiratory treatment of preterm infants.

**What changes in current practice are likely to improve outcomes?**

Using SNIPPV to wean infants from invasive mechanical ventilation significantly decreases extubation failure and the incidence of BPD

Using SNIPPV as primary mode for RDS decreases the need for invasive ventilation

Flow-trigger and NAVA-trigger seems to be the best tools for synchronization

**Major Recommendations**

SNIPPV is the most effective noninvasive technique after extubation and as primary mode, even if the evidence is less strong for its use as primary mode

**Summary statement**

SNIPPV should be used in NICUs as it is the best way to reduce the need for invasive ventilation and the most effective physiological noninvasive ventilation mode for the newborn infant

**Bibliographic Source(s):** *Lemyre B, Laughon M, Bose C, et al.* Early nasal intermittent positive pressure ventilation (NIPPV) versus early nasal continuous positive airway pressure (NCPAP) for preterm infants. Cochrane Database Syst Rev 2016;12:CD005384. *Lemyre B, Davis PG, De Paoli AG, et al.* Nasal intermittent positive pressure ventilation (NIPPV) versus nasal continuous positive airway pressure (NCPAP) for preterm neonates after extubation. Cochrane Database Syst Rev 2017;2:CD003212. 10. *Ramaswamy VV, Bandyopadhyay T, Nanda D, et al.* Efficacy of non-invasive respiratory support modes as post-extubation respiratory support in preterm neonates: a systematic review and network meta-analysis. Pediatr Pulmonology 2020;55:2924–39.

## CLINICS CARE POINTS

- Synchronization reduces work of breathing by improving transpulmonary pressure and decreasing thoracoabdominal asynchrony.

- Early SNIPPV for the treatment of RDS decreases the incidence of respiratory failure and the need for invasive ventilation. In moderate-to-severe RDS, the success of SNIPPV is augmented by early use of surfactant and caffeine.

- Extubation to SNIPPV significantly decreases failure rate and the incidence of BPD.

- The parameters indicated for SNIPPV are very similar to those for invasive ventilation: peak inspiratory pressure 10-25 cmH$_2$O, PEEP 4-8 cmH$_2$O, inspiratory time (Ti) 0.33-0.40 sec, and flow generally in the range of 6-10 L/min.

- The resistance of nasal interfaces affects the pressure transmission to the lungs. Interfaces with low resistance are recommended for effective SNIPPV.

## ACKNOWLEDGMENTS

The authors are grateful to Paolo Marchionni for his contribution.

## DISCLOSURE

C. Moretti is a consultant for GINEVRI Medical Technologies. GINEVRI Medical Technologies has not contributed any financial support for this paper or had any part in the authorship. C. Gizzi has nothing to disclose.

## REFERENCES

1. Dargaville PA, Gerber A, Johansson S, et al. Incidence and outcome of CPAP failure in preterm infants. Pediatrics 2016;138:e20153985.

2. Praud JP, Samson N, Moreau-Bussiere F. Laryngeal function and nasal ventilatory support in the neonatal period. Paediatr Respir Rev 2006;7:S180-2.

3. Owen LS, Morley CJ, Dawson JA, et al. Effects of non-synchronized nasal intermittent positive pressure ventilation on spontaneous breathing in preterm infants. Arch Dis Child Fetal Neonatal Ed 2011;96:F422-8.

4. de Waal CG, van Leuteren RW, de Jongh FH, et al. Patient-ventilator asynchrony in preterm infants on nasal intermittent positive pressure ventilation. Arch Dis Child Fetal Neonatal Ed 2019;104:F280-4.

5. Moretti C, Gizzi C, Papoff P, et al. Comparing the effects of nasal synchronized intermittent positive pressure ventilation (nSIPPV) and nasal continuous positive airway pressure (nCPAP) after extubation in very low birth weight infants. Early Hum Dev 1999;56:167-77.

6. Huang L, Mendler MR, Waitz M, et al. Effects of synchronization during non-invasive intermittent mandatory ventilation in preterm infants with respiratory distress syndrome immediately after extubation. Neonatology 2015;108:108-14.

7. Lemyre B, Laughon M, Bose C, et al. Early nasal intermittent positive pressure ventilation (NIPPV) versus early nasal continuous positive airway pressure (NCPAP) for preterm infants. Cochrane Database Syst Rev 2016;12:CD005384.

8. Ramaswamy VV, More K, Roehr CC, et al. Efficacy of non-invasive respiratory support modes for primary respiratory support in preterm neonates with respiratory distress syndrome: systematic review and network meta-analysis. Pediatr Pulmonol 2020;55:2940-63.

9. Lemyre B, Davis PG, De Paoli AG, et al. Nasal intermittent positive pressure ventilation (NIPPV) versus nasal continuous positive airway pressure (NCPAP) for preterm neonates after extubation. Cochrane Database Syst Rev 2017;2:CD003212.

10. Ramaswamy VV, Bandyopadhyay T, Nanda D, et al. Efficacy of non-invasive respiratory support modes as post-extubation respiratory support in preterm neonates: a systematic review and network meta-analysis. Pediatr Pulmonology 2020;55:2924-39.

11. Friedlich P, Lecart C, Posen R, et al. A randomized trial of nasopharyngeal-synchronized intermittent mandatory ventilation versus nasopharyngeal continuous positive airway pressure in very low birth weight infants after extubation. J Perinatol 1999;19:413-8.

12. de Waal CG, Kraaijenga JV, Hutten GJ, et al. Breath detection by transcutaneous electromyography of the diaphragm and the Graseby capsule in preterm infants. Pediatr Pulmonol 2017;52:1578-82.

13. Owen LS, Morley CJ, Davis PG. Effects of synchronization during SiPAP-generated nasal intermittent positive pressure ventilation (NIPPV) in preterm infants. Arch Dis Child Fetal Neonatal Ed 2015;100:F24-30.

14. Moretti C, Gizzi C, Montecchia F, et al. Synchronized nasal intermittent positive pressure ventilation of the newborn: technical Issues and clinical results. Neonatology 2016;109:359-65.

15. Gizzi C, Papoff P, Giordano I, et al. Flow-synchronized nasal intermittent positive pressure ventilation for infants <32 weeks' gestation with respiratory distress syndrome. Crit Care Res Pract 2012;2012:301818.

16. Ramos-Navarro C, Sanchez-Luna M, Sanz-López E, et al. Effectiveness of synchronized noninvasive ventilation to prevent intubation in preterm infants. AJP Rep 2016;6:e264–71.

17. Moretti C, Giannini L, Fassi C, et al. Nasal flow-synchronized intermittent positive pressure ventilation to facilitate weaning in very low-birthweight infants: unmasked randomized controlled trial. Pediatr Int 2008;50:85–91.

18. Gizzi C, Montecchia F, Panetta V, et al. Is synchronized NIPPV more effective than NIPPV and NCPAP in treating apnoea of prematurity (AOP)? A randomized crossover trial. Arch Dis Child Fetal Neonatal 2015;100:F17–23.

19. Beck J, Reilly M, Grasselli G, et al. Patient-ventilator interaction during neurally adjusted ventilatory assist in low birth weight infants. Pediatr Res 2009;65:663–8.

20. Firestone KS, Beck J, Stein H. Neurally adjusted ventilatory assist for noninvasive support in neonates. Clin Perinatol 2016;43:707–24.

21. Nam SK, Lee J, Jun YH. Neural feedback is insufficient in preterm infants during neurally adjusted ventilatory assist. Ped Pulmonol 2019;54:1277–83.

22. Goel D, Oei JL, Smyth J, et al. Diaphragm-triggered non-invasive respiratory support in preterm infants. Cochrane Database Syst Rev 2020;3:CD012935.

23. Warren RH, Horan SM, Robertson PK. Chest wall motion in preterm infants using respiratory inductive plethysmography. Eur Respir J 1997;10:2295–300.

24. Hammer J, Newth CJL. Assessment of thoraco-abdominal asynchrony. Paediatr Respir Rev 2009;10:75–80.

25. Kiciman NM, Andreasson B, Bernstein G, et al. Thoracoabdominal motion in newborns during ventilation delivered by endotracheal tube or nasal prongs. Pediatr Pulmonol 1998;25:175–81.

26. Eichenwald EC, Howell RG, Kosch PC, et al. Developmental changes in sequential activation of laryngeal abductor muscle and diaphragm in infants. J Appl Physiol 1992;73:1425–31.

27. Aghai ZH, Saslow JG, Nakhla T, et al. Synchronized nasal intermittent positive pressure ventilation (SNIPPV) decreases work of breathing (WOB) in premature infants with respiratory distress syndrome (RDS) compared to nasal continuous positive airway pressure (NCPAP). Pediatr Pulmonol 2006;41:875–81.

28. Chang HY, Claure N, D'Ugard C, et al. Effects of synchronization during nasal ventilation in clinically stable preterm infants. Pediatr Res 2011;69:84–9.

29. Charles E, Hunt KA, Rafferty GF, et al. Work of breathing during HHHFNC and synchronised NIPPV following extubation. Eur J Pediatr 2019;178:105–10.

30. Ricci F, Casiraghi C, Storti M, et al. Surfactant replacement therapy in combination with different non-invasive ventilation techniques in spontaneously breathing, surfactant-depleted adult rabbits. PLoS One 2018;13:e0200542.

31. Green EA, Dawson JA, Davis PG, et al. Assessment of resistance of nasal continuous positive airway pressure interfaces. Arch Dis Child Fetal Neonatal Ed 2019; 104:F535–9.

32. Singh N, McNally MJ, Darnall RA. Does the RAM cannula provide continuous positive airway pressure as effectively as the Hudson prongs in preterm neonates? Am J Perinatol 2019;36:849–54.

33. Matlock DN, Bai S, Weisner MD, et al. Tidal volume transmission during non-synchronized nasal intermittent positive pressure ventilation via RAM cannula. J Perinatol 2019;39:723–9.

34. Moretti C, Lista G, Carnielli V, et al. Flow-Synchronized NIPPV with double-inspiratory loop cannula (DILC): an in vitro study. Ped Pulmunol 2020;56(2): 400–8.

35. Santin R, Brodsky N, Bhandari V. A prospective observational pilot study of synchronized nasal intermittent positive pressure ventilation (SNIPPV) as a primary mode of ventilation in infants > or =28 weeks with respiratory distress syndrome (RDS). J Perinatol 2004;24:487–93.
36. Ricotti A, Salvo V, Zimmermann LJ, et al. N-SIPPV versus bi-level N-CPAP for early treatment of respiratory distress syndrome in preterm infants. J Matern Fetal Neonatal Med 2013;26:1346–51.
37. Bhandari V, Gavino RG, Nedrelow JH, et al. A randomized controlled trial of synchronized nasal intermittent positive pressure ventilation in RDS. J Perinatol 2007; 27:697–703.
38. Kugelman A, Feferkorn I, Riskin A, et al. Nasal intermittent mandatory ventilation versus nasal continuous positive airway pressure for respiratory distress syndrome: a randomized, controlled, prospective study. J Pediatr 2007;150:521–6.
39. Salvo V, Lista G, Lupo E, et al. Noninvasive ventilation strategies for early treatment of RDS in preterm infants: an RCT. Pediatrics 2015;135:444–51.
40. Yagui AC, Meneses J, Zólio BA, et al. Nasal continuous positive airway pressure (NCPAP) or noninvasive neurally adjusted ventilatory assist (NIV-NAVA) for preterm infants with respiratory distress after birth: a randomized controlled trial. Pediatr Pulmonol 2019;54:1704–11.
41. Kallio M, Mahlman M, Koskela U, et al. NIV NAVA versus nasal CPAP in premature infants: a randomized clinical trial. Neonatology 2019;116:380–4.
42. Yonehara K, Ogawa R, Kamei Y, et al. NIV-NAVA versus NIPPV in preterm infants born before 30 weeks of GA. Pediatr Int 2018;60:957–61.
43. Yagui ACZ, Gonçalves P, Murakami SH, et al. Is noninvasive neurally adjusted ventilatory assistance (NIV-NAVA) an alternative to NCPAP in preventing extubation failure in preterm infants? J Matern Fetal Neonatal Med 2019;24:1–151.
44. Lee BK, Shin SH, Jung YH, et al. Comparison of NIV-NAVA and NCPAP in facilitating extubation for very preterm infants. BMC Pediatr 2019;19:298.
45. Barrington KJ, Bull D, Finer NN. Randomized trial of nasal synchronized intermittent mandatory ventilation compared with continuous positive airway pressure after extubation of very low birth weight infants. Pediatrics 2001;107:638–41.
46. Gao WW, Tan S, Chen Y, et al. Randomized trail of nasal synchronized intermittent mandatory ventilation compared with nasal continuous positive airway pressure in preterm infants with respiratory distress syndrome. Zhongguo Dang Dai Er Ke Za Zhi 2010;12(7):524–6.
47. Tabacaru CR, Moores RR Jr, Khoury J, et al. NAVA-synchronized compared to nonsynchronized noninvasive ventilation for apnea, bradycardia, and desaturation events in VLBW infants. Pediatr Pulmonol 2019;54:1742–6.
48. Bai XM, Bian J, Zhao YL, et al. The application of nasal synchronized intermittent mandatory ventilation in primary apnea of prematurity. Turk J Pediatr 2014;56: 150–3.

# Nasal High-Frequency Ventilation

Daniele De Luca, MD, PhD[a,b,*], Roberta Centorrino, MD[a,b]

**KEYWORDS**

- Neonate • Noninvasive • Oscillation • Percussive • Rescue • Respiratory support
- Interface • Newborn infant

**KEY POINTS**

- The role of interface during noninvasive high-frequency ventilatory modes is very important and physical characteristics of different interfaces must be known to optimize their use.
- NHFOV needs to be used within a physiology-driven protocol with accurate mini-invasive multimodal monitoring and adequate nurse training. A protocol proposal is enclosed.
- NHFOV may be useful to reduce Paco$_2$ and spare intubation and invasive ventilation in neonates with CPIP (ie, evolving BPD).
- Future trials about NHFOV need to be more explanatory and physiology-based.
- There is less experience with NHFPV, although it might be useful for TTN.

## INTRODUCTION

The term "noninvasive high-frequency ventilation" designates a nonconventional ventilatory technique with supraphysiologic frequencies applied through an external noninvasive interface (nasal prongs, helmet, or various types of mask), thus without endotracheal intubation or tracheostomy. It is out of our scope to discuss whether conventional or nonconventional modalities are generally preferable but we will review the data regarding noninvasive high-frequency ventilations available in neonatology and their possible benefits.

Within this technique, we may recognize 2 modalities:

- Noninvasive high-frequency oscillatory ventilation (NHFOV),
- Noninvasive high-frequency percussive ventilation (NHFPV).

[a] Division of Pediatrics and Neonatal Critical Care, "A.Beclere" Medical Center, Paris Saclay University Hospitals, APHP, Paris - France; [b] Physiopathology and Therapeutic Innovation Unit-INSERM U999, Paris Saclay University, Paris - France
* Corresponding author. Service de Pédiatrie et Réanimation Néonatale, Hôpital "A. Béclère"-GHU Paris Saclay, APHP, 157 rue de la Porte de Trivaux, Clamart Paris-IDF 92140, France.
*E-mail address:* dm.deluca@icloud.com

Clin Perinatol 48 (2021) 761–782
https://doi.org/10.1016/j.clp.2021.07.006
0095-5108/21/© 2021 Elsevier Inc. All rights reserved.

Only scanty exist about NHFPV, whereas NHFOV is quite often used in some countries.[1] The diffusion of NHFOV is likely due to the wide experience about the use of endotracheal high-frequency oscillatory ventilation (HFOV) and nasal continuous positive airway pressure (CPAP) in preterm neonates. The experience in HFOV and CPAP has pushed clinicians to combine them to maximize their advantages (such as noninvasive interface, increase in functional residual capacity determining oxygenation improvement, no need for synchronization, efficient $CO_2$ removal).

## PHYSIOLOGY OF NON-INVASIVE HIGH-FREQUENCY OSCILLATORY VENTILATION
### General Characteristics

NHFOV is based on the application of a continuous flow, generating a constant distending positive pressure with superimposed oscillations, delivered all over the spontaneous breathing cycle. NHFOV could be applied either in a restrictive (eg,: respiratory distress syndrome [RDS]) or in a mixed (eg, evolving bronchopulmonary dysplasia [BPD] or BPD plus acute-on-chronic respiratory failure) respiratory insufficiency. NHFOV has the same basic principles and peculiar physiology in both cases: **Fig. 1** shows similar flow, volume, and pressures tracings recorded from active neonatal lung models of restrictive or mixed pattern ventilated with NHFOV.

Oscillations have constant frequency and may be seen as somehow similar to those of bubble CPAP, which provides a positive pressure with oscillations although the latter are smaller, irregular, and with inconstant amplitude.[2] Furthermore, NHFOV can produce much higher mean airway pressure (Paw) than bubble CPAP, as it is generated by a ventilator rather than a simple water valve.

A first interesting characteristic of NHFOV is that it can be easily used for alveolar recruitment increasing Paw, without the risk of gas trapping-induced $CO_2$ retention,

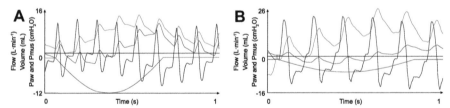

**Fig. 1.** NHFOV during spontaneous breathing in an active lung model of neonatal restrictive (model A) and mixed (model B) respiratory failure. Blue, green, red, and orange lines represent flow, volume, airway pressure (measured at the lung), and inspiratory muscle pressure (spontaneously generated by the patient), respectively. Data have been generated using a bench model modified from adult setting consisting of a neonatal mannequin ventilated through a nasal mask and whose trachea had been connected to an electronic active test lung (ASL5000; Ingmar Medical, Pittsburgh, Pennsylvania, USA). A Sensormedics SM3100A oscillator (Vyaire, San Diego, California, USA) was used. Data were filtered at 100 Hz and measured at the lung simulator using a specific software (ICU Lab rel.2.3; KleisTEK Advanced Electronic System, Bari, Italy). Model A mimics a preterm neonate with RDS (birth weight: 1.5 kg, resistances: 100 $cmH_2O/L/s$, compliance: 0.5 mL/$cmH_2O$/kg, respiratory rate: 40 breaths/min, Paw: 8 $cmH_2O$, amplitude 30 $cmH_2O$; frequency 9 Hz, IT 50%). Model B mimics an infant with BPD and acute worsening of respiratory function (acute-on-chronic respiratory failure) (birth weight: 2 kg, resistances: 300 $cmH_2O/L/s$, compliance: 0.4 mL/$cmH_2O$/kg, respiratory rate: 50 breaths/min, Paw: 10 $cmH_2O$, amplitude 50 $cmH_2O$; frequency 6 Hz, IT 50%); notice how the inspiratory effort is weaker in this example, as the patients are experiencing relevant work of breathing. A single spontaneous breath is shown in both panels. Paw, airway pressure measured at the lung; Pmus, negative spontaneously generated inspiratory muscle pressure.

as this is avoided by the superimposed oscillations. Alveolar recruitment in NHFOV can be performed in a patient with restrictive respiratory failure in the same manner as it is performed in endotracheal HFOV, following the well-known principles of the optimum lung volume strategy.[3] Compared to endotracheal HFOV, however, NHFOV is generally accompanied by relevant pressure leaks that should be considered.[4]

If the effects on oxygenation are quite well known, the mechanisms of gas exchange during NHFOV are incompletely understood. They partially correspond to the ones occurring in endotracheal HFOV[5] albeit with some peculiarities. During NHFOV, a tidal volume is spontaneously generated, but at the same time, a small oscillatory volume is provided by the cyclic pressure oscillations and delivered all along the respiratory cycle.[1] These oscillations may be variably transmitted along the respiratory tree and this adds to the complexity of gas exchange, which is based on several physical phenomena.[6]

Oscillation transmission seems to be the most important variable influencing ventilation, although both tidal and oscillatory volumes actually contribute to gas exchange.[7,8] This dual contribution has been initially hypothesized in *in vitro* measurements, but recent *in vivo* studies in preterm infants have provided consistent results.[9] Bench data have also initially shown that NHFOV is able to washout $CO_2$ from the upper airways' dead space.[10] Subsequently, $CO_2$ clearance has been also demonstrated at lung level in similar bench models.[11] However, recent *in vivo* data demonstrated that during binasal prongs-delivered NHFOV, oscillations are not only transmitted to the upper airways but also to the alveolar tissue, especially in the nongravity dependent and right-sided lung regions; this effect was noticed at relatively low oscillatory amplitude values.[9] Nonetheless, these data may be significantly influenced by several factors. For instance, oscillation transmission is more efficient through stiff structures,[12] thus the amount of oscillatory volume reaching the alveoli may be different between babies with mainly restrictive and homogeneous (ie, RDS) and those with mixed and nonhomogeneous patterns (ie, evolving BPD). Furthermore, type, size, and material of interfaces may significantly influence the oscillation transmission and the resulting volume delivery (see below).[1] These can also be influenced by alveolar recruitment which changes the regional compliance.[12] Patients' position could also have an effect, as neonates are often turned and this changes the non–gravity-dependent lung zones. In adults, this shift has been associated with increased regional compliance and pulmonary perfusion and subsequent effects on volume delivery and oxygenation.[13,14] An useful tool to summarize the interplay of factors influencing oscillation transmission is the oscillatory pressure ratio, that is, the ratio between the oscillation amplitude set at the ventilator and that actually measured at a given level (eg, at the interface or the pharynx).[12]

### Non-invasive High-Frequency Oscillatory Ventilation and Patient-Ventilator Interaction

Noninvasive ventilation is difficult to synchronize in neonates because of their high respiratory rate, low tidal volume, and irregular breathing pattern. NHFOV bypasses this problem as all ventilations at supraphysiological frequencies, by definition, do not require synchronization. Furthermore, NHFOV could provide benefits over conventional noninvasive ventilations, because it does not induce phasic inspiratory glottal constriction, or decrease inspiratory glottal dilatation in newborn lambs.[15] This may allow a more constant pressure/volume transmission to the distal airways.[16] However, animal data also showed suppression of respiratory drive when nasal mask-delivered NHFOV was applied with a very low frequency (4 Hz).[15] This effect has been confirmed in various models and is not mediated by hypocarbia, but rather by an increased vagal pulmonary stretch receptor or thoracic wall afferent activity.[17,18] However, such low frequencies are not used in neonatology and an increased respiratory drive with consequent diaphragmatic activation has also been observed in animals: this depends on the ventilation parameters and is mediated by pulmonary rapidly adapting receptors.[19,20] Conversely, in adults with central sleep apnea, nasal mask-delivered high-frequency oscillations stimulate respiratory effort in adult patients.[21] In neonates, other mechanisms also influence the spontaneous respiratory drive, such as inflammation, pain, or discomfort and the choice of NHFOV interface may play a relevant role (see below).[22] Finally, as patients are spontaneously breathing during NHFOV, an increment in their work of breathing (WOB) could be observed, although this is lower in smaller patients.[23] WOB increment depends on many factors such as lung compliance and resistances, patients' size, ventilator type (see below), and parameters. Regarding these latter, lower frequencies seem to be associated with lower additional WOB[24]: this should be considered for long-lasting NHFOV, but also balanced with the need to deliver adequate ventilation. *Therefore, the interactions between high-frequency oscillations and spontaneous respiratory drive are complex and opposite effects might be observed in different patients or in different moments: tailoring ventilation with close patient monitoring is crucial.*

### Effect of Different Interfaces for Non-invasive High-Frequency Oscillatory Ventilation

NHFOV can be provided using different interfaces and each has its own mechanical characteristics and multiples effects on NHFOV physiology. Moreover, interfaces may significantly affect patients' comfort and the combination of these mechanisms can considerably change the effect of NHFOV in terms of oxygenation and gas exchange.

The first clinical experiences on NHFOV used single, long, high-resistive nasopharyngeal tubes.[25] As demonstrated for CPAP, these interfaces were unsuitable and should not be used; in fact, they are associated with large leaks occurring through the contralateral nostril and with a relevant resistive load increasing the patients' WOB.[26] As short binasal prongs should be preferred over nasopharyngeal tubes,[27] and nasal masks seem even better than short prongs,[28] we have investigated them in dedicated NHFOV bench studies finding efficient oscillation transmission and volume delivery.[4,29,30] Finally, the use of prongs occluding only a small portion of the nostril cross-sectional area and connected via a long and resistive tubing (RAMCannula) is currently spreading. These interfaces are particularly comfortable; however, they provide high resistance, which increases the patients' WOB,[31] and significant leaks when used to deliver CPAP[32,33] or conventional noninvasive ventilation.[34] Despite these negative mechanical characteristics, a case series described the use of RAMCannula-delivered NHFOV in 3 neonates ventilated with relatively low Paw.[35]

Our knowledge on the different interfaces for NHFOV and their effects on physiology can be resumed as follows:

1. The diameter of binasal prongs is important to guarantee an efficient ventilation (ie, the larger the probe, the greater the volume delivery); for a given amplitude and frequency, increasing the inspiratory time from 33% to 50%, allows a greater volume delivery, but increasing the amplitude beyond 50 to 60 cmH$_2$O does not significantly increase ventilation.[29,30] Thus, when binasal prong-delivered NHFOV is provided with maximal parameters (ie, with amplitude of approximately 50–60 cmH$_2$O, a frequency of 8–10 Hz, and 50% inspiratory time), a suitable oscillatory volume might be provided to neonates up to 1 to 1.5 kg[29,30] (if we consider 1–2 mL/kg as an ideal target alike in invasive HFOV[36]).
2. Nasal masks can efficaciously deliver NHFOV but provide lower oscillation transmission, due to the dampening occurring on the skin tissue and the mask soft

material.[4] This seems consistent with what happens during full-face mask-delivered NHFOV in infants beyond neonatal age.[7] More aggressive parameters (particularly lower frequency) may be needed to deliver the same oscillatory volume provided through binasal prongs.[4] Nasal masks are associated with lower pressure leaks compared to nasal prongs[33] and these leaks ($\approx$30%-35%) seem similar during NHFOV and other types of noninvasive support.[4] Bench data have demonstrated that moderate leakage may increase $CO_2$ clearance during NHFOV, probably facilitating the washout from the upper airways dead space and reducing gas trapping; thus, moderate leaks may be allowed, on a case-by-case evaluation.[37,38]

3. RAMCannula should not be used to deliver NHFOV, if it is applied in cases of severe respiratory failure (for instance, when intubation is pending) or for long periods or when the added resistance may have negative consequences (for instance, in extremely low birth weight neonates).

These mechanical data do not advocate for universal use of a single interface. In fact, patients' comfort, ventilatory parameters, integrity of skin, and also nonrespiratory factors should be considered, as well. Moreover, the severity of respiratory failure may vary from one patient to the other and between different moments during the clinical course; thus, sometimes less aggressive parameters may be sufficient to compensate respiratory failure. Mechanical characteristics of interfaces, patients' comfort, and severity have a complex interplay on NHFOV physiology; therefore, the choice of NHFOV interface should be based on all these aspects and aim to find the best compromise between ventilation efficiency and patients' comfort.[1] This latter remains to be evaluated in specifically dedicated studies and, therefore, *interfaces should be tailored on a case-by-case basis evaluation and interchanged to reduce the risk of skin lesions and according to patients' needs.*[39] **Table 1** resumes the factors influencing gas exchange during NHFOV.

### Different Devices Producing Non-invasive High-Frequency Oscillatory Ventilation

NHFOV may be applied with any ventilator able to provide the HFOV mode: several technologies are available.[1] From a formal point of view, an actual "oscillatory"

**Table 1**
**Factors influencing gas exchange during NHFOV**

| Variable | Effect on Gas Exchange |
| --- | --- |
| Oscillation amplitude | ↑ |
| Inspiratory time | ↑ |
| Frequency | ↓ |
| Leaks | ↓ [a] |
| Interface | Variable |
| Mean airway pressure | Variable |
| Gravity (patient positioning) | Variable |

Effect of interface is variable because different interfaces may facilitate or reduce oscillation transmission through an improved patients' comfort and/or changing pressure leaks and/or oscillation dampening.

[a] Leaks are generally reducing gas exchange through decreased oscillation transmission, but moderate leaks have been demonstrated to increase $CO_2$ clearance under certain experimental conditions.[37,38] The effects of Paw or gravity are variable because increasing constant distending pressure, or positioning the infant prone or supine may change regional compliance and affect oscillation transmission.

ventilation should have an active expiratory phase produced by a vibrating piston or membrane over a continuous gas flow or by an electronically controlled, cyclic flow reversal. These 2 ways to produce active oscillations have not been compared with respect to the application of NHFOV. Other technologies to produce HFOV (although without an active expiratory phase) are represented by the flow interruption because of the cyclic opening-closure of one or more pressure valves. Some neonatal ventilators are technically able to provide NHFOV using this technology, but their performance to provide invasive HFOV can be suboptimal at extreme settings or for late preterm/term neonates.[40,41] As NHFOV is usually proposed for preterm infants, and, as bench studies have demonstrated an adequate ventilation for neonates up to 1 to 1.5 kg,[29,30] this is not likely to represent a significant problem. Another ventilator produces oscillations based on the inertia of gas in the circuit when the pressure at airway opening is rapidly changing: this technology is combined with fast responding inspiratory valves and high-flow capability but it has not been formally tested for NHFOV yet. There are also hybrid systems based on positive pressure generated by high-flow nasal cannula with superimposed high-frequency oscillations provided by a solenoid valve: they have been shown to provide efficacious $CO_2$ clearance in bench models.[42,43] Finally, a new technology based on electronically controlled blower and valve has been specifically proposed for NHFOV.[44] So far, hybrid high flow or blower and valve technologies have not been incorporated in any commercially available ventilator.

The active oscillation is considered important for the $CO_2$ clearance; however, the wide experience accumulated on invasive HFOV seems to indicate that this is not actually affecting clinical outcomes.[45] Nonetheless, at least in some patients, the kind of NHFOV-producing device may have an impact on its short-term efficiency.[40,41] This problem may be less relevant in NHFOV, as this is supposed to be used in neonates below 1 to 1.5 kg. It is also important to note that, as patients are spontaneously breathing during NHFOV, a certain WOB may theoretically be superimposed by NHFOV application. This WOB increment is relatively low for preterm infants, but seems significantly different between ventilators based on the above-described technologies, with tendency to a lower WOB for ventilators with an active expiration.[24]

### Humidification During Non-invasive High-Frequency Oscillatory Ventilation

Heating and humidification during noninvasive respiratory support seem to improve comfort in adults, although we do not have specific neonatal data.[46] An European survey identified viscous secretions and consequent upper airway obstructions as specific side effects of NHFOV[47] and this seems logical as NHFOV is usually applied as rescue, when other noninvasive respiratory techniques have failed. The American Association for Respiratory Care suggests to use active humidification during noninvasive ventilation, although there are still open questions about the type of active humidifier to prefer.[46] Ullrich and colleagues have studied humidification during NHFOV and found that aggressive NHFOV settings (ie, low frequency, high amplitude, and IT) significantly reduced oropharyngeal gas conditioning.[48] This is consistent with data on $CO_2$ pharyngeal washout[10]; thus, it seems reasonable to think that aggressive NHFOV removes water through physical mechanisms similar to those of HFOV gas exchange.[5] The presence of leakage might also contribute, as gas particles can be mixed by thermodiffusion, and heat may be lost by thermal conduction or with the entry of cool dry gas particles from the room air. The clinical relevance of these phenomena is unknown, but probably limited if NHFOV is not used for a long time.

## BIOLOGY OF NON-INVASIVE HIGH-FREQUENCY OSCILLATORY VENTILATION

Reddy and colleagues showed that superimposing oscillations over tidal volume excursions in a surfactant bubble lowers surface tension significantly more than tidal volume excursion alone.[49] Minimum surface tension decreased with increasing frequencies and reached a value of $\approx 7$ mN/m at extreme frequencies (70–80 Hz), not attainable in clinical care. Conversely, minimum surface tension of 15 to 30 mN/m was measured with frequencies usually applied when using NHFOV. Similar values have been measured in neonates and infants with neonatal or pediatric ARDS.[50,51] Invasive HFOV improves lung mechanics and histology in surfactant-depleted rabbits.[52] Consistent findings, as well as larger surfactant aggregates, have been reported in animal models mimicking different types of lung injury.[53,54] These data allow to hypothesize that NHFOV could improve surfactant function, although this only remains a working hypothesis.

## EVIDENCE-BASED REVIEW OF CLINICAL DATA ON NON-INVASIVE HIGH-FREQUENCY OSCILLATORY VENTILATION

### Uncontrolled Studies

In 2016, we have analyzed the clinical data on NHFOV available at that time and these were mainly represented by uncontrolled small case series, showing globally promising results.[1] Because of the neonatal experience on HFOV and wide availability of this ventilatory mode, NHFOV spread in the last 5 years led to the publication of other similar studies. These latest uncontrolled studies were consistent with the earlier data, reporting that: (1) NHFOV may reduce the extubation failure or the need of invasive ventilation in infants with pending intubation; (2) NHFOV may improve gas exchange; (3) NHFOV may reduce the number of apneic spells; and (4) NHFOV did not cause any severe adverse event.[55–58] The absence of these had also been suggested by a European survey of physicians using NHFOV.[47]

### Randomized Controlled Trials

After these studies, randomized controlled trials finally started to be published. We performed a systematic review of these trials. A literature search was performed on PubMed (on November 7, 2020), using "nasal" or "noninvasive high-frequency oscillatory ventilation" or "NHFOV", as words or MeSH terms, without year or language restrictions. We also hand-searched references cited in the studies identified through the initial search, review articles, and the authors' personal archives. We excluded "gray" literature, unpublished or non–peer-reviewed reports. Non-English manuscripts were translated using Google translator. We used a data extraction sheet based on the Cochrane Review Group template adapted from our previous work.[59] Data from included trials were extracted and cross-verified independently by the 2 authors. We analyzed data applying the Sidik-Jonkman method[60] with random-effects models. Consistency was evaluated using the $I2$ statistics and $\chi^2$ test for heterogeneity. Meta-regressions were performed adjusting for gestational age and prenatal steroids as confounders. We inserted one covariate in each model to reduce false-positive results.[59] Analyses were performed with Open-MetaAnalyst 10.1.[61]

### Meta-Analysis of Randomized Controlled Trials

To date, there are 11 trials comparing NHFOV against single-level or biphasic CPAP, either with parallel or crossover design, mainly having short-term events or gas exchange as primary outcomes.[62–72] **Table 2** shows essential trials' characteristics. All but 2 trials[63,68] recruited relatively small populations and 3 enrolled extremely

**Table 2**
Randomized clinical trials comparing NHFOV versus single-level or bilevel CPAP

| Author/Year | No. of Patients | GA (wk) | Prenatal Steroids (%) | Primary Outcomes | Secondary Outcomes | Maximum Paw and Amplitude | Enrolled Population |
|---|---|---|---|---|---|---|---|
| Bottino et al,[62] 2018 | 30 | 26.4 | N.A. | $Paco_2$ | N.A. | 8/10[a] | Stable preterm neonates |
| Chen et al,[63] 2020 | 206 | 32.6 | 89.8 | Need for IMV and $Paco_2$ | Complications of prematurity | 16/40 | Preterm neonates with RDS or NARDS as postextubation support |
| Iranpour et al,[64] 2019 | 68 | 33 | 26.4 | Duration of CPAP or NHFOV | Need for reintubation; Complications of prematurity | 8/20[a] | Preterm neonates with RDS as primary support |
| Klotz et al,[65] 2018 | 26 | 26.7 | 100 | $Paco_2$ | Apneas, bradycardia, and safety data | 8/N.A.[a] | Stable preterm neonates |
| Lou & Zhang,[66] 2017 | 65 | 32.4 | 38.4 | Need for IMV | Oxygenation and $Paco_2$, complications of prematurity | N.A. | Preterm neonates with RDS as postextubation support |
| Lou et al,[67] 2018 | 65 | 33.8 | 35.3 | Oxygenation and $Paco_2$ | IMV duration, apneas, complications of prematurity | 12/35 | Preterm neonates with RDS as postextubation support |
| Malakian et al,[68] 2018 | 124 | 31.1 | 53.9 | Need for IMV | IMV duration, complications of prematurity | 8/7[a] | Preterm neonates with RDS as primary support |
| Mukerji et al,[69] 2017 | 39 | 28.8 | 80.9 | Feasibility | IMV duration, $Paco_2$, complications of prematurity | 10/N.A.[a] | Preterm neonates with RDS as postextubation support |
| Rüegger et al,[70] 2018 | 40 | 26.5 | 90 | Bradycardia and/or desaturation | Vital parameters and safety data | 7/40[a] | Stable extremely preterm neonates |
| Zhu et al,[71] 2017 | 76 | 31.8 | 36.7 | Need for IMV | Complications of prematurity | 6/N.A.[a] | Preterm neonates with RDS as postextubation support |
| Zhu et al,[72] 2017 | 38 | 31.8 | 36.6 | Oxygenation and $Paco_2$ | Complications of prematurity | 10/10[a] | Preterm neonates with RDS as postextubation support |

Gestational age and prenatal steroids were considered as the weighted mean of the 2 trial arms. Three studies had a crossover design[62,65,70], the remaining were parallel trials. Values have been rounded to the closest decimal.

Abbreviations: GA, gestational age; IMV, invasive mechanical ventilation; N.A., not available; NARDS, neonatal acute respiratory distress syndrome; $Paco_2$, carbon dioxide levels; Paw, mean airway pressure; RDS, respiratory distress syndrome.

[a] Asterisks indicate that patients in trial arms have equivalent Paw.

preterm neonates.[62,65,70] Most of the primary outcomes were represented by short-term need for intubation and invasive ventilation (IMV)[63,66,68,71] or $Paco_2$/oxygenation.[62,63,65,67,72] Although authors should be commended for the efforts, there are important problems behind these outcomes' choice:

1. The need for IMV can be a sensible outcome; however, some studies investigated NHFOV in preterm neonates with RDS as primary respiratory support (ie, before surfactant administration, if any)[64,68] and others as secondary support after extubation or surfactant administration.[63,66,67,69,71,72] This lack of homogeneity prevents to draw any conclusion: although it seems logical that a higher Paw would reduce the risk of extubation failure as demonstrated for other noninvasive respiratory support techniques,[73,74] we need larger trials focused on the postextubation phase, comparing NHFOV with other noninvasive techniques. More and above this, we need to actually use higher Paw during NHFOV; in the majority of trials, Paw was equivalent in the 2 arms,[62,64,65,68–72] and this would prevent NHFOV to provide an actual alveolar recruitment. Furthermore, it is unclear what might be the advantage of NHFOV in the early phase of RDS. In fact, it is known that CPAP works very well for most of the patients in this phase[75] and, when CPAP fails, that is usually for worsening oxygenation. Oxygenation impairment in a purely restrictive and homogeneous condition (such as RDS) is easily overcome by alveolar recruitment. However, as trials investigating NHFOV as a primary mode always used an equivalent Paw in the 2 arms,[64,68] no alveolar recruitment was provided and it was logical to observe no difference. Moreover, if alveolar recruitment through NHFOV would be applied in this phase, this might delay surfactant replacement, reducing its efficacy, which is optimal only within the first 3 hours of life.[76,77]

2. HFOV is known to be very powerful in washing out $CO_2$. Because NHFOV has some peculiar physiologic characteristics, it was interesting to evaluate its carbon dioxide clearance capacity, although it would have been unlikely to see NHFOV failing in this regard. In fact, face mask-delivered NHFOV has been found to effectively washout $CO_2$ also in a small crossover trial enrolling adults.[78] However, $CO_2$ clearance has been tested in trials enrolling stable preterm neonates or anyway with relatively low $Paco_2$ levels and no respiratory acidosis.[62,63,65–67,69,72] This choice has led to less meaningful and possibly biased results, since, in the daily NICU care, no one would shift a patient from CPAP to NHFOV if there is no hypercarbia. Moreover, having $CO_2$ clearance as outcome also presents a problem similar to the aforementioned issue about Paw and oxygenation. In fact, some trials used a flow interruption device, generating very low amplitudes, which are unlikely to be transmitted downstream[62,68,71,72]; the generation of a very little oscillatory volume and its actual contribution to gas exchange is doubtful.

Two large well-designed physiology-driven multicenter trials are currently ongoing.[1] These trials aim to verify if NHFOV provides any benefit, compared to CPAP or noninvasive positive pressure ventilation, either as primary respiratory support or in the postextubation phase for preterm neonates with RDS.[79,80]

The trials published so far had a panoply of secondary outcomes, among which, there are some difficult to improve, but also several vital parameters and safety data. NHFOV reduced the number of desaturations and bradycardia in one trial,[70] although there was no difference in any safety data in the other trials.[62–69,71,72] Therefore, we can reasonably state that NHFOV is essentially safe or can even be beneficial in reducing bradycardia, desaturations, and/or apneas, at least in some patients. However, due to the complex effects of NHFOV on the spontaneous breathing (see above), these results cannot be generalized as they can change according to the patient's clinical condition, cointerventions, NHFOV interfaces, and parameters.

We present here the meta-analysis of trials focusing on the 2 more commonly studied outcomes: (1) need for intubation and mechanical ventilation; (2) $Paco_2$ levels after NHFOV application (**Fig. 2**). *NHFOV significantly reduces the risk or intubation and need of IMV (odds ratio: 0.29; 95% confidence interval: 0.2–0.4; P<.001) compared to single-level or biphasic CPAP. These results are confirmed if we only analyze the trials using NHFOV as postextubation support (odds ratio: 0.3; 95% confidence interval: 0.18–0.5; P<.001). NHFOV also tends to reduce $CO_2$ compared to single-level or biphasic CPAP (mean difference: −4.6 mm Hg; 95% confidence interval: −9.3 to 0.08; P = .05);* significant heterogeneity is seen for this outcome and this may be related to the different times and techniques to measure $Paco_2$ and to the different ventilatory strategies described earlier.

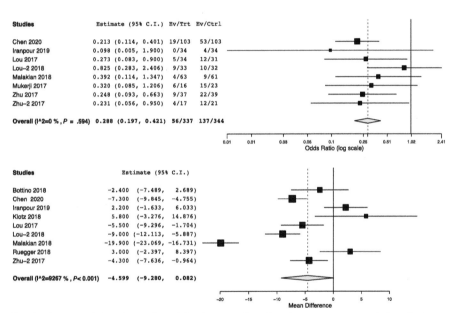

**Fig. 2.** *Meta-analysis of NHFOV trials: Forrest plots for the more commonly studied outcomes.* Panels A and B show the need for intubation and mechanical ventilation (681 patients) and $Paco_2$ levels after NHFOV application (662 patients), respectively. NHFOV and the single-level or biphasic CPAP are considered as treatment (Trt) and control (Ctrl) arm, respectively; events per arm and odds ratio or mean difference (95% confidence interval) are reported in panels A and B, respectively. Square size is proportional to trial weight. Diamond width indicates the 95% confidence interval of the final effect size. The need for intubation and invasive ventilation was considered at any timepoint after intervention (some trials defined this outcome within 72 hours, others within a 7-day time-window). $Paco_2$ levels were considered at any timepoint after intervention (trials defined this outcome by measuring $Paco_2$ at various times after the intervention). Trials weight for the outcome intubation were as follows: Chen: 36.138%, Iranpour: 1.636%, Lou: 10.087%, Lou-2: 12.530%, Malakian: 9.406%, Mukerji: 8.153%, Zhu: 14.882%, Zhu-2: 7.167%. Trials weight for the outcome $Paco_2$ levels were as follows: Bottino: 10.820%, Chen: 11.968%, Iranpour: 11.454%, Klotz: 8.461%, Lou: 11.471%, Lou-2: 11.762%, Malakian: 11.740%, Rüegger: 10.651%, Zhu-2: 11.672%. 95% CI, 95% confidence interval; Ctrl, control arm (ie, single-level or biphasic CPAP); $Paco_2$, carbon dioxide levels; Trt, treatment arm (ie, NHFOV).

We further studied the effect of possible confounders: for the outcome intubation, neither gestational age (coefficient: 0.104 [95% confidence interval: −0.2; 0.4]; $P$ = .527), nor prenatal steroids (coefficient: −0.007 [95% confidence interval: −0.02; 0.007]; $P$ = .327), were associated with the effect size; same results were found for $Paco_2$ levels, regarding gestational age (coefficient: −1.1 [95% confidence interval: −2.7; 0.4]; $P$ = .137) and prenatal steroids (coefficient: 0.07 [95% confidence interval: −0.1; 0.2]; $P$ = .424).

These results, and particularly those issued by subgroup analyses and metaregressions, should be cautiously seen also in light of the above-described problems in trial design and outcome choice. The NHFOV trials published so far have been affected by significant intrinsic biases and these have been reported in comment letters.[81,82] We do not analyse here all the biases, as this would be beyond our scope. *Nonetheless, future trials shall investigate NHFOV with a physiology-driven management, in homogeneous populations, with a clearly defined lung mechanics and restricted,*

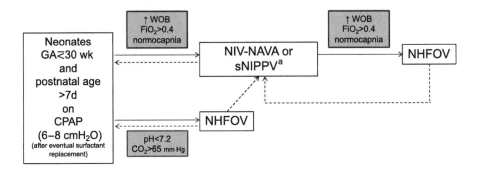

**Fig. 3.** Proposal for a tailored protocol to apply NHFOV in extremely preterm infants with developing BPD (ie, chronic pulmonary insufficiency of prematurity).[86] This is the protocol in use at Paris Saclay University Hospitals NICU. Different types of noninvasive respiratory techniques are used after the first week of life in extremely preterm infants if they experience a worsening of their respiratory function. NHFOV is integrated into the strategy with the other techniques based on a physiology-driven approach. Hypoxic respiratory failure (*blue lines*) is defined with an increased work of breathing (Silverman score >4) without hypercarbia and with $Fio_2$ greater than 0.4 to achieve peripheral saturation between 90% and 95% and is treated with synchronized conventional noninvasive ventilations (NIV-NAVA or sNIPPV); NHFOV is used if these fail. Hypercapnic respiratory failure (*red lines*) is defined with hypercarbia ($CO_2$ >65 mm Hg) and acidosis (pH<7.20), irrespective of the oxygenation deficit, and treated with NHFOV as first line. NHFOV is managed by applying alveolar recruitment maneuvers and with a close multimodal monitoring. Definition criteria should be fulfilled for at least 4 to 6 h before instigating NIV-NAVA, sNIPPV, or NHFOV and patients are monitored over time with several noninvasive techniques (see text for more details). As the patient is improving, the respiratory support can be de-escalated. Full and hatched lines indicate deterioration and improvement of respiratory conditions, respectively. [a]The choice between NIV-NAVA and sNIPPV depends on the availability of ventilators. EDIN, *"Echelle et Inconfort du Nouveau-né"* score; $Fio_2$, inspired oxygen fraction; LUS, lung ultrasound score; NIV-NAVA, noninvasive ventilation with neurally adjusted ventilator assist; PI, perfusion index; SatO_2, peripheral hemoglobin saturation; sNIPPV, synchronized noninvasive positive pressure ventilation; WOB, work of breathing.

*physiopathologically sound objectives.* NHFOV shall be compared to a well-defined "control" technique and both shall be applied with a strict protocol. In other words, future trials should have an explanatory design and tend to recruit only from well-experienced sites. More pragmatic inclusive approaches are unsuitable because they seek a "real world" answer for a more widely used and well-known intervention.[83] On the contrary, NHFOV is a relatively new technique and, by mixing different populations or leaving ventilatory management too free, we risk to lose important information.[84]

To date, according to the available clinical data and the physiology background, NHFOV can be considered as an additional technique for infants with severe respiratory failure. It may be suitable in preterm patients with pending reintubation or in those with evolving BPD, where one may want to spare oxygen exposure and invasive ventilation as much as possible. In these cases, NHFOV can be used, if there is enough expertise, after careful evaluation on a case-by-case scenario and with accurate patients' monitoring and physiology-based management.

## PERSONAL EXPERIENCE AND PROTOCOL TO MANAGE NON-INVASIVE HIGH-FREQUENCY OSCILLATORY VENTILATION

As NHFOV represents another "brick in the wall" of the noninvasive respiratory support,[85] we have been using it for extremely preterm infants with evolving BPD to reduce invasive ventilation as much as possible. These patients are comprised under the definition of chronic pulmonary insufficiency of prematurity (CPIP), recently issued by the International Neonatal Consortium, which spans as a *continuum* from the end of the first week of life to 36 weeks' postconceptional age.[86] During this period, in our experience, some extremely preterm infants show a worsening of their respiratory function around 14 days of postnatal age and this can be easily visualized with semiquantitative lung ultrasound.[87]

Our NHFOV protocol follows a physiology-based approach, with alveolar recruitment maneuvers alike in endotracheal HFOV[3] and close multimodal monitoring, based on semiquantitative lung ultrasound,[88] transcutaneous blood gas measurements, peripheral saturation, and perfusion index.[89] Lung ultrasound is used to assess lung aeration and guide the alveolar recruitment in real-time, as described in critically ill adults.[90] Nurses are specifically trained to care for these infants who are considered at high risk: nonpharmacological sedation is widely given, hydrocolloid gels are used, and interfaces are swapped to change the pressure points and reduce the risk of skin injuries. COMFORT[91] and/or EDIN[92] scores are serially used to evaluate

**Table 3**
**Suggested parameter boundaries of NHFOV for extremely preterm infants with developing BPD (ie, chronic pulmonary insufficiency of prematurity)**

|  | Minimum | Maximum |
|---|---|---|
| Mean airway pressure (cmH$_2$O) | 10 | 18 |
| Amplitude (cmH$_2$O) | 30 | 55 |
| Frequency (Hz) | 8 | 12 |

These suggestions have been modified from those previously proposed,[1] based on accumulated clinical experience. Inspiratory time should be fixed at 50%. Parameters may require serial adjustments according to patients' monitoring. Paw should be titrated on oxygenation and/or ultrasound assessed lung aeration. Oscillation amplitude and frequency should be titrated according to transcutaneous CO$_2$ levels. Interfaces might also impact the NHFOV performance and patients' comfort needing to be changed and requiring parameters adjustments.
*Data from* Steinhorn R, Davis JM, Göpel W, et al.Chronic Pulmonary Insufficiency of Prematurity: Developing Optimal Endpoints for Drug Development.J Pediatr 2017;191:15-21.e1.

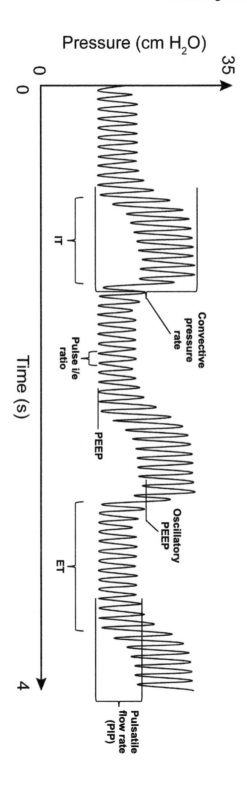

patients' comfort. Our proposal also integrates different respiratory techniques and respiratory support in personalized fashion.

As shown in **Fig. 3**, the respiratory management is initially based on gas exchange traits. Owing to its capability to washout $CO_2$, NHFOV is used as first intention in extremely preterm infants experiencing hypercapnic respiratory failure. Conventional noninvasive respiratory support is initially used in infants with hypoxemic respiratory failure and NHFOV is regarded as rescue intervention in case of failure; conventional noninvasive ventilation is synchronized, either using neurally adjusted ventilator assist[93] or flow/pressure-sensors to increase its efficacy and optimize patient-ventilator interaction (more details in the figure legend). Point-of-care echocardiography is also performed according to international guidelines[94]: when there are signs of pulmonary hypertension and this significantly influences hypoxia, nebulized iloprost is started,[95] using modern vibrating-mesh nebulizers inserted on the inspiratory limb.[96] Thus, intubation and inhaled nitric oxide are only considered as last resource. When the monitoring shows consistent signs of improvement, the respiratory support is de-escalated and can go back to CPAP, which is usually weaned between 33 and 34' weeks postconceptional age. An illustrative case of a patient managed with this respiratory strategy has been described in our previous review on NHFOV.[1]

This is obviously just a proposal for a respiratory management protocol integrating NHFOV for neonates with evolving BPD. **Table 3** shows suggested boundaries for NHFOV in our strategy. Other possible strategies exist and, for example, NHFOV has been proposed also as first-line technique in neonates with RDS.[1] However, the use of NHFOV later in life for neonates with CPIP seems to us more reasonable and well-grounded. It is actually difficult to design randomized controlled trials for these patients, but in absence of these studies, the respiratory care should be tailored to the patients' characteristics as much as possible.

## EXPERIENCES WITH NON-INVASIVE HIGH-FREQUENCY PERCUSSIVE VENTILATION

High-frequency percussive ventilation is a pneumatic, pressure-limited, time-cycled, high-frequency ventilation providing subphysiological volumes generated by Venturi's effect through a sliding device (called Phasitron®) powered by high-flow compressed gas inlet. Thus, the high-frequency volume delivery is provided as gas "percussions" into the airways. Between 90 and 650 percussions per minute can be provided. These percussions are superimposed to a pressure-limited, conventional respiratory support with physiologic rate and volume: conventional frequency, IT, and positive end-expiratory pressure need to be set as usual. An end-expiratory pressure for the gas percussions must be set, while the peak pressure is decided through the value of pulsatile gas flow (the greater the flow, the higher is the peak pressure reached all along the conventional respiratory cycle). A typical pressure waveform during this modality is shown in **Fig. 4**: conventional breaths are drawn with superimposed percussions. As the percussions are generated through the Venturi effect, the ventilator circuit has an

---

**Fig. 4.** *Illustrative time-pressure waveform during neonatal NHFPV.* Conventional breaths are drawn with superimposed percussions. Ventilatory parameters to be decided by clinicians are indicated in the figure. Pressure rates for conventional breaths and flow rates for the pulsatile percussions must also be set to decide the maximum delivered pressures. ET, conventional breath expiratory time; i/e ratio, inspiratory/expiratory ratio for the gas percussions; IT, conventional breath inspiratory time; PEEP, positive end-expiratory pressure; PIP, peak inspiratory pressure.

open expiratory limb and the patient may spontaneously breathe without any added WOB. Only one ventilator can provide this modality, which can be delivered both endotracheally or as NHFPV. This modality has the physical capability to improve secretions clearance and to move secretions toward upper airways. Because of these characteristics, this modality has been mainly used for aspiration-induced lung injuries and acute RDS, both in adults and children.[97]

In neonatology, NHFPV has been investigated in a randomized controlled trial to treat transient tachypnoea of the neonate (TTN): NHFPV was superior to CPAP in improving oxygenation and reducing the duration of TTN.[98] In a second work, the same authors showed that NHFPV is safe in terms of cerebral oxygenation in neonates with TTN or moderate RDS.[99] As TTN is due to a lack of lung fluid reabsorption, these results seem physiopathologically plausible as NHFPV may have facilitated the lung fluid clearance. Given its physical characteristics, NHFPV might also be theoretically useful in meconium aspiration, alike for other inhalation syndromes in older patients. Interestingly, endotracheal high-frequency percussive ventilation compared to HFOV resulted in a better oxygenation in the animal model of meconium aspiration,[100] while the two techniques resulted equivalent in a model of lung injury caused by depleting lung lavages.[101] Furthermore, 2 other animal studies compared the long-term effect of NHFPV and invasive ventilation in preterm lambs mimicking infants with CPIP (ie, evolving BPD). The animals ventilated with NHFPV for 3 weeks showed improved alveolarization with increased surfactant protein-B expression and better oxygenation.[102,103] These findings may be at least partially explained by an enhanced PTHrP-PPAR$\gamma$-mediated epithelial/mesenchymal signaling of alveolarization.[102] These results allow to hypothesize that long-term respiratory support with NHFPV, or a strategy integrating different noninvasive nonconventional respiratory supports, might be useful to improve long-term respiratory outcomes in preterm infants. In conclusion, the use of NHFPV for TTN seems interesting, but given its complexity, the mildness of TTN and the effectiveness of CPAP, it is unclear if NHFPV may be really useful.

## ACKNOWLEDGMENTS

Authors are grateful to Alejandro Alonso for the artwork and to Prof. Giorgio Conti, for the modeling of NHFOV.

## CONFLICTS OF INTEREST

Prof. D. De Luca has received research grants, technical assistance, and travel grants from Vyaire Inc. He also served as a lecturer for Getinge Inc. Dr R. Centorrino received a travel grant from Vyaire Inc. These companies produce ventilators that are able to provide noninvasive high-frequency ventilations but had no role in the conception, writing, or decision to submit this article.

## REFERENCES

1. De Luca D, Dell'Orto V. Non-invasive high-frequency oscillatory ventilation in neonates: review of physiology, biology and clinical data. Arch Dis Child Fetal Neonatal Ed 2016;101:F565–70.

2. Pillow JJ, Hillman N, Moss TJM, et al. Bubble continuous positive airway pressure enhances lung volume and gas exchange in preterm lambs. Am J Respir Crit Care Med 2007;176:63–9.

3. De Jaegere A, van Veenendaal MB, Michiels A, et al. Lung recruitment using oxygenation during open lung high-frequency ventilation in preterm infants. Am J Respir Crit Care Med 2006;174:639–45.

4. Centorrino R, Dell'Orto V, Gitto E, et al. Mechanics of nasal mask-delivered HFOV in neonates: a physiologic study. Pediatr Pulmonol 2019;54:1304–10.

5. Pillow JJ. High-frequency oscillatory ventilation: mechanisms of gas exchange and lung mechanics. Crit Care Med 2005;33(3 Suppl):S135–41.

6. Boynton BR, Hammond MD, Fredberg JJ, et al. Gas exchange in healthy rabbits during high-frequency oscillatory ventilation. J Appl Physiol 1989;66:1343–51.

7. De Luca D, Costa R, Visconti F, et al. Oscillation transmission and volume delivery during face mask-delivered HFOV in infants: bench and in vivo study: noninvasive HFOV Feasibility in Infants. Pediatr Pulmonol 2016;51:705–12.

8. De Luca D, Costa R, Spinazzola G, et al. Oscillation transmission and ventilation during face mask-delivered high frequency oscillatory ventilation in infants: a bench study with active lung simulator. Arch Dis Child 2012;97(Suppl 2): A117–8.

9. Gaertner VD, Waldmann AD, Davis PG, et al. Transmission of oscillatory volumes into the preterm lung during noninvasive high-frequency ventilation. Am J Respir Crit Care Med 2020. https://doi.org/10.1164/rccm.202007-2701OC.

10. Mukerji A, Finelli M, Belik J. Nasal high-frequency oscillation for lung carbon dioxide clearance in the newborn. Neonatology 2013;103:161–5.

11. Sivieri EM, Eichenwald EC, Rub DM, et al. An in-line high frequency flow interrupter applied to nasal CPAP: improved carbon dioxide clearance in a premature infant lung model. Pediatr Pulmonol 2019;54:1974–81.

12. van Genderingen HR, Versprille A, Leenhoven T, et al. Reduction of oscillatory pressure along the endotracheal tube is indicative for maximal respiratory compliance during high-frequency oscillatory ventilation: a mathematical model study. Pediatr Pulmonol 2001;31:458–63.

13. Prisk GK, Yamada K, Henderson AC, et al. Pulmonary perfusion in the prone and supine postures in the normal human lung. J Appl Physiol 2007;103:883–94.

14. Nyrén S, Radell P, Lindahl SGE, et al. Lung ventilation and perfusion in prone and supine postures with reference to anesthetized and mechanically ventilated healthy volunteers. Anesthesiology 2010;112:682–7.

15. Hadj-Ahmed MA, Samson N, Nadeau C, et al. Laryngeal muscle activity during nasal high-frequency oscillatory ventilation in nonsedated newborn lambs. Neonatology 2015;107:199–205.

16. Owen LS, Morley CJ, Dawson JA, et al. Effects of non-synchronised nasal intermittent positive pressure ventilation on spontaneous breathing in preterm infants. Arch Dis Child Fetal Neonatal Ed 2011;96:F422–8.

17. Kohl J, Freund U, Koller EA. Reflex apnea induced by high-frequency oscillatory ventilation in rabbits. Respir Physiol 1991;84:209–22.

18. England SJ, Onayemi A, Bryan AC. Neuromuscular blockade enhances phrenic nerve activity during high-frequency ventilation. J Appl Physiol 1984;56:31–4.

19. Kohl J, Scholz U, Glowicki K, et al. Discharge of pulmonary rapidly adapting stretch receptors during HFO ventilation. Respir Physiol 1992;90:115–24.

20. Kohl J, Koller EA. Blockade of pulmonary stretch receptors reinforces diaphragmatic activity during high-frequency oscillatory ventilation. Pflugers Arch 1988; 411:42–6.

21. Henke KG, Sullivan CE. Effects of high-frequency pressure waves applied to upper airway on respiration in central apnea. J Appl Physiol 1992;73:1141–5.

22. Di Fiore JM, Martin RJ, Gauda EB. Apnea of prematurity-Perfect storm. Respir Physiol Neurobiol 2013;189:213–22.

23. van Heerde M, van Genderingen H, Leenhoven T, et al. Imposed work of breathing during high-frequency oscillatory ventilation: a bench study. Crit Care 2006; 10:R23.

24. Bordessoule A, Piquilloud L, Lyazidi A, et al. Imposed work of breathing during high-frequency oscillatory ventilation in spontaneously breathing neonatal and pediatric models. Respir Care 2018;63:1085–93.

25. van der Hoeven M, Brouwer E, Blanco CE. Nasal high frequency ventilation in neonates with moderate respiratory insufficiency. Arch Dis Child Fetal Neonatal Ed 1998;79:F61–3.

26. De Paoli AG, Lau R, Davis PG, et al. Pharyngeal pressure in preterm infants receiving nasal continuous positive airway pressure. Arch Dis Child Fetal Neonatal Ed 2005;90:F79–81.

27. De Paoli AG, Davis PG, Faber B, et al. Devices and pressure sources for administration of nasal continuous positive airway pressure (NCPAP) in preterm neonates. Cochrane Database Syst Rev 2002;4:CD002977.

28. Jasani B, Ismail A, Rao S, et al. Effectiveness and safety of nasal mask versus binasal prongs for providing continuous positive airway pressure in preterm infants-A systematic review and meta-analysis. Pediatr Pulmonol 2018;53: 987–92.

29. De Luca D, Carnielli VP, Conti G, et al. Noninvasive high frequency oscillatory ventilation through nasal prongs: bench evaluation of efficacy and mechanics. Intensive Care Med 2010;36:2094–100.

30. De Luca D, Piastra M, Pietrini D, et al. Effect of amplitude and inspiratory time in a bench model of non-invasive HFOV through nasal prongs. Pediatr Pulmonol 2012;47:1012–8.

31. Green EA, Dawson JA, Davis PG, et al. Assessment of resistance of nasal continuous positive airway pressure interfaces. Arch Dis Child Fetal Neonatal Ed 2019;104:F535–9.

32. Gerdes JS, Sivieri EM, Abbasi S. Factors influencing delivered mean airway pressure during nasal CPAP with the RAM cannula: factors Affecting MAP during NCPAP with RAM Cannula. Pediatr Pulmonol 2016;51:60–9.

33. Sharma D, Murki S, Maram S, et al. Comparison of delivered distending pressures in the oropharynx in preterm infant on bubble CPAP and on three different nasal interfaces. Pediatr Pulmonol 2020;55:1631–9.

34. Mukerji A, Belik J. Neonatal nasal intermittent positive pressure ventilation efficacy and lung pressure transmission. J Perinatol 2015;35:716–9.

35. Aktas S, Unal S, Aksu M, et al. Nasal HFOV with binasal cannula appears effective and Feasible in ELBW newborns. J Trop Pediatr 2016;62:165–8.

36. Ventre KM, Arnold JH. High frequency oscillatory ventilation in acute respiratory failure. Paediatr Respir Rev 2004;5:323–32.

37. Klotz D, Schaefer C, Stavropoulou D, et al. Leakage in nasal high-frequency oscillatory ventilation improves carbon dioxide clearance-A bench study. Pediatr Pulmonol 2017;52:367–72.

38. Schäfer C, Schumann S, Fuchs H, et al. Carbon dioxide diffusion coefficient in noninvasive high-frequency oscillatory ventilation. Pediatr Pulmonol 2019;54: 759–64.

39. De Luca D, Servel AC, de Klerk A. Noninvasive ventilation interfaces and equipment in neonatology. In: Noninvasive mechanical ventilation and difficult

weaning in critical care. New York: Springer-Verlag International; 2015. p. 393–400. https://doi.org/10.1007/978-3-319-04259-6.

40. Tingay DG, John J, Harcourt ER, et al. Are all oscillators created equal? In vitro performance characteristics of Eight high-frequency oscillatory ventilators. Neonatology 2015;108:220–8.

41. Grazioli S, Karam O, Rimensberger PC. New generation neonatal high frequency ventilators: effect of oscillatory frequency and working principles on performance. Respir Care 2015;60:363–70.

42. Sivieri EM, Eichenwald E, Bakri SM, et al. Effect of high frequency oscillatory high flow nasal cannula on carbon dioxide clearance in a premature infant lung model: a bench study. Pediatr Pulmonol 2019;54:436–43.

43. Rub DM, Sivieri EM, Abbasi S, et al. Effect of high-frequency oscillation on pressure delivered by high flow nasal cannula in a premature infant lung model. Pediatr Pulmonol 2019;54:1860–5.

44. Yuan Y, Sun J, Wang B, et al. A noninvasive high frequency oscillation ventilator: achieved by utilizing a blower and a valve. Rev Sci Instrum 2016;87:025113.

45. Cools F, Offringa M, Askie LM. Elective high frequency oscillatory ventilation versus conventional ventilation for acute pulmonary dysfunction in preterm infants. Cochrane Database Syst Rev 2015;3:CD000104.

46. Restrepo RD, Walsh BK. Humidification during invasive and noninvasive mechanical ventilation:2012. Respir Care 2012;57:782–8.

47. Fischer HS, Bohlin K, Bührer C, et al. Nasal high-frequency oscillation ventilation in neonates: a survey in five European countries. Eur J Pediatr 2015;174:465–71.

48. Ullrich TL, Czernik C, Bührer C, et al. Nasal high-frequency oscillatory ventilation impairs heated humidification: a neonatal bench study. Pediatr Pulmonol 2017;52:1455–60.

49. Reddy PI, Al-Jumaily AM, Bold GT. Dynamic surface tension of natural surfactant extract under superimposed oscillations. J Biomech 2011;44:156–63.

50. Autilio C, Echaide M, De Luca D, et al. Controlled hypothermia may improve surfactant function in asphyxiated neonates with or without meconium aspiration syndrome. PLoS One 2018;13:e0192295.

51. De Luca D, Lopez-Rodriguez E, Minucci A, et al. Clinical and biological role of secretory phospholipase A2 in acute respiratory distress syndrome infants. Crit Care 2013;17:R163.

52. Simma B, Luz G, Trawöger R, et al. Comparison of different modes of high-frequency ventilation in surfactant-deficient rabbits. Pediatr Pulmonol 1996;22:263–70.

53. Kerr CL, Veldhuizen RAW, Lewis JF. Effects of high-frequency oscillation on Endogenous surfactant in an acute lung injury model. Am J Respir Crit Care Med 2001;164:237–42.

54. Aspros AJ, Coto CG, Lewis JF, et al. High-frequency oscillation and surfactant treatment in an acid aspiration model. Can J Physiol Pharmacol 2010;88:14–20.

55. Ali YAH, Seshia MM, Ali E, et al. Noninvasive high-frequency oscillatory ventilation: a Retrospective chart review. Am J Perinatol 2020. https://doi.org/10.1055/s-0040-1718738.

56. Thatrimontrichai A, Sirianansopa K, Janjindamai W, et al. Comparison of endotracheal Reintubation between nasal high-frequency oscillation and continuous positive airway pressure in neonates. Am J Perinatol 2020;37:409–14.

57. Łoniewska B, Tousty J, Michalczyk B, et al. The use of noninvasive ventilation with high frequency in newborns—a single-center experience. Am J Perinatol 2019;36:1362–7.

58. Binmanee A, el Helou S, Shivananda S, et al. Use of high noninvasive respiratory support pressures in preterm neonates: a single-center experience. J Matern Fetal Neonatal Med 2017;30:2838–43.

59. Tridente A, De Martino L, De Luca D. Porcine vs bovine surfactant therapy for preterm neonates with RDS: systematic review with biological plausibility and pragmatic meta-analysis of respiratory outcomes. Respir Res 2019;20:28.

60. Inthout J, Ioannidis JP, Borm GF. The Hartung-Knapp-Sidik-Jonkman method for random effects meta-analysis is straightforward and considerably outperforms the standard DerSimonian-Laird method. BMC Med Res Methodol 2014;14:25.

61. Wallace BC, Schmid CH, Lau J, et al. Meta-Analyst: software for meta-analysis of binary, continuous and diagnostic data. BMC Med Res Methodol 2009;9:80.

62. Bottino R, Pontiggia F, Ricci C, et al. Nasal high-frequency oscillatory ventilation and CO2 removal: a randomized controlled crossover trial. Pediatr Pulmonol 2018;53:1245–51.

63. Chen L, Wang L, Ma J, et al. Nasal high-frequency oscillatory ventilation in preterm infants with respiratory distress syndrome and ARDS after extubation. Chest 2019;155:740–8.

64. Iranpour R, Armanian AM, Abedi AR, et al. Nasal high-frequency oscillatory ventilation (nHFOV) versus nasal continuous positive airway pressure (NCPAP) as an initial therapy for respiratory distress syndrome (RDS) in preterm and near-term infants. BMJ Paediatr Open 2019;3:e000443.

65. Klotz D, Schneider H, Schumann S, et al. Non-invasive high-frequency oscillatory ventilation in preterm infants: a randomised controlled cross-over trial. Arch Dis Child Fetal Neonatal Ed 2018;103:F1–5.

66. Lou W, Zhang W. Noninvasive high-frequency oscillatory ventilation versus nasal continuous positive airway pressure in premature infants with respiratory distress syndrome after weaning: a randomized controlled trial. Guangdong Med J 2017;38:2037–40.

67. Lou W, Zhang W, Yuan L, et al. Comparative study of noninvasive high-frequency oscillatory ventilation and bilevel positive airway pressure ventilation for preterm infants with respiratory distress syndrome. Chin Gen Pract 2018;21:1983–8.

68. Malakian A, Bashirnezhadkhabaz S, Aramesh MR, et al. Noninvasive high-frequency oscillatory ventilation versus nasal continuous positive airway pressure in preterm infants with respiratory distress syndrome: a randomized controlled trial. J Mater Fetal Neonatal Med 2020;33:2601–7.

69. Mukerji A, Sarmiento K, Lee B, et al. Non-invasive high-frequency ventilation versus bi-phasic continuous positive airway pressure (BP-CPAP) following CPAP failure in infants<1250g: a pilot randomized controlled trial. J Perinatol 2017;37:49–53.

70. Rüegger CM, Lorenz L, Kamlin COF, et al. The effect of noninvasive high-frequency oscillatory ventilation on desaturations and bradycardia in very preterm infants: a randomized crossover trial. J Pediatr 2018;201:269–73.e2.

71. Zhu XW, Zhao JN, Tang SF, et al. Noninvasive high-frequency oscillatory ventilation versus nasal continuous positive airway pressure in preterm infants with

moderate-severe respiratory distress syndrome: a preliminary report. Pediatr Pulmonol 2017;52:1038–42.

72. Zhu X, Yan J, Ran Q, et al. Noninvasive high-frequency oscillatory ventilation versus for respiratory distress syndrome in preterm infants: a preliminary report. Chin J Neonatol 2017;32:291–4.

73. Buzzella B, Claure N, D'Ugard C, et al. A randomized controlled trial of two nasal continuous positive airway pressure levels after extubation in preterm infants. J Pediatr 2014;164:46–51.

74. Lemyre B, Davis PG, De Paoli AG, et al. Nasal intermittent positive pressure ventilation (NIPPV) versus nasal continuous positive airway pressure (NCPAP) for preterm neonates after extubation. Cochrane Database Syst Rev 2017;2: CD003212.

75. Subramaniam P, Ho JJ, Davis PG. Prophylactic nasal continuous positive airway pressure for preventing morbidity and mortality in very preterm infants. Cochrane Database Syst Rev 2016;6:CD001243.

76. Raschetti R, Yousef N, Vigo G, et al. Echography-guided surfactant therapy to improve Timeliness of surfactant replacement:A Quality improvement project. J Pediatr 2019;212:137–43.

77. Bahadue FL, Soll R. Early versus delayed selective surfactant treatment for neonatal respiratory distress syndrome. Cochrane Database Syst Rev 2012; 11:CD001456.

78. Esquinas A, Mantellini E, Benitez Leon F, et al. International study use of high frequency chest wall oscillation (HFCWO) in secretion management in the mechanically ventilated patient. Proceedings of ESICM 2010 Congress. Barcelona (Spain): Intensive Care Med 2010;36(S2):105(n.0080). https://doi.org/10.1007/s00134-010-1999-x.

79. Zhu XW, Shi Y, Shi LP, et al, NHFOV Study Group. Non-invasive high-frequency oscillatory ventilation versus nasal continuous positive airway pressure in preterm infants with respiratory distress syndrome: study protocol for a multicenter prospective randomized controlled trial. Trials 2018;19:319.

80. Shi Y, De Luca D. NASal OscillatioN post-Extubation (NASONE) study group.-Continuous positive airway pressure (CPAP) vs noninvasive positive pressure ventilation (NIPPV) vs noninvasive high frequency oscillation ventilation (NHFOV) as post-extubation support in preterm neonates: protocol for an assessor-blinded, multicenter, randomized controlled trial. BMC Pediatr 2019; 19:256.

81. De Luca D. Noninvasive high-frequency ventilation and the errors from the past: designing simple trials neglecting complex respiratory physiology. J Perinatol 2017;37:1065–6.

82. Fischer HS, Rimensberger PC. Early noninvasive high-frequency oscillatory ventilation in the primary treatment of respiratory distress syndrome. Pediatr Pulmonol 2018;53:126–7.

83. Thorpe KE, Zwarenstein M, Oxman AD, et al. A pragmatic–explanatory continuum indicator summary (PRECIS): a tool to help trial designers. J Clin Epidemiol 2009;62:464–75.

84. De Luca D, Harrison D, Peters MJ. 'Lumping or splitting' in paediatric acute respiratory distress syndrome (PARDS). Intensive Care Med 2018;44:1548–50.

85. Gregoretti C, Cortegiani A, Maggiore SM. Noninvasive oscillatory ventilation (NHFOV) in infants: another brick in the wall of paediatric noninvasive ventilation? Pediatr Pulmonol 2016;51:663–4.

86. Steinhorn R, Davis JM, Göpel W, et al. Chronic pulmonary insufficiency of prematurity: developing optimal Endpoints for Drug development. J Pediatr 2017; 191:15–21.e1.

87. Loi B, Vigo G, Baraldi E, et al. LUSTRE study group.Lung ultrasound to monitor extremely preterm infants and predict BPD: multicenter longitudinal cohort study. Am J Respir Crit Care Med 2020. https://doi.org/10.1164/rccm.202008-3131OC.

88. Brat R, Yousef N, Klifa R, et al. Lung ultrasonography score to evaluate oxygenation and surfactant need in neonates treated with continuous positive airway pressure. JAMA Pediatr 2015;169:e151797.

89. De Luca D, Romain O, Yousef N, et al. Monitorages physiopathologiques en réanimation néonatale. J Pediatrie Puericulture 2015;28:276–300.

90. Tusman G, Acosta CM, Costantini M. Ultrasonography for the assessment of lung recruitment maneuvers. Crit Ultrasound J 2016;8:8.

91. van Dijk M, Peters JWB, van Deventer P, et al. The COMFORT Behavior Scale: a tool for assessing pain and sedation in infants. Am J Nurs 2005;105:33–6.

92. Debillon T, Zupan V, Ravault N, et al. Development and initial validation of the EDIN scale, a new tool for assessing prolonged pain in preterm infants. Arch Dis Child Fetal Neonatal Ed 2001;85:F36–41.

93. Piastra M, De Luca D, Costa R, et al. Neurally adjusted ventilatory assist vs pressure support ventilation in infants recovering from severe acute respiratory distress syndrome: nested study. J Crit Care 2014;29:312.e1–5.

94. Singh Y, Tissot C, Fraga MV, et al. International evidence-based guidelines on point of care ultrasound (POCUS) for critically ill neonates and children issued by the POCUS working group of the European society of paediatric and neonatal Intensive care (ESPNIC). Crit Care 2020;24(1):65.

95. Piastra M, De Luca D, De Carolis MP, et al. Nebulized iloprost and noninvasive respiratory support for impending hypoxaemic respiratory failure in formerly preterm infants: a case series. Pediatr Pulmonol 2012;47:757–62.

96. DiBlasi RM, Crotwell DN, Shen S, et al. Iloprost Drug delivery during infant conventional and high-frequency oscillatory ventilation. Pulm Circ 2016;6:63–9.

97. Allan PF, Osborn EC, Chung KK, et al. High-frequency percussive ventilation Revisited. J Burn Care Res 2010;31:510–20.

98. Dumas De La Roque E, Bertrand C, Tandonnet O, et al. Nasal high frequency percussive ventilation versus nasal continuous positive airway pressure in transient tachypnea of the newborn: a pilot randomized controlled trial (NCT00556738): NHFPV versus NCPAP in Transient Tachypnea of the Newborn. Pediatr Pulmonol 2011;46:218–23.

99. Renesme L, Dumas de la Roque E, Germain C, et al. Nasal high-frequency percussive ventilation vs nasal continuous positive airway pressure in newborn infants respiratory distress: a cross over clinical trial. Pediatr Pulmonol 2020;55: 2617–23.

100. Renesme L, Elleau C, Nolent P, et al. Effect of high-frequency oscillation and percussion versus conventional ventilation in a piglet model of meconium aspiration: Hi-Frequency vs. Conventional Ventilation in MAS. Pediatr Pulmonol 2013;48:257–64.

101. Messier SE, DiGeronimo RJ, Gillette RK. Comparison of the Sensormedics® 3100A and Bronchotron® transporter in a neonatal piglet ARDS model. Pediatr Pulmonol 2009;44:693–700.

102. Rehan VK, Fong J, Lee R, et al. Mechanism of reduced lung injury by high-frequency nasal ventilation in a preterm lamb model of neonatal chronic lung disease. Pediatr Res 2011;70:462–6.
103. Null DM, Alvord J, Leavitt W, et al. High-frequency nasal ventilation for 21d maintains gas exchange with lower respiratory pressures and promotes alveolarization in preterm lambs. Pediatr Res 2014;75:507–16.

# Neurally Adjusted Ventilatory Assist in Newborns

Jennifer Beck, PhD[a,b,c,*], Christer Sinderby, PhD[a,c,d]

## KEYWORDS

- Diaphragm electrical activity • Mechanical ventilation
- Neurally adjusted ventilatory assist (NAVA) • Non-invasive (NIV) NAVA
- Patient-ventilator interaction • Control of breathing

## KEY POINTS

- The Edi is a physiological signal representative of central respiratory output and is normally present in spontaneously breathing subjects. The Edi allows monitoring of neural breathing activity, central apnea, diaphragm function, and patient-ventilator interaction.
- NAVA is a neurally-controlled mode of mechanical ventilation. It uses the Edi waveform to control both the timing and the level of assist provided.
- Because it is pneumatically-independent, leaks do not affect patient-ventilator synchrony during non-invasive NAVA, allowing truly synchronized non-invasive positive pressure ventilation.
- Besides improved patient-ventilator interaction, ventilating with NAVA shows less oxygen and sedation requirements, less apnea, lower peak pressures, improved comfort, and possibly improved extubation success.

## INTRODUCTION

Neurally adjusted ventilatory assist (NAVA) is a mode available on the Servo-i, Servo-n, and Servo-u ventilator systems (Maquet Critical Care AB, Solna, Sweden) and is intended for patients who are spontaneously breathing. Different from other modes of partial ventilatory assist, NAVA uses the electrical activity of the diaphragm (Edi) to control triggering, cycling, and the magnitude of assist[1] (**Fig. 1**). Based on this concept of neurally controlled mechanical ventilation, NAVA can be considered to

[a] Department of Critical Care, St. Michael's Hospital, 30 Bond Street, Toronto, Ontario M5B1W8, Canada; [b] Department of Pediatrics, University of Toronto, Toronto, Canada; [c] Institute for Biomedical Engineering and Science Technology (iBEST) at Ryerson University and St-Michael's Hospital, Toronto, Canada; [d] Department of Medicine and Interdepartmental Division of Critical Care Medicine, University of Toronto, Toronto, Canada
* Corresponding author.
*E-mail address:* jennifer.beck@rogers.com
Twitter: @jennava (J.B.)

Clin Perinatol 48 (2021) 783–811
https://doi.org/10.1016/j.clp.2021.07.007
0095-5108/21/© 2021 Elsevier Inc. All rights reserved.

have two purposes: (1) to provide synchronized and proportional support, both with invasive and noninvasive interfaces, and (2) to monitoring the neural respiratory drive and neural breathing pattern, via the Edi waveform, with or without NAVA.

The purpose of this review is to provide a summary of the physiologic concepts related to Edi and NAVA, with an update on publications since 2016. The authors have previously published a detailed review up to 2016.[2]

## UNIQUE FEATURES ABOUT INFANTS RELEVANT TO NEURALLY ADJUSTED VENTILATORY ASSIST

In all patient groups and all ages, conventional modes of mechanical ventilation are limited in their ability to provide synchronized assist and to accurately monitor respiratory drive. In infants, the challenges are increased because of small tidal volumes and high respiratory rates. In addition, owing to the frequent use of uncuffed endotracheal tubes, leaks are present and affect ventilator control—in turn interfering with patient-ventilator synchrony. The same applies to noninvasive positive pressure ventilation (the preferred mode in neonates), where leaky interfaces are often used. Leaks also cause unreliable monitoring of pneumatic forms of respiratory rate.[3] Furthermore, ventilator adjustment must take into account that infants have strong vagal reflexes[4] and demonstrate central apnea[5] and periodic breathing, with a high variability in breathing pattern.[5] Surfactant deficiency and a compliant chest wall means that the lung has a tendency to derecruit. All these characteristic features suggest a "one-size-fits-all" approach to mechanical ventilation is not suitable for neonates.

## PHYSIOLOGY OF SPONTANEOUS BREATHING

Breathing is a complex process and is often oversimplified as being only involved with movement of air in and out of the lungs. Breathing is actually *neurally* controlled by specialized centers in the brainstem, a part of the central nervous system sitting at the base of the brain. The brainstem automatically regulates the rate and depth of breathing depending on the respiratory demand and the feedback it receives from various organs in the body.

As shown in **Fig. 2**, the chain of events for spontaneous breathing can be simplified to involve the following course, beginning with a signal transmitted from the respiratory centers via the phrenic nerves, which then electrically activates the diaphragm. After

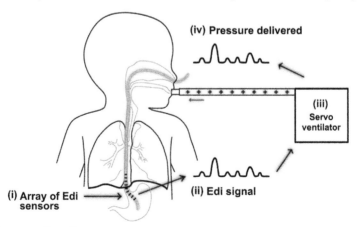

**(iv) Pressure delivered**

**(iii) Servo ventilator**

**(ii) Edi signal**

**(i) Array of Edi sensors**

**Fig. 1.** Concept of NAVA.

electrical activation, the diaphragm contracts, resulting in chest wall and lung expansion, lowered thoracic pressures, and generation of flow and volume at the airway. Depending on the respiratory rate and the amount of dead space, alveolar ventilation and gas exchange will occur. This in turn affects the acid-base balance of the arterial and venous blood. The following factors provide strong feedback to the respiratory centers on a continuous basis: lung distension, arterial CO2, and the diaphragmatic force generated. During noninvasive NAVA (NIV-NAVA), the upper airways also influence neural breathing pattern.

## ELECTRICAL ACTIVITY OF THE DIAPHRAGM

NAVA depends on the Edi. The Edi is the closest signal we can record noninvasively to represent the neural respiratory drive originating in the respiratory centers. The Edi is measured with an array of small sensors on the patient's feeding tube ("Edi catheter") at the level of the gastroesophageal junction.[6] Sensors in this position pick up the Edi signals from the crural diaphragm, which forms a scarf-like structure around the lower esophageal sphincter. Appropriate positioning of the sensors is required to obtain a reliable Edi signal. An array of sensors is used to automatically track (and account for) the displacement of the diaphragm during spontaneous breathing.[7–10]

## EDI = ELECTROMYOGRAM OF THE DIAPHRAGM

The Edi signal is in fact an electromyogram (EMG signal). During spontaneous breathing, activation of the diaphragm motor units is achieved by increases in the discharge frequency of phrenic motoneurons and/or by recruitment of new motoneurons. When several motor units are recruited, and/or their firing rate increases, this yields spatial and/or temporal summation of the motor unit action potentials, resulting in an interference pattern EMG signal. This chaotic, "noisy" *EMG signal* can be processed with filters and signal-conditioning techniques to yield a waveform.[6,7] Note that for the waveform to be reliable for physiologic interpretation, the EMG signal of the diaphragm must be recorded with electrodes of an appropriate configuration, maintenance of electrode positioning and orientation with respect to the muscle fiber

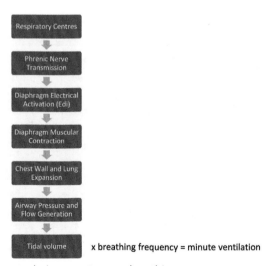

**Fig. 2.** Chain of events during spontaneous breathing.

direction, and avoidance of signal disturbances, such as motion artifacts (for review of signal processing, see the study by Sinderby and Beck[6]).

## METHOD FOR EDI CATHETER POSITIONING

NAVA requires an accurate Edi signal with the catheter positioned appropriately. Initially, an insertion distance is calculated and predicted based on an "NEX" measurement (nose-ear-xyphoid) with an adjustment factor added. Depending on the ventilator platform, this is performed manually by the clinician according to the manufacturer's formula (Servo-i) or is implemented automatically based on inputting the NEX measurement (Servo-U, Servo-N). Note: The manufacturers' recommendations for catheter insertion and verification should be followed.

After initial insertion, verification of the position is achieved by a dedicated window on the Servo ventilators (**Fig. 3**). The positioning window displays 4 of the leads (top to bottom representing proximal to distal) as well as the processed Edi waveform. Verification is accomplished by observing an expected retrocardiac ECG pattern (P waves large on top leads, getting smaller and/or disappearing toward the bottom). Finally, position can be verified by confirmation of the highlighting of the leads closest to the diaphragm, as determined by the cross-correlation method. Ideally, the two middle leads should be highlighted during inspiration.[6] An inspiratory occlusion (end-expiratory "hold") can be performed if connected to the ventilator and no leaks are present. If the catheter is in the correct position, the Edi waveform should increase as the airway pressure becomes more negative during the occlusion.

## CHARACTERISTICS OF THE EDI WAVEFORM

As mentioned previously, the Edi waveform contains the afferent information about lung stretch and deflation, arterial blood gases ($CO_2$ and $O_2$), and diaphragm force but is also influenced as well by sedation and voluntary inputs (in adults). The Edi waveform has a characteristic cyclic pattern, with varying peak and minimum values that can be used to interpret neural inspiratory effort ("phasic Edi") and postinspiratory

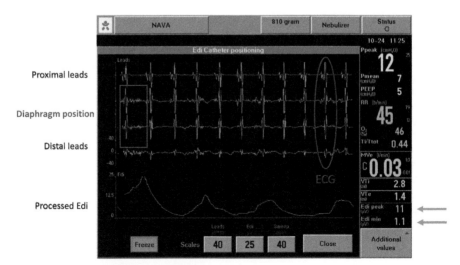

**Fig. 3.** Edi catheter positioning window.

activity ("tonic Edi"), respectively.[5] **Fig. 3** demonstrates an Edi-waveform, with corresponding display of Edi peak and Edi min.

Monitoring the Edi waveform also provides accurate information on respiratory metrics (neural breathing frequency), as well central apnea (flat Edi waveform).[5] Because of the critical information it provides, the Edi waveform can be considered a respiratory vital sign, and monitoring its activity is often referred to as the "neural breathing pattern" to incorporate all the information (phasic, tonic, neural respiratory rate, and central apnea). The Edi in combination with various other pneumatic variables (such as occlusion pressure or tidal volume) can provide indices of respiratory muscle function.[6]

When the Edi waveform is increasing (upwards deflection), it is representative of neural inspiration, and when the waveform is decreasing back to baseline, it is representative of neural expiration. Both the highest value reached (Edi peak) and the lowest value (Edi min) can be quantified for each breath and given a numerical value. Because of the distinct pattern of the waveform increasing and decreasing, the Edi peak is often referred to as the *phasic Edi*, whereas the baseline (between breaths) is often referred to as the *tonic Edi*. The Edi waveform can be characterized by its timing to calculate *neural respiratory rate*, that is, the number of neural respiratory efforts per minute. The *neural inspiratory time* can be defined as the period from onset of the increase in Edi to the peak Edi. The *neural expiratory time* can be defined as the time from the peak Edi to the onset of the next increase in Edi. The Edi waveform in infants can be characterized by larger variability in timing and Edi peak, with a distinct amount of changes in the Edi min value. The Edi waveform in adults is generally less variable with low and stable Edi min.

When a subject's ability to generate a tidal breath decreases because of disease, this may increase the demand for increased diaphragm activity and, hence, will demand a higher Edi peak. For example, if a resistive load is applied, the immediate result, if neural respiratory output does not change, is a reduction in tidal volume. After several breaths, the respiratory centers will compensate for this reduced tidal volume by increasing respiratory drive, and hence, the Edi peak, restoring tidal volume.

Other factors which can result in increased Edi peak include worsening of respiratory status, dynamic hyperinflation (shortened diaphragm), reduced ventilator assist, reduced sedation, increased demand for ventilation such as exercise, and increased dead space. The opposite holds true: Edi decreases within a given subject with respiratory improvement, increased sedation, increasing levels of ventilator assist, and reducing arterial CO2.

The Edi waveform can sometimes remain elevated at the end of neural expiration (does not return to baseline), sometimes referred to as "tonic Edi". The tonic Edi can be quantified by the Edi min value. If end-expiratory lung volume is lowered artificially (eg, removing positive end-expiratory pressure [PEEP] while intubated), the deflation-sensitive receptors in the lungs will send signals to the respiratory centers about the derecruitment of alveoli and will stimulate activation of the diaphragm. Even during neural expiration, the diaphragm remains active so as not to "relax" in between respiratory cycles. The maintained diaphragm activity prevents further derecruitment or even recruits lung units to restore end-expiratory lung volume. In intubated infants, application of PEEP helps the baby to keep the lung recruited and minimizes the tonic Edi.[11]

## REPORTED EDI VALUES

Over the last 12 years, 15 studies in 525 babies have reported Edi peak and min values (**Table 1**) during various conditions. These studies show mean Edi peaks in the range of 6 to 13 uV and Edi min in the range of 1 to 4 uV.

**Table 1**
**Reported Edi peak and Edi min values for infants under different conditions**

|  |  | Edi Peak (uV) |  | Edi Min (uV) |  |
|---|---|---|---|---|---|
| Invasive NAVA | Mean | 8.7 | n = 282 | 2.5 | n = 149 |
|  | SD | 1.9 |  | 1 |  |
|  | min | 6 |  | 1 |  |
|  | max | 11.4 |  | 4 |  |
| NIV-NAVA | Mean | 9.1 | n = 258 | 2.5 | n = 211 |
|  | SD | 2.1 |  | 1 |  |
|  | min | 6 |  | 4 |  |
|  | max | 12.6 |  | 0.8 |  |
| No assist | Mean | 11.3 | n = 72 | 2.8 | n = 72 |
|  | SD | 1.2 |  | 0.2 |  |
|  | min | 10.2 |  | 2.5 |  |
|  | max | 13 |  | 3 |  |

## PATIENT-VENTILATOR INTERACTION

The term *patient-ventilator interaction* refers to the ability of a mechanical ventilator to deliver respiratory assist in tandem with patient effort. Patient-ventilator interaction (PVI) can be monitored by comparing the Edi waveform to the ventilator pressure waveform during any mode of ventilation. Overlay of the Edi and pressure curves permits immediate visualization of how well (or poor) the ventilator is synchronized with the patient.[6]

Briefly, there are several types of poor PVIs and can be classified as "asynchrony" or "dys-synchrony."[12]

### Asynchrony

1. Wasted efforts: Also known as *ineffective triggering*, this is the type of asynchrony where the patient makes a neural inspiratory effort (upward increase in Edi waveform) and the ventilator fails to trigger.
2. Auto-triggering: Auto-triggering represents a situation where assist is initiated in the absence of inspiratory effort, indicating that the ventilator delivered a breath that was not triggered by the patient.

### Dys-synchrony

1. Delayed triggering: Delayed triggering represents a situation where the ventilator starts delivering a breath later than the onset of neural inspiratory effort.
2. Delayed cycling-off: When a patient has finished their neural inspiratory effort and switches to neural exhalation, if the ventilator does not cycle into expiration, it will continue to deliver air.
3. Premature cycling-off: This type of dys-synchrony is characterized by the ventilator terminating the breath before the end of neural inspiration.
4. Double triggering: Double triggering is characterized as two ventilator-delivered breaths for one neural inspiratory effort.

## APNEA

Apnea is defined as a period where there is a cessation of inspiratory flow. *Central apneas* are characterized by no respiratory drive (a flat Edi waveform) and can be characterized by their duration.[5] *Obstructive apneas* occur when respiratory drive is present (Edi curve shows its characteristic phasic inspiration and expiration), but owing to an airway obstruction, no flow can occur. A *tonic apnea* can occur when the Edi curve is continuously elevated (at a high Edi min value), without any phasic deflection in the curve, and no flow is generated.[5]

## NEURALLY ADJUSTED VENTILATORY ASSIST AND NON-INVASIVE-NEURALLY ADJUSTED VENTILATORY ASSIST

In the NAVA mode, the Edi waveform is used as the controller signal (see **Fig. 1**; **Fig. 4**). Ventilator breaths are triggered when a threshold change in Edi is reached (typically 0.5 uV). The ventilator then delivers assist (pressure) in proportion to the Edi throughout neural inspiration. After the Edi has reached its peak, and decreases by 30%, the ventilator cycles-off the breath. Therefore, during the NAVA mode, the ventilator delivers assist in a synchronized and proportional fashion (see **Fig. 4**).

## NEURALLY ADJUSTED VENTILATORY ASSIST SETTINGS

The assist level during NAVA must be set by the clinician (so-called "NAVA level"), which determines the proportionality between the Edi and the ventilator pressure during the inspiratory phase. PEEP and $Fio_2$ are fixed and set by the clinician. While some recommend targeting Edi values, other methods to adjust the NAVA level include simply targeting peak inspiratory pressures (PIPs). If the target is 10 cm H2O, and the phasic Edi is 12 (peak 14, min 2), then the NAVA level would be set to 0.8 cm H2O/ uV (10 cm H2o/12 uV). With respect to safety, upper pressure limits are in place,

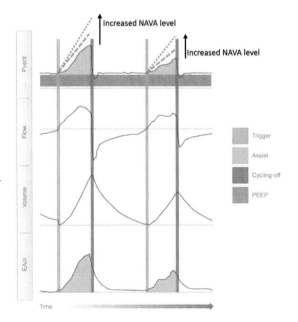

Settings in NAVA:

- NAVA level (cm H2O/uV)
- PEEP (cm H2O)
- FIO2
- Apnea time
- Backup ventilation
- Upper pressure limits

**Fig. 4.** How NAVA works. Demonstrates schematically the Edi and ventilator pressure waveforms during NAVA and demonstrates the synchrony between the patient (Edi) and the ventilator (Pvent), both in terms of timing and proportionality.

and backup ventilation is provided in the case of no Edi (central apnea or accidental catheter removal). NAVA is available for both invasive and noninvasive ventilation.

The reader is referred to two recent reviews for more details on clinical settings during NAVA.[13,14] In addition, there are educational videos by Stein & Firestone published in video format:

http://www.NeonatologyToday.net/NAVA/4.html for Edi catheter insertion;
http://www.NeonatologyToday.net/NAVA/2.html for NAVA level;
http://www.NeonatologyToday.net/NAVA/5.html for Peak pressure limit;
http://www.NeonatologyToday.net/AVA/3.html for Edi trigger.

NAVA is a mode of ventilation that is neurally integrated with the inherent lung protective reflexes. During spontaneous breathing, as lung inflation progresses, stretch receptors in the lungs will eventually sense an adequate inspired volume and "switch off" inspiration. For a patient on NAVA, where the neural inspiration also controls the assist delivery, the ventilator breath will be cycled-off when neural exhalation begins. Several studies have demonstrated that patients spontaneously choose lower PIP and tidal volume during NAVA than conventional ventilation (targeted by the clinician).[2] (This of course does not include those studies where peak pressures were intentionally matched as part of the protocol.)

## INDICATIONS AND CONTRAINDICATIONS

NAVA requires the presence of Edi; hence, if the Edi is absent (for whatever reason), NAVA cannot be applied. As the Edi measurement relies on placement of orogastric/nasogastric tube, NAVA cannot be used if such catheter placement is contraindicated.

The authors have previously published a detailed review up to 2016.[2] **Table 2** (refer to the study by Mally and colleagues[12] and others[15–31,32–61]) and the summaries provided in this article complement those studies up until the present date.

## STUDIES ABOUT CATHETER POSITIONING

In children, 7 studies have evaluated the Edi catheter, the Edi signal quality, and its ease of insertion and positioning.[62–64] A review on the safety of catheter insertion was provided in the study by Beck and colleagues,[2] with only one study commenting on this since that publication,[54] and they report no adverse effects of catheter positioning.

## STUDIES ABOUT CHARACTERIZATION OF NEURAL BREATHING PATTERN

A flat Edi waveform indicates central apnea (provided there is a functional Edi catheter which can be confirmed by presence of ECG waveforms on the positioning window). Several studies have used Edi waveform to quantify central apnea during different feeding methods,[61] caffeine administration,[65] ventilation modes,[12] or body position.[37,66] Refer to the study by Beck and colleagues[2] for a complete review. Garcia-Munoz Rodrigo and colleagues[51] recently reported a method (similar to that of Beck and colleagues[5]) to characterize neural breathing pattern during NIV-NAVA in 19 preterms (average gestational age, GA, at birth = 27 weeks) and also found a high variability in Edi with a fair amount of tonic activity.

## STUDIES ABOUT EDI VALUES OVER THE COURSE OF INTENSIVE CARE UNIT STAY

Most of the studies on Edi values over the course of intensive care unit (ICU) stay have been described in the review by Beck and colleagues[2] and include that of Stein and colleagues.[62,67,68]

**Table 2**
Studies published about Edi or NAVA since 2016

| First Author, Ref, Year | NAVA or Edi Study? | n | Type of Study | Type of Patient | Intervention | Outcome |
|---|---|---|---|---|---|---|
| Soukka et al,[15] 2021 | NAVA | 60 pre-NAVA vs 76 post-NAVA | Retrospective | Extremely low birth weight (ELBW) | NAVA vs Conventional | Equivalent brain growth No other outcome differences |
| Bordessoule et al,[16] 2021 | Edi | 20 | Crossover physiologic | Preterm (<2500 g) | IF, nCPAP Servo-i, MedinCNO | No difference in Edi between CPAP devices |
| Meinen et al,[17] 2021 | NAVA, NIV-NAVA | 10 | Physiologic | Postsurgical CDH | Postsurgical application NAVA and NIV-NAVA | Lower pk P, lower $Fio_2$, lower mean airway P with NAVA |
| Protain,[25] 2021 | NAVA | 56 | Retrospective, ventilator data review | Preterm (862 g at study) | None, observational | Mean pk pressure was 16 in both NAVA and NIV-NAVA Mean VT was $3.5 \pm 2.7$ mL/kg |
| Latremouille,[18] 2020 | Edi | 13 | Prospective Observational | Preterm (median bw 800 g) | Edi variables during ET CPAP | Edi peak and Edi variability increased during ET CPAP, and variability was higher for failure group |
| Goel,[19] 2020 | NAVA | 23 (from 2 trials) | Meta-analysis | Preterm (<1000 g or <28 wk) | NIV-NAVA vs NIPPV, NCPAP, HFNC | Unable to conclude due to limited data/strict study inclusion |
| McKinney,[20] 2020 | NAVA | 112 | Multi-centre experience | Preterm, BPD | NAVA | NAVA was successful in 67% of patients |
| Rong,[21] 2020 | NAVA | 30 | Retrospective, matched cohort | Preterm (<1500 g) with evolving or established BPD | NAVA after 2 wk CV vs staying on CV | No difference in duration of resp support Sedation was less in NAVA group |

*(continued on next page)*

**Table 2**
*(continued)*

| First Author, Ref, Year | NAVA or Edi Study? | n | Type of Study | Type of Patient | Intervention | Outcome |
|---|---|---|---|---|---|---|
| Rochon,[22] 2020 | NAVA | 20 | New technology (NeuroPAP) | Preterm (<28 wk) | NeuroPAP | Feasible and safe |
| Firestone,[23] 2020 | NAVA | 17 | Retrospective | Preterm (26 wk GA) | NIV-NAVA, level 0 vs NCPAP | Apnea less with NIV-NAVA set to 0 cm H20/uV |
| Hunt,[24] 2020 | NAVA | 18 | Prospective, crossover | Preterm (<32 wk) evolving or established BPD | NAVA vs PAV vs CV | Improved oxygenation with NAVA and PAV Better A-a gradient with NAVA |
| Makker et al,[26] 2020 | NAVA | 30 | Pilot, prospective, randomized | Preterm ready for extubation (<1000 g) | Extubation to NIV-NAVA or NIPPV | Initial extubation success was higher with NIV-NAVA, lower pIPs with Niv-NAVA |
| Iwasaki,[28] 2020 | Edi | 14 | Retrospective, observational | Preterm (<28 wk, almost all BPD) | Postnatal follow-up of Edi | Frequency and amplitude of Edi sighs increased with age. Edi pk and Edi min did not change with age. |
| Matlock,[29] 2020 | NAVA | 15 | Prospective, crossover, physiologic | Preterm (mean study weight 1472 g) | NIV-NAVA vs NIV | No difference in phase angle determined by RIP Improved synchrony with NAVA |
| Gupta,[27] 2019 | Edi and NAVA | 10 | Pilot, prospective, crossover | Preterm (mean 29 wk) | 12 h each of CPAP/NIPPV vs NIV-NAVA | Edi pk was lower in NIV-NAVA |
| Nam et al,[30] 2019 | NAVA | 14 | Prospective physiologic | Preterm (<32 wk) | NAVA titration | Inc NAVA levels showed down-regulation of Edi Improved comfort (dec PIPP score) with inc NAVA |

| Study | Modality | n | Study type | Population | Comparison | Findings |
|---|---|---|---|---|---|---|
| Morgan et al,[31] 2019 | NAVA | 14 | Prospective, physiologic | Preterm (26 wk) | Change apnea time in NAVA (2s vs 5s) | Shorter apnea times led to more time in backup, but less clinically significant events |
| Tabacaru et al,[32] 2019 | NAVA | 108 | Retrospective, nursing records | Preterm (<1500 g) | NIV-NAVA vs NIPPV | Less clinical apnea with NIV-NAVA |
| Kallio et al,[33] 2019 | NAVA | 40 | Pilot RCT | Preterm (<28 wk, 5 h old) | NIV-NAVA vs nCPAP | Equal oxygen requirements No diff in intubation rate |
| Yagui et al,[34] 2019 | NAVA | 213 | Randomized, unblinded | Preterm (<1500 g, <48 h NIV) | NIV-NAVA vs nCPAP | Similar intubation, use of surfactant, BPD, death Longer duration of ventilation in CPAP |
| Yagui et al,[35] 2019 | NAVA | 49 | Retrospective chart review | Preterm (bw <1000 g) at risk of failing NIV | NIV-NAVA vs nCPAP | Reintubation rate until 72 h after extubation was less for NAVA |
| Lee et al,[36] 2019 | NAVA | 32 | Retrospective | Preterm (<30 wk, inv vent for at least 24 h) | Extubation to NIV-NAVA or nCPAP | Extubation failure lower in NIV-NAVA |
| Baudin et al,[37] 2019 | Edi | 14 | Prospective | Bronchiolitis (1 month old) | Prone vs supine during CPAP | Edi peak and NME were improved in prone position |
| Miyahara et al,[38] 2019 | NAVA | 15 | Prospective | Preterm (GA 30 wk, bw 1300 g) | Safety of NIV-NAVA after INSURE surfactant | No adverse events or complications, two infants failed INSURE |
| Cosi et al,[39] 2019 | NAVA | 34 | Prospective | Preterm (GA 33 wk, bw 2 kg) | Ventilation and wean with NAVA (compared to prior SIMV period) | All infants weaned and extubated with NAVA. Significant improvements in $Fio_2$, SF ratio and PIPs, less sedation, lower pain |

(continued on next page)

**Table 2**
*(continued)*

| First Author, Ref, Year | NAVA or Edi Study? | n | Type of Study | Type of Patient | Intervention | Outcome |
|---|---|---|---|---|---|---|
| Baudin et al,[40] 2019 | NAVA | 11 | Prospective | Bronchiolitis, PICU (35 days old) | nasal CPAP vs NIV-NAVA | Lower WOB on NIV-NAVA |
| Bonacina et al,[41] 2019 | NAVA | 14 | Randomized crossover trial | Intubated, hypoxemic, postcardiac surgery | PSV vs NAVA vs PSV-sigh | NAVA had higher coefficient of variability in respiratory parameters and decrease in asynchrony index |
| Baez Hernandez et al,[42] 2019 | NAVA | 81 | Retrospective review | Postcardiac surgery PICU | SIMV transition to NAVA | Lower PIP, lower sedation requirements |
| Oda et al,[43] 2019 | Edi | 8 | Prospective | Preterms (31 wk) | Edi measured during high-flow nasal therapy and no support | Edi peak decreased from no support to High-flow nasal cannula (HFNC) 6 lpm. Number of sighs were lower during HFNC. |
| Singh et al,[44] 2018 | Edi | 21 | Prospective, physiologic | Preterm (28 wk, 1200 g) | Edi before and after extubation | Edi peak before extubation did not predict extubation success vs failure |
| Longhini et al,[45] 2018 | NAVA | 10 | Prospective, physiologic | Term babies (3 kg) | NAVA before and after extubation | Similar patient-ventilator interaction despite leak during NIV-NAVA |
| Crulli et al,[46] 2018 | NAVA | 28 | Retrospective | Postcardiac surgery (3 mo old PICU) | NAVA after surgery | PIP and MAP decreased progressively during NAVA |
| Sood et al,[47] 2018 | NAVA | 75 | Nonrandomized, pilot trial comparing NAVA prospectively to historical controls | Postcardiac surgery PICU | Invasive NAVA vs CV until extubation | Extubation success was higher in NAVA than conventional. Less sedation and days on MV in NAVA |

| Study | Measure | N | Study design | Population | Comparison | Findings |
|---|---|---|---|---|---|---|
| Oda et al,[48] 2018 | Edi | 8 | Prospective, observational | Preterms at birth (30 wk, 1377 g) | Edi measured during first few hours after birth | Edi changes described over time after birth (19 uV to 11 uV at 1 h of life) |
| Oda et al,[49] 2018 | NAVA | 35 | Retrospective, NAVA compared to historical controls | Preterm (<27 wk) | NAVA vs CV | Less sedation requirements with NAVA |
| Mally et al,[12] 2018 | NAVA | 23 | Prospective, crossover | Preterm (27 wk) | Invasive NAVA vs SIMV | Asynchrony reduced during NAVA. Central apneas (defined as absent Edi>5 s) reduced during NAVA |
| Yonehara et al,[50] 2018 | NAVA | 15 | Retrospective | Preterm (<30 wk GA) | NAVA vs NIPPV | Treatment failure (change to the other mode or reintubation <7 d after extubation) with NAVA was less than NIPPV |
| Garcia-Muñoz Rodrigo et al,[51] 2018 | Edi | | Prospective, methodological | Preterm | Edi monitoring | Characterization of neural breathing pattern |
| Brenne et al,[52] 2018 | Edi | 21 | Prospective | Preterm | CPAP vs HFNC | Similar Edi pk (8.8 HFNC vs 7.8 uV CPAP) |
| Rosterman,[53] 2018 | NAVA | 24 | Randomized, crossover trial | Preterm (1293 g) | NAVA vs SIMV + PS | Respiratory severity score and resting energy expenditure were not different. PIP and WOB were less with NAVA |
| Gibu,[54] 2017 | NAVA | 11 | Prospective pilot | Preterm (840–2200 g) | NIV-NAVA vs NIV | No catheter complications NIV-NAVA reduced PIP, $FiO_2$, frequency and length of desaturations, caretaker and infant movement |

(continued on next page)

**Table 2**
*(continued)*

| First Author, Ref, Year | NAVA or Edi Study? | n | Type of Study | Type of Patient | Intervention | Outcome |
|---|---|---|---|---|---|---|
| Shetty et al,[55] 2017 | NAVA | 9 | Randomized, cross-over trail | Preterm with evolving BPD | NAVA vs AC | Lower OI, PIP, $Fio_2$, MAP with NAVA |
| Lee et al,[56] 2017 | NAVA | 14 | Retrospective | Tracheotomized >6 mo ventilation | NAVA (min 2 mo) vs triggered modes | NAVA could reduce cyanotic episodes and the need for sedatives and dexamethasone |
| Mortamet et al,[57] 2017 | Edi | 52 | Prospective | PICU | Asynchrony during CV | No association between asynchrony and ventilator-free days at day 28 |
| Iyer et al,[58] 2017 | Edi | 25 | Prospective | Preterm | Neural breathing pattern before and after extubation | Extubation failure was associated with a smaller increase in Edi after extubation |
| Colaizy et al,[59] 2017 | NAVA | 24 | Retrospective | Preterm <1500 g | NIV-NAVA after extubation | NIV-NAVA was successful in 83% of the subjects with 5 mm Hg reduction in $Pco_2$ |
| Jung et al,[60] 2016 | NAVA | 29 | Retrospective | BPD (25 wk GA, 680 g bw; 1 month old at study.) | Transition from SIMV to NAVA | Peak and mean airway pressures, blood gases, WOB improved with NAVA |
| Ng et al,[61] 2016 | Edi | 10 | Prospective | Preterm <1250 g | Edi during continuous or bolus feeds | Neural breathing pattern is not affected by enteral feeding or the feeding method. |

Earlier studies can be found in the review by Beck and colleagues.[2]

More recently, Oda and colleagues[48] described the Edi values within the first few hours after birth. In 8 preterms (median GA 30 weeks, median body weight [bw] 1377 g), they measured the Edi peak and Edi min every minute with a Servo-N while on CPAP (EasyFlow CPAP interface) directly in the delivery room. The Edi catheter was inserted at 3 to 6 minutes of life. Edi peak was high at birth (19 uV) and down to 11 uV after 1 hour. For Edi min, birth values were 4.5 uV down to 1.6 after 85 minutes. Neural respiratory rate increased from 24 to 39 breaths per minute after 1 hour of Edi monitoring.

In a retrospective, observational study, Iwasaki and colleagues[28] evaluated Edi peak and Edi min in 14 preterm infants born at less than 28 weeks GA. Median values were collected every week over the course of the Neonatal intensive care unit (NICU) stay. The authors also reported the Edi peak values obtained during sighs (defined as Edi peak twice as large as the median Edi peak for the same period) as well as the frequency of neural sighs per hour. Measurements were taken weekly. From 26 to 35 postmenstrual weeks, the median values of Edi-sigh significantly increased as postmenstrual weeks increased ($P<.001$). In contrast, there were no significant changes in the median Edi peak and median Edi minimum at each postmenstrual week. In the whole observation period, the median Edi peak value was 6.9 $\mu V$ (6.6-7.0), and the median Edi minimum value was 1.5 $\mu V$ (1.4-1.6).

## STUDIES ABOUT EDI MONITORING FOR DETECTING PATIENT-VENTILATOR ASYNCHRONY

The studies that describe the use of Edi to detect asynchrony are mainly discussed in the "Studies about NAVA and Synchrony" section which have shown the use of the Edi waveform to detect and quantify asynchrony during conventional modes compared with NAVA.

Only one study has specifically used the Edi during conventional ventilation to analyze PVI. Mortamet and colleagues[57] performed a prospective study describing the characteristics of patient-ventilator asynchrony and the impact it has on ventilator-free days at day 28. During conventional ventilation, data were acquired and analyzed in 52 children (Children of median age 6 months were included in the study.). Eighteen patients had too low respiratory drive to evaluate PVI. In the remaining patients, the NeuroSync index revealed high asynchrony (45%, range 32%–70%), with a total proportion of time spent in asynchrony of 27% (22%–39%). The authors did not find any association between the level of asynchrony and ventilator-free days, or any of the other secondary outcomes.

## STUDIES ABOUT EDI MONITORING AND BODY POSITION

Since 2016, only one study has evaluated how the Edi is affected by body position.

Baudin and colleagues[37] studied 14 infants (33 days old) with bronchiolitis breathing on CPAP during the supine position (SP) and prone position (PP) for 1 hour each. From the SP, the investigators found significant reductions in Edi peak (22 uV to 16 uV), delta Edi, and Edi min (3.5 uV to 2.1 uV) in the PP, which was accompanied by a higher neuro-muscular efficiency (NME), evaluated by the ratio of transdiaphragmatic pressure per Edi.

## STUDIES ABOUT EDI MONITORING FOR PREDICTING EXTUBATION READINESS

Several new studies since 2016 have used Edi monitoring to predict extubation success.

Iyer and colleagues[58] described the Edi (timings and amplitudes) before and after extubation in a group of 25 preterm infants. Intubated infants were considered for extubation when they were breathing spontaneously on minimal support and not sedated. Before extubation, 30 minutes of Edi was recorded, followed by the extubation period and 2 hours after extubation. The infants were then divided into 2 groups: success (n = 19 events) versus failure (n = 10 events, defined as >2 significant apneic events/h or pH<7.2 or $Pco_2$>65 mm Hg or desaturations despite increasing $Fio_2$). Edi values before extubation were similar for the 2 groups. Edi peak increased in both groups immediately after extubation but was different for the 2 groups: success from 10 to 20 uV, and less of an increase in the failure group 9 to 16 uV.

To answer the question about whether Edi monitoring can predict extubation success, Singh and colleagues[44] studied 21 preterm infants (mean GA 28 weeks, bw 1208 g) with respiratory distress syndrome (RDS) breathing on volume guarantee 24 hours before extubation. Fourteen infants were successfully extubated, and 7 failed. The investigators found no differences in preextubation Edi to predict extubation success. The authors suggest that ventilator settings (specifically the VG mode) before extubation may have affected their results.

One case report[69] demonstrates in a 6-month-old tracheotomized child how the Edi and Neuro-ventilatory efficiency (NVE) were valuable for deciding extubation readiness.

Mortamet and colleagues[70] used Edi monitoring in a child with tetraplegia to demonstrate lack of Edi activity which could return by lowering the amount of assist and subsequent weaning with NAVA until successful extubation.

Not exactly an extubation-readiness study, but the one by Oda and colleagues[43] compared Edi during 6 L/min HFNC to no respiratory support in eight preterm infants (corrected GA 31 weeks) and found a reduction in Edi peak from 7 to 6 uV, as well as a reduction in the number of neural sighs.

In a prospective crossover pilot study of 10 premature infants requiring NIV,[29] the babies were randomized to initially receive either CPAP/biphasic or NIV-NAVA and then switched over. Continuous Edi signals were recorded for 24 hours, with 12 hours on each mode. Edi peak on the biphasic/CPAP group (15.6 ± 7 mcV) was significantly higher ($P$<.005) than that on the NIV-NAVA group (10.8 ± 3.3 mcV). The Edi min values were 3.23 ± 1.1 mcV and 3.07 ± 0.5 mcV on CPAP/biphasic and NIV-NAVA ($P$ = .69), respectively.

Latremouille and colleagues[18] studied ELBW infants during a 5-minute endotracheal intubation CPAP trial (ETT-CPAP for extubation readiness) and found that Edi peak increased from about 7 uV (on mechanical ventilation) to 11 UV, but more importantly, the variability of the Edi parameters increased, and more for the extubation failure group.

The reader is referred to the review of Ducharme-Crevier and colleagues[71] for an excellent review on the importance of Edi monitoring in newborns.

## STUDIES ABOUT NEURALLY ADJUSTED VENTILATORY ASSIST AND SYNCHRONY

Since 2009 — when a prototype version of NAVA was introduced to neonates[72] — there have been 17 published studies in 253 neonatal and pediatric patients that evaluated the synchrony during NAVA compared to a conventional mode (for both invasive and noninvasive ventilation) (**Table 3**). Similar to the studies conducted in adults, all pediatric and neonatal studies showed that PVI is improved during both invasive NAVA and noninvasive NAVA. Although the methodology for calculating the asynchrony index varies between studies, a review of these articles shows on average

**Table 3**
Studies pertaining to patient-ventilator interaction during NAVA

| Author, Reference, Year | Number of Patients | Type | INV or NIV? | Asynchrony Index NAVA (%) | Asynchrony Index NAVA (%) | Asynchrony Index Conventional (%) |
|---|---|---|---|---|---|---|
| Beck et al,[72] 2009 | 7 | NICU | INV and NIV | | | |
| Bengtsson and Edberg,[73] 2010 | 21 | PICU | INV | | | |
| Breatnach et al,[74] 2010 | 16 | PICUNICU | INV | | | |
| Clement et al,[75] 2011 | 23 | PICU | INV | | | |
| Bordessoule et al,[76] 2012 | 10 | PICU mixed | INV | 11 | | 25 |
| De la Oliva et al,[77] 2012 | 12 | PICU mixed | INV | 2 | | 12 |
| Alander et al,[78] 2012 | 18 | PICUNICU | INV | 9 | | 28 |
| Vignaux et al,[79] 2013 | 19 | PICU | INV | 4 | | 29 |
| Vignaux et al,[80] 2013 | 6 | PICU | NIV | 2 | | 40 |
| Longhini et al,[3] 2015 | 12 | NICU | INV | 0 | | 22 |
| Baudin et al,[81] 2015 | 11 | PICU | NIV | 3 | | 38 |
| Ducharme-Crevier et al,[82] 2015 | 13 | PICU | NIV | 8 | | 27 |
| Lee et al,[83] 2015 | 15 | NICU | NIV | 20 | | 73 |
| Chidini et al,[84] 2016 | 18 | PICU | NIV | 0 | | 16 |
| Mally et al,[12] 2018 | 23 | NICU | INV | 18 | | 47 |
| Bonacina et al,[41] 2019 | 14 | PICU | INV | 2 | | 22 |
| Matlock et al,[29] 2020 | 15 | NICU | NIV | 21 | | 78 |
| | 253 | | Mean | 8 | | 35 |

35% asynchrony during conventional modes, compared to 8% during NAVA[2] and updated in **Table 3**.

The review by Beck and colleagues[2] summarizes the studies pertaining to PVI during NAVA versus conventional modes and will not be repeated here. Updates since 2016 are presented in the following sections and in **Table 3**.

The NeuroSync index was evaluated in 23 preterms (median GA 27 weeks, bw 780 g) by Mally and colleagues,[12] in a crossover study comparing conventional ventilation and NAVA. The automated and standardized "NeuroSync index" was lower (improved synchrony) during NAVA (18%) than during SIMV (47%). Optimizing SIMV guided by the Edi (increased inspiratory time) did not improve the NeuroSync index (46%).

In 14 hypoxemic intubated children (after cardiac surgery), Bonacina and colleagues[41] performed a randomized crossover trial to compare PSV (1 hour) to NAVA (1 hour) and PSV SIGH (1 hour). The PSV SIGH mode is a PSV mode adapted to deliver one pressure-control breath per minute (30 cm $H_2O$ for 3 seconds). $Pao_2/Fio_2$ and oxygenation index improved in PSV SIGH compared with PSV ($P<.05$) but not in NAVA compared with PSV. PSV SIGH showed increased tidal volumes and lower respiratory rate than PSV ($P<.05$), as well as a significant improvement in compliance with respiratory system indexed to bw when compared with both PSV and NAVA ($P<.01$). No changes in mean airway pressure were registered among steps. Inspiratory time prolonged for both PSV SIGH and NAVA compared with that for PSV ($P<.05$). NAVA showed higher coefficient of variability in respiratory parameters and a significative decrease in asynchrony index than both PSV and PSV SIGH ($P<.01$).

Chidini and colleagues[84] studied 18 children with acute respiratory failure needing noninvasive ventilation upon admission to the PICU. The children were randomized to undergo 60 minutes of NIV-PSV or NIV-NAVA first and then undergo the other mode for an additional 60 minutes. A full-face mask was used throughout both modes. The results were measured as an asynchrony index, which was significantly lower during the NIV-NAVA mode. All types of asynchrony measures were lower with NIV-NAVA, but they found the majority of asynchrony was mainly due to ineffective efforts.

Matlock and colleagues[29] used respiratory inductance plethysmography and Edi to quantify the work of breathing (WOB) and neural effort, respectively, in 15 preterm infants (mean GA at birth 27 weeks, mean birth weight 908 g). They compared NIV-NAVA to conventional noninvasive positive pressure ventilation (NIPPV) and found improved synchrony with NIV-NAVA compared with NIPPV (NeuroSync 21% in NAVA compared to 78% in NIPPV).

Although not a comparison to a conventional mode, Longhini and colleagues[45] studied term infants (n = 10, mean weight 2.9 kg) breathing on NAVA before and after extubation, without changing the NAVA level. No differences in synchrony were observed between invasive and noninvasive NAVA, despite the leak.

Two recent meta-analyses have reported that NAVA improves PVI compared with conventional modes[2] in infants; Pettenuzzo and colleagues[85] reported the same in adults.

## STUDIES DESCRIBING DOWNREGULATION OF EDI, PROTECTION OF PEAK INSPIRATORY PRESSURES, AND VT DURING NEURALLY ADJUSTED VENTILATORY ASSIST

Beck and colleagues[2] reviewed all studies up until 2016 showing that NAVA limits PIP or VT by downregulation of Edi. The following sections discuss a summary of the studies since 2016.

## Titration Studies

Evidence of patient downregulation of the Edi to avoid lung overdistension was shown by LoVerde and colleagues,[86] who performed a NAVA-level titration and NIV-NAVA titrations in 15 premature neonates (mean birthweight was 950 g). Beginning at a low NAVA level (0.5 cm H2O), the NAVA level was systematically increased by 0.5 cm H2O every 3 minutes until a NAVA level of 4 cm H2O. Similar to adults, in the early portion of the titration, the peak inspiratory pressure increased with increasing NAVA levels, until a certain NAVA level where the pressure did not further increase, due to downregulation of Edi. The authors termed this NAVA level, the "breakpoint" (visually determined plateau in PIP), similar to the "adequate NAVA level" (described by Brander and colleagues[87]). Tidal volume also followed the same pattern as PIP, with an initial increase until a point where the subject no longer allowed Vt to increase and downregulates Edi to avoid overdistension.

Despite the negative title of the publication "Neural feedback is insufficient in preterm infants during neurally adjusted ventilatory assist", Nam and colleagues[30] demonstrate in an original way the physiologic responses to increasing *and decreasing* NAVA levels (previous studies only showed responses to increasing NAVA levels). They studied 14 preterm infants (<32 weeks) during increasing and decreasing NAVA levels (from 0.5 to 4.0 cm H2O/μV with an interval of 0.5 cm H2O/μV) applied for 10 minutes each. Comfort increased with increasing NAVA levels, as demonstrated using the PIPP scale. Edi was downregulated with increasing NAVA levels (showing in-fact that neural feedback is sufficient) and reached a plateau; PIP and VT showed a "breakpoint"; however, because the authors continued to increase to supra-high NAVA levels, the variables became "erratic" with increased variability. A letter to the Editor was published[88] pointing out that NAVA levels greater than 2.5 cm H2O/μV are probably excessive for preterm infants. The 8-fold increase in ventilatory assistance would not likely be applied during conventional modes and should also be avoided in NAVA (personal observations).

## Crossover and Randomized Studies

The findings of lower PIPs (compared to SIMV or PC) have been confirmed in randomized crossover designs (eg, the mean GA was 26 weeks in a study by Rosterman and colleagues[54]) or during a switch from CV to NAVA.[49] In extremely low-birth-weight preterms with established or evolving BPD (n = 9), Shetty and clleagues[55] found the peak and mean airway pressure to be lower during NAVA than during ACV. In the same patient population (evolving BPD: mean weight 680 g, GA 25 weeks), over 24 hours of NAVA versus SIMV, Jung and colleagues[60] reported that PIPs dropped from 20 cm H2O down to 14 cm H2O (n = 29). Kallio and colleagues,[89] in a larger trial (n = 60), demonstrated the same lower PIP in preterm infants (GA 31 weeks, bw ~1700 g). During NIV-NAVA, Gibu and colleagues[53] reported a 13% reduction in PIP compared to conventional NIV in preterms (n = 11).

Five studies (Zhu and colleagues[90]; Liet and colleagues[91]; Crulli and colleagues[46]; Baez-Hernandez and colleagues[42]; Meinen and colleagues[17]) have demonstrated in patients after cardiac surgery that PIP was lower with NAVA than conventional modes (n = 136 for all 5 studies).

In a retrospective review of 56 preterm infants on NAVA and NIV-NAVA, Protain[18] performed a distributional assessment of peak pressure and tidal volume, overall and per NAVA level. Over 1 million breaths were evaluated, and they found mean peak pressure was 16.4 ± 6.4 in the NAVA group and 15.8 ± 6.4 in the NIV-NAVA group (t test, $P<.001$). Mean tidal volume was 3.5 ± 2.7 mL/kg.

## STUDIES ABOUT NEURALLY ADJUSTED VENTILATORY ASSIST PERFORMANCE DURING SEDATION

One group demonstrated in the PICU that propofol administration reduces the Edi by 32%, in as short a time as 310 seconds[92] which affected the tidal volumes and pressures during NAVA, requiring backup ventilation. There are no new publications on this topic since 2016.

## STUDIES ABOUT NEURALLY ADJUSTED VENTILATORY ASSIST AND SEDATION REQUIREMENTS

In infants, 5 studies have demonstrated less sedation requirements.[3,39,42,49,56,93] One study demonstrated equivalence in opiate use,[89] NAVA versus PSV.

In a non-randomized study, Sood[47] evaluated 75 patients (n=35 NAVA vs, n= 40 in conventional ventilation) who were post-op from congenital heart disease. They evaluated initial extubation success utilizing neurally adjusted ventilatory assist (NAVA) compared with pressure-regulated volume controlled, synchronized intermittent mandatory ventilation with pressure support (SIMV-PRVC + PS) for ventilatory weaning in patients who required prolonged mechanical ventilation (MV). Also, total days on MV, inotropes, sedation, analgesia, and pediatric intensive care unit (PICU) length of stay (LOS) between both groups were compared. Ninety-seven percent of the NAVA group were successfully extubated on the initial attempt, while it was 80% in the SIMV-PRVC + PS group ($P = .0317$). Patients placed on NAVA were eight times more likely to have successful initial extubation (odds ratio [OR]: 8.50, 95% confidence interval [CI]: 1.01, 71.82). The NAVA group demonstrated a shorter median duration on MV (9.0 vs 11.0 days, $P = .032$), PICU LOS (9.0 vs 13.5 days, $P<.0001$), and shorter median duration of days on dopamine (8.0 vs 11.0 days, $P = .0022$), milrinone (9.0 vs 12.0 days, $P = .0002$), midazolam (8.0 vs 12.0 days, $P<.0001$), and fentanyl (9.0 vs 12.5 days, $P<.0001$) than the SIMV-PRVC + PS group. Hernandez and colleagues (2019) later confirmed the findings of less sedation in postcardiac surgery babies (n = 81), when transitioned from SIMV to NAVA.[42]

Rong and colleagues[21] did a retrospective study in babies weighing less than 1500 g with established or evolving BPD and matched with historical controls (total n = 30). The primary outcome was to compare the total duration of respiratory support between the NAVA group and the control group. The secondary outcomes were comparisons of duration of invasive and noninvasive support, oxygen therapy, length of stay, severity of BPD, weight gain, and sedation need between the groups. There were no significant differences between NAVA group and control group in the primary and most of the secondary outcomes (all $P>.05$). There was a decrease in the need of sedation ($P = .012$) after switching to NAVA.

## STUDIES ABOUT NEURALLY ADJUSTED VENTILATORY ASSIST AND GAS EXCHANGE

In children, 19 studies in 528 patients have reported gas exchange during NAVA compared to a conventional mode. Three studies reported an improvement in $Paco_2$.[60,90] Seven studies reported less oxygenation requirements or improved oxygenation.[25,39,55,90,94–96] The remainder of the studies demonstrated equivalence.[33]

## STUDIES ABOUT NEURALLY ADJUSTED VENTILATORY ASSIST AND COMFORT

Three studies in infants reported results about comfort, two of which showed improved comfort with NAVA[77,94] in the pediatric population. Nam and colleagues[30] reported increased comfort with increasing NAVA levels in preterms.

## STUDIES ABOUT NEURALLY ADJUSTED VENTILATORY ASSIST AND APNEA

In 14 intubated preterm infants (mean GA 32 weeks, study weight 1741 g), Longhini and colleagues[3] compared 12 hours of ventilation with PRVC to 12 hours of ventilation with NAVA, in a crossover trial. Central apnea, defined as no Edi for more than 15 seconds, was reduced with NAVA.

### Since 2016

In a crossover study comparing conventional ventilation (SIMV + PSV) and NAVA, Mally and colleagues[12] demonstrated in 23 preterms (median GA 27 weeks, bw 780 g) that central apneas (defined as absent Edi>5 sec) were significantly reduced during NAVA.

Gibu and colleagues,[53] in the second of a two-part study, perfomed a randomized crossover study to compare NIV-NAVA and NIMV (n = 8). After 2 hours each of NIV-NAVA and NIPPV, the authors found reductions in the number of and length of desaturations (by 42% and 32%, respectively).

Yonehara and colleagues[50] in a retrospective study in 15 preterm infants born before 30-week gestation compared postextubation NIV-NAVA to NIPPV. Their primary outcome was treatment failure, defined as a change to the other mode or reintubation less than 7 days after extubation. Treatment failure occurred in 40% of the NIV-NAVA group and in 47% of the NIPPV group (no significant difference), with apnea (defined as >20s or accompanying bradycardia and desaturation) being the main cause of treatment failure and not different between the groups. This is in contrast to a retrospective study by Tabacaru and colleagues[32] who found less clinically relevant apneas during NAVA.

Morgan and colleagues[31] evaluated various apnea times in neonates on NIV-NAVA (n = 15, 26 weeks gestational age, birthweight 893 g). When compared to the 5-second apnea time, the 2-second apnea time showed increased switches into backup ventilation from 0.5 switches/min to 2.5 switches/min ($P<.001$), and time spent in backup ventilation increased from 2%/min to 9%/min ($P<.001$). Clinically important events decreased from 7 per hour to 2 per hour ($P<.001$).

## STUDIES ABOUT WEANING, EXTUBATION SUCCESS, DURATION OF VENTILATION, AND LENGTH OF STAY WITH NEURALLY ADJUSTED VENTILATORY ASSIST
### Since 2016

In very-low-birthweight preterm infants, Colaizy and colleagues[59] in a retrospective study of 24 newly extubated preterm neonates (mean birth weight 814 g) describe the capacity of NIV NAVA to provide efficient ventilator support, as defined by a reduction in $P_{CO_2}$, with an increase in NAVA levels. In 83% of the babies, an increase in the NAVA level demonstrated a decrease in $P_{CO_2}$ ("responders" n = 20); while in the remaining patients, the increase in assist had no impact ("non-responders" n = 4).

Yonehara and colleagues,[50] as discussed previously, compared postextubation support with either NIV-NAVA or NIPPV. Their primary outcome was treatment failure, defined as a change to the other mode or reintubation less than 7 days after extubation. Treatment failure occurred in 40% of the NIV-NAVA group and in 47% of the NIPPV group (no significant difference).

Kallio and colleagues,[89] in a randomized study, did not find any difference in the duration of invasive ventilation in a group of 60 infants (bw 1700 g, GA 32 weeks) when NAVA was compared to conventional ventilation.

Sood and colleagues,[47] in postcardiac surgery PICU (n = 35 NAVA, vs n = 40 SIMV historical controls) studied weaning: 97% of the NAVA group was successfully extubated on the initial attempt, while 80% were in the SIMV-PRVC + PS group (P = .0317). Patients placed on NAVA were eight times more likely to have successful initial extubation (OR: 8.50, 95% CI: 1.01, 71.82). The NAVA group demonstrated a shorter median duration on MV (9.0 vs 11.0 days, P = .032) and PICU LOS (9.0 vs 13.5 days, P<.0001).

Two studies by Yagui and colleagues,[34,35] one retrospective and one RCT demonstrated in ELBW preterms that when compared to CPAP, NIV-NAVA decreased reintubation rate until 72 hours after extubation (retrospective study) and shorter duration of ventilation (RCT).

Lee and colleagues[36] compared NIV-NAVA and NCPAP for the postextubation stabilization of preterm infants in a retrospective study (n = 14 NCPAP, 16 NIV-NAVA). Extubation failure within 72 hours after extubation was observed in 6.3% of the NIV-NAVA group and 37.5% of the NCPAP group (P = .041).

Makker and colleagues[26] randomized 30 mechanically ventilated preterm infants at the time of initial elective extubation to NI-NAVA or NIPPV. Primary study outcome was initial extubation success. Rates of continuous extubation for 120 hours were 92% in the NI-NAVA group and 69% in the NIPPV group (12/13 vs 9/13, respectively, P = .14). Infants extubated to NI-NAVA remained extubated longer (median 18 vs 4 days, P = .02) and experienced lower peak inspiratory pressures (PIP) than infants managed with NIPPV throughout the first 3 days after extubation. Survival analysis through 14 days after extubation showed a sustained difference in the primary study outcome until 12 days after extubation.

## NON-INVASIVELY-NEURALLY ADJUSTED VENTILATORY ASSIST AND SAFETY OF SURFACTANT ADMINISTRATION

In a prospective study in 15 preterm infants (median GA 30 wks, bw 1301 g), Miyahara and colleagues[38] evaluated the efficacy and safety of noninvasive neurally adjusted ventilatory assist used after INtubation-SURfactant-Extubation in preterm infants with respiratory distress syndrome. NIV-NAVA was applied immediately after temporary intubation and surfactant administration, using Medin prongs or face mask, depending on patient size. Two of the infants failed the INSURE protocol while on NIV-NAVA (13%) (similar to the failure rate of flow-synchronized NIPPV, and less than the nCPAP failure rate). No infants experienced adverse events or complications, such as pneumothorax, PDA, severe IVH, abdominal distension, or Edi catheter-related events.

Two systematic reviews in neonates found no significant differences between NAVA and other forms of triggered ventilation[97] or NIV-NAVA versus other modes of NIV.[19]

## SUMMARY

- NAVA uses the Edi to control the timing and level of assist.
- Both NIV- and INV-NAVA improves synchrony.
- Both NIV- and INV-NAVA show less apnea.
- NAVA provides improved comfort.

- Both NIV- and INV-NAVA show lower PIP.
- Both NIV- and INV-NAVA have lower oxygen and sedation requirements.

## CLINICS CARE POINTS

- Monitoring the diaphragm electrical activity (Edi) is important to interpret neural respiratory effort, and how the baby is interacting with the ventilator.
- The Edi waveform is obtained from miniaturized sensors embedded in the baby's nasogastric feeding tube and imposes no additional level of invasiveness.
- NAVA uses the Edi waveform to control the timing and magnitude of pressure delivery.
- Use of Neurally Adjusted Ventilatory Assist synchronizes the ventilator to the baby, and can be delivered invasively or non-invasively.

## DISCLOSURE

Drs J. Beck and C. Sinderby have made inventions related to neural control of mechanical ventilation that are patented. The patents are assigned to the academic institution(s) where inventions were made. The license for these patents belongs to Maquet Critical Care. Future commercial uses of this technology may provide financial benefit to Dr J. Beck and Dr C. Sinderby through royalties. Dr J. Beck and Dr C. Sinderby each own 50% of Neurovent Research Inc (NVR). NVR is a research and development company that builds the equipment and catheters for research studies. NVR has a consulting agreement with Maquet Critical Care.

## REFERENCES

1. Sinderby C, Navalesi P, Beck J, et al. Neural control of mechanical ventilation in respiratory failure. Nat Med 1999;5(12):1433–6.
2. Beck J, Emeriaud G, Liu Y, et al. Neurally-adjusted ventilatory assist (NAVA) in children: a systematic review. Minerva Anestesiol 2016;82(8):874–83.
3. Longhini F, Ferrero F, De Luca D, et al. Neurally adjusted ventilatory assist in preterm neonates with acute respiratory failure. Neonatology 2015;107(1):60–7.
4. Cross KW, Klaus M, Tooley WH, et al. The response of the new-born baby to inflation of the lungs. J Physiol 1960;151(3):551–65.
5. Beck J, Reilly M, Grasselli G, et al. Characterization of neural breathing pattern in spontaneously breathing preterm infants. Pediatr Res 2011;70(6):607–13.
6. Sinderby C, Beck J. Neurally adjusted ventilatory assist. In: Tobin MJ, editor. Principles and practice of mechanical ventilation. 3rd edition. New York: McGraw Hill; 2012. Chapter 13. p. 351-75.
7. Aldrich TK, Sinderby C, McKenzie DK, et al. Electrophysiological techniques for the assessment of respiratory muscle function. Am J Respir Crit Care Med 2002; 166:518–624.
8. Sinderby CA, Beck JC, Lindström LH, et al. Enhancement of signal quality in esophageal recordings of diaphragm EMG. J Appl Physiol (1985) 1997;82(4): 1370–7.
9. Beck J, Sinderby C, Weinberg J, et al. Effects of muscle-to-electrode distance on the human diaphragm electromyogram. J Appl Physiol (1985) 1995;79(3):975–85.
10. Beck J, Sinderby C, Lindström L, et al. Influence of bipolar esophageal electrode positioning on measurements of human crural diaphragm electromyogram. J Appl Physiol (1985) 1996;81(3):1434–49.

11. Emeriaud G, Beck J, Tucci M, et al. Diaphragm electrical activity during expiration in mechanically ventilated infants. Pediatr Res 2006;59(5):705–10.

12. Mally PV, Beck J, Sinderby C, et al. Neural breathing pattern and patient-ventilator interaction during neurally adjusted ventilatory assist and conventional ventilation in newborns. Pediatr Crit Care Med 2018;19(1):48–55.

13. Stein H, Firestone K, Beck J. Neurally adjusted ventilatory assist (NAVA). In: Donn SM, Mammel MC, Van Kaam AH, editors. Manual of neonatal respiratory care. 5th edition. New York: Springer Science; 2021, in press.

14. Shi Y, Muniraman H, Biniwale M, et al. A review on non-invasive respiratory support for management of respiratory distress in extremely preterm infants. Front Pediatr 2020;8:270.

15. Soukka H, Parkkola R, Lehtonen L. Brain growth in extremely preterm infants before and after implementing NAVA ventilation. Acta Paediatr 2021;110(6): 1812–4.

16. Bordessoule A, Moreira A, Felice Civitillo C, et al. Comparison of inspiratory effort with three variable-flow nasal continuous positive airway pressure devices in preterm infants: a cross-over study. Arch Dis Child Fetal Neonatal Ed 2021;106(4): 404–7.

17. Meinen RD, Alali YI, Al-Subu A, et al. Neurally-adjusted ventilatory assist can facilitate extubation in neonates with congenital diaphragmatic hernia. Respir Care 2021;66(1):41–9.

18. Latremouille S, Bhuller M, Rao S, et al. Diaphragmatic activity and neural breathing variability during a 5-min endotracheal continuous positive airway pressure trial in extremely preterm infants. Pediatr Res 2021;89(7):1810–7.

19. Goel D, Oei JL, Smyth J, et al. Diaphragm-triggered non-invasive respiratory support in preterm infants. Cochrane Database Syst Rev 2020;(3):CD012935.

20. McKinney RL, Keszler M, Truog WE, et al. Experience with Neurally Adjusted Ventilatory Assist in Infants with Severe Bronchopulmonary Dysplasia. Am J Perinatol 2020. [Epub ahead of print].

21. Rong X, Liang F, Li YJ, et al. Application of neurally adjusted ventilatory assist in premature neonates less than 1,500 grams with established or evolving bronchopulmonary dysplasia. Front Pediatr 2020;8:110.

22. Rochon ME, Lodygensky G, Tabone L, et al. Continuous neurally adjusted ventilation: a feasibility study in preterm infants. Arch Dis Child Fetal Neonatal Ed 2020;105(6):640–5.

23. Firestone K, Horany BA, de Leon-Belden L, et al. Nasal continuous positive airway pressure versus noninvasive NAVA in preterm neonates with apnea of prematurity: a pilot study with a novel approach. J Perinatol 2020;40(8):1211–5.

24. Hunt KA, Dassios T, Greenough A. Proportional assist ventilation (PAV) versus neurally adjusted ventilator assist (NAVA): effect on oxygenation in infants with evolving or established bronchopulmonary dysplasia. Eur J Pediatr 2020; 179(6):901–8.

25. Protain AP, Firestone KS, McNinch NL, et al. Evaluating peak inspiratory pressures and tidal volume in premature neonates on NAVA ventilation. Eur J Pediatr 2021;180(1):167–75.

26. Makker K, Cortez J, Jha K, et al. Comparison of extubation success using noninvasive positive pressure ventilation (NIPPV) versus noninvasive neurally adjusted ventilatory assist (NI-NAVA). J Perinatol 2020;40(8):1202–10.

27. Gupta A, Lumba R, Bailey S, et al. Electrical activity of the diaphragm in a small cohort of preterm infants on noninvasive neurally adjusted ventilatory assist and

continuous positive airway pressure: a prospective comparative pilot study. Cureus 2019;11(12):e6291.

28. Iwasaki E, Hirata K, Morikawa K, et al. Postnatal physiological changes in electrical activity of the diaphragm in extremely preterm infants. Pediatr Pulmonol 2020; 55(8):1969–73.

29. Matlock DN, Bai S, Weisner MD, et al. Work of breathing in premature neonates: noninvasive neurally-adjusted ventilatory assist versus noninvasive ventilation. Respir Care 2020;65(7):946–53.

30. Nam SK, Lee J, Jun YH. Neural feedback is insufficient in preterm infants during neurally adjusted ventilatory assist. Pediatr Pulmonol 2019;54(8):1277–83.

31. Morgan EL, Firestone KS, Schachinger SW, et al. Effects of changes in apnea time on the clinical status of neonates on NIV-NAVA. Respir Care 2019;64(9): 1096–100.

32. Tabacaru CR, Moores RR Jr, Khoury J, et al. NAVA-synchronized compared to nonsynchronized noninvasive ventilation for apnea, bradycardia, and desaturation events in VLBW infants. Pediatr Pulmonol 2019;54(11):1742–6.

33. Kallio M, Mahlman M, Koskela U, et al. NIV NAVA versus nasal CPAP in premature infants: a randomized clinical trial. Neonatology 2019;116(4):380–4.

34. Yagui AC, Meneses J, Zólio BA, et al. Nasal continuous positive airway pressure (NCPAP) or noninvasive neurally adjusted ventilatory assist (NIV-NAVA) for preterm infants with respiratory distress after birth: a randomized controlled trial. Pediatr Pulmonol 2019;54(11):1704–11.

35. Yagui ACZ, Gonçalves PA, Murakami SH, et al. Is noninvasive neurally adjusted ventilatory assistance (NIV-NAVA) an alternative to NCPAP in preventing extubation failure in preterm infants? J Matern Fetal Neonatal Med 2019;1–151 [Epub ahead of print].

36. Lee BK, Shin SH, Jung YH, et al. Comparison of NIV-NAVA and NCPAP in facilitating extubation for very preterm infants. BMC Pediatr 2019;19(1):298.

37. Baudin F, Emeriaud G, Essouri S, et al. Physiological effect of prone position in children with severe bronchiolitis: a randomized cross-over study (BRONCHIO-DV). J Pediatr 2019;205:112–9.

38. Miyahara J, Sugiura H, Ohki S. The evaluation of the efficacy and safety of noninvasive neurally adjusted ventilatory assist in combination with INtubation-SURfactant-Extubation technique for infants at 28 to 33 weeks of gestation with respiratory distress syndrome. SAGE Open Med 2019;7. 2050312119838417.

39. Nam SK, Lee J, Jun YH, et al. Neural feedback is insufficient in preterm infants during neurally adjusted ventilatory assist. Pediatr Pulmonol 2019;54(8):1277–83.

40. Baudin F, Emeriaud G, Essouri S, et al. Neurally adjusted ventilatory assist decreases work of breathing during non-invasive ventilation in infants with severe bronchiolitis. Crit Care 2019;23(1):120.

41. Bonacina D, Bronco A, Nacoti M, et al. Pressure support ventilation, sigh adjunct to pressure support ventilation, and neurally adjusted ventilatory assist in infants after cardiac surgery: a physiologic crossover randomized study. Pediatr Pulmonol 2019;54(7):1078–86.

42. Baez Hernandez N, Milad A, Li Y, et al. Utilization of neurally adjusted ventilatory assist (NAVA) mode in infants and children undergoing congenital heart surgery: a retrospective review. Pediatr Cardiol 2019;40(3):563–9.

43. Oda A, Parikka V, Lehtonen L, et al. Nasal high-flow therapy decreased electrical activity of the diaphragm in preterm infants during the weaning phase. Acta Paediatr 2019;108(2):253–7.

44. Singh N, McNally MJ, Darnall RA. Does diaphragmatic electrical activity in preterm infants predict extubation success? Respir Care 2018;63(2):203–7.

45. Longhini F, Scarlino S, Gallina MR, et al. Comparison of neurally-adjusted ventilator assist in infants before and after extubation. Minerva Pediatr 2018;70(2): 133–40.

46. Crulli B, Khebir M, Toledano B, et al. Neurally adjusted ventilatory assist after pediatric cardiac surgery: clinical experience and impact on ventilation pressures. Respir Care 2018;63(2):208–14.

47. Sood SB, Mushtaq N, Brown K, et al. Neurally adjusted ventilatory assist is associated with greater initial extubation success in postoperative congenital heart disease patients when compared to conventional mechanical ventilation. J Pediatr Intensive Care 2018;7(3):147–58.

48. Oda A, Parikka V, Lehtonen L, et al. Rapid respiratory transition at birth as evaluated by electrical activity of the diaphragm in very preterm infants supported by nasal CPAP. Respir Physiol Neurobiol 2018;258:1–4.

49. Oda A, Kamei Y, Hiroma T, et al. Neurally adjusted ventilatory assist in extremely low-birthweight infants. Pediatr Int 2018;60(9):844–8.

50. Yonehara K, Ogawa R, Kamei Y, et al. Non-invasive neurally adjusted ventilatory assist versus nasal intermittent positive-pressure ventilation in preterm infants born before 30 weeks' gestation. Pediatr Int 2018;60(10):957–61.

51. García-Muñoz Rodrigo F, Urquía Martí L, Galán Henríquez G, et al. Neural breathing patterns in preterm newborns supported with non-invasive neurally adjusted ventilatory assist. J Perinatol 2018;38(9):1235–41.

52. Brenne H, Grunewaldt KH, Follestad T, et al. A randomised cross-over study showed no difference in diaphragm activity during weaning from respiratory support. Acta Paediatr 2018;107(10):1726–32.

53. Gibu CK, Cheng PY, Ward RJ, et al. Feasibility and physiological effects of noninvasive neurally adjusted ventilatory assist in preterm infants. Pediatr Res 2017; 82(4):650–7.

54. Rosterman JL, Pallotto EK, Truog WE, et al. The impact of neurally adjusted ventilatory assist mode on respiratory severity score and energy expenditure in infants: a randomized crossover trial. J Perinatol 2018;38(1):59–63.

55. Shetty S, Hunt K, Peacock J, et al. Crossover study of assist control ventilation and neurally adjusted ventilatory assist. Eur J Pediatr 2017;176(4):509–13.

56. Lee J, Kim HS, Jung YH, et al. Neurally adjusted ventilatory assist for infants under prolonged ventilation. Pediatr Int 2017;59(5):540–4.

57. Mortamet G, Larouche A, Ducharme-Crevier L, et al. Patient-ventilator asynchrony during conventional mechanical ventilation in children. Ann Intensive Care 2017;7(1):122.

58. Iyer NP, Dickson J, Ruiz ME, et al. Neural breathing pattern in newborn infants pre- and postextubation. Acta Paediatr 2017;106(12):1928–33.

59. Colaizy TT, Kummet GJ, Kummet CM, et al. Noninvasive neurally adjusted ventilatory assist in premature infants postextubation. Am J Perinatol 2017;34(6): 593–8.

60. Jung YH, Kim HS, Lee J, et al. Neurally adjusted ventilatory assist in preterm infants with established or evolving bronchopulmonary dysplasia on high-intensity mechanical ventilatory support: a single-center experience. Pediatr Crit Care Med 2016;17(12):1142–6.

61. Ng E, Schurr P, Reilly M, et al. Impact of feeding method on diaphragm electrical activity and central apnea in preterm infants (FEAdi study). Early Hum Dev 2016; 101:33–7.

62. Stein H, Hall R, Davis K, et al. Electrical activity of the diaphragm (Edi) values and Edi catheter placement in non-ventilated preterm neonates. J Perinatol 2013; 33(9):707–11.

63. Green ML, Walsh BK, Wolf GK, et al. Electrocardiographic guidance for the placement of gastric feeding tubes: a pediatric case series. Respir Care 2011; 56(4):467–71.

64. Duyndam A, Bol BS, Kroon A, et al. Neurally adjusted ventilatory assist: assessing the comfort and feasibility of use in neonates and children. Nurs Crit Care 2013;18(2):86–92.

65. Parikka V, Beck J, Zhai Q, et al. The effect of caffeine citrate on neural breathing pattern in preterm infants. Early Hum Dev 2015;91(10):565–8.

66. Soukka H, Grönroos L, Leppäsalo J, et al. The effects of skin-to-skin care on the diaphragmatic electrical activity in preterm infants. Early Hum Dev 2014;90(9): 531–4.

67. Emeriaud G, Larouche A, Ducharme-Crevier L, et al. Evolution of inspiratory diaphragm activity in children over the course of the PICU stay. Intensive Care Med 2014;40(11):1718–26.

68. Kallio M, Peltoniemi O, Anttila E, et al. Electrical activity of the diaphragm during neurally adjusted ventilatory assist in pediatric patients. Pediatr Pulmonol 2015; 50(9):925–31.

69. Naito Y, Shimizu Y, Hatachi T, et al. Predicting extubation readiness by monitoring the electrical activity of the diaphragm after prolonged mechanical ventilation: a pediatric case report. JA Clin Rep 2018;4(1):76.

70. Mortamet G, Proulx F, Crulli B, et al. Diaphragm electrical activity monitoring as a breakpoint in the management of a tetraplegic child. Crit Care 2017;21(1):116.

71. Ducharme-Crevier L, Du Pont-Thibodeau G, Emeriaud G. Interest of monitoring diaphragmatic electrical activity in the pediatric intensive care unit. Crit Care Res Pract 2013;2013:384210.

72. Beck J, Reilly M, Grasselli G, et al. Patient-ventilator interaction during neurally adjusted ventilatory assist in low birth weight infants. Pediatr Res 2009;65(6): 663–8.

73. Bengtsson JA, Edberg KE. Neurally adjusted ventilatory assist in children: an observational study. Pediatr Crit Care Med 2010;11(2):253–7.

74. Breatnach C, Conlon NP, Stack M, et al. A prospective crossover comparison of neurally adjusted ventilatory assist and pressure-support ventilation in a pediatric and neonatal intensive care unit population. Pediatr Crit Care Med 2010; 11(1):7–11.

75. Clement KC, Thurman TL, Holt SJ, et al. Neurally triggered breaths reduce trigger delay and improve ventilator response times in ventilated infants with bronchiolitis. Intensive Care Med 2011;37(11):1826–32.

76. Bordessoule A, Emeriaud G, Morneau S, et al. Neurally adjusted ventilatory assist improves patient–ventilator interaction in infants as compared with conventional ventilation. Pediatr Res 2012;72(2):194–202.

77. De la Oliva P, Schüffelmann C, Gómez-Zamora A, et al. Asynchrony, neural drive, ventilatory variability and COMFORT: NAVA versus pressure support in pediatric patients. A non-randomized cross-over trial. Intensive Care Med 2012;38(5): 838–46.

78. Alander M, Peltoniemi O, Pokka T, et al. Comparison of pressure-, flow-, and NAVA-Triggering in pediatric and neonatal ventilatory care. Pediatr Pulmonol 2012;47(1):76–83.

79. Vignaux L, Grazioli S, Piquilloud L, et al. Optimizing patient-ventilator synchrony during invasive ventilator assist in children and infants remains a difficult task*. Pediatr Crit Care Med 2013;14(7):e316–25.

80. Vignaux L, Grazioli S, Piquilloud L, et al. Patient-ventilator asynchrony during noninvasive pressure support ventilation and neurally adjusted ventilatory assist in infants and children. Pediatr Crit Care Med 2013;14(8):e357–64.

81. Baudin F, Pouyau R, Cour-Andlauer F, et al. Neurally adjusted ventilator assist (NAVA) reduces asynchrony during non-invasive ventilation for severe bronchiolitis. Pediatr Pulmonol 2015;50(12):1320–7.

82. Ducharme-Crevier L, Beck J, Essouri S, et al. Neurally adjusted ventilatory assist (NAVA) allows patient-ventilator synchrony during pediatric noninvasive ventilation: a crossover physiological study. Crit Care 2015;19:44.

83. Lee J, Kim HS, Jung YH, et al. Non-invasive neurally adjusted ventilatory assist in preterm infants: a randomised phase II crossover trial. Arch Dis Child Fetal Neonatal Ed 2015;100(6):F507–13.

84. Chidini G, De Luca D, Conti G, et al. Early noninvasive neurally adjusted ventilatory assist versus noninvasive flow-triggered pressure support ventilation in pediatric acute respiratory failure: a physiologic randomized controlled trial. Pediatr Crit Care Med 2016;17(11):e487–95.

85. Pettenuzzo T, Aoyama H, Englesakis M, et al. Effect of neurally adjusted ventilatory assist on patient-ventilator interaction in mechanically ventilated adults: a systematic review and meta-analysis. Crit Care Med 2019;47(7):e602–9.

86. LoVerde B, Firestone KS, Stein HM. Comparing changing neurally adjusted ventilatory assist (NAVA) levels in intubated and recently extubated neonates. J Perinatol 2016;36(12):1097–100.

87. Brander L, Leong-Poi H, Beck J, et al. Titration and implementation of neurally adjusted ventilatory assist in critically ill patients. Chest 2009;135(3):695–703.

88. Bridier A, François T, Baudin F, et al. Neural feedback is effective in preterm infants during neurally adjusted ventilatory assist, when using clinically relevant settings. Pediatr Pulmonol 2019;54(12):1878–9.

89. Kallio M, Koskela U, Peltoniemi O, et al. Neurally adjusted ventilatory assist (NAVA) in preterm newborn infants with respiratory distress syndrome-a randomized controlled trial. Eur J Pediatr 2016;175(9):1175–83.

90. Zhu L, Xu Z, Gong X, et al. Mechanical ventilation after bidirectional superior cavopulmonary anastomosis for single-ventricle physiology: a comparison of pressure support ventilation and neurally adjusted ventilatory assist. Pediatr Cardiol 2016;37(6):1064–71.

91. Liet JM, Barrière F, Gaillard-Le Roux B, et al. Physiological effects of invasive ventilation with neurally adjusted ventilatory assist (NAVA) in a crossover study. BMC Pediatr 2016;16(1):180.

92. Amigoni A, Rizzi G, Divisic A, et al. Effects of propofol on diaphragmatic electrical activity in mechanically ventilated pediatric patients. Intensive Care Med 2015; 41(10):1860–1.

93. Kallio M, Peltoniemi O, Anttila E, et al. Neurally adjusted ventilatory assist (NAVA) in pediatric intensive care-A randomized controlled trial. Pediatr Pulmonol 2015; 50(1):55–62.

94. Piastra M, De Luca D, Costa R, et al. Neurally adjusted ventilatory assist vs pressure support ventilation in infants recovering from severe acute respiratory distress syndrome: nested study. J Crit Care 2014;29(2):312.e1-5.

95. Durrani NU, Chedid F, Rahmani A. Neurally adjusted ventilatory assist mode used in congenital diaphragmatic hernia. J Coll Physicians Surg Pak 2011;21(10): 637–9.
96. Firestone KS, Fisher S, Reddy S, et al. Effect of changing NAVA levels on peak inspiratory pressures and electrical activity of the diaphragm in premature neonates. J Perinatol 2015;35(8):612–6.
97. Rossor TE, Hunt KA, Shetty S, et al. Neurally adjusted ventilatory assist compared to other forms of triggered ventilation for neonatal respiratory support. Cochrane Database Syst Rev 2017;(10):CD012251.

# Synchronized Invasive Mechanical Ventilation

Ilia Bresesti, MD[a,b], Massimo Agosti, MD[b], Satyan Lakshminrusimha, MD[c],
Gianluca Lista, MD, PhD[a,*]

## KEYWORDS

- Respiratory care • Ventilation technique • Neonatal population
- Mechanical ventilation • Synchronized invasive ventilation

## KEY POINTS

- Neonatal ventilation has witnessed substantial advances in the last decades, leading to a decreased early mortality rate
- Synchronization have shown to be feasibile in neonatal ventilation, with positive impact on long-term outcomes
- There are several modalities to synchronize mechanical ventilation in preterm infants, but there is still uncertainty about the superiority of one method over the others.

## INTRODUCTION

Respiratory care of premature neonates has witnessed substantial advances in the last decades and has played a crucial role in decreasing early mortality in this population.[1] This review outlines advances in techniques of synchronization and modes of synchronized invasive mechanical ventilation in neonates.

Since the mid-1960s, assisted ventilation was mostly available in the form of intermittent mandatory ventilation (IMV), which provided mechanical breaths irrespective of the patient's spontaneous effort (**Fig. 1**). However, most of the infants breathe while they are mechanically ventilated; thus, synchronization during IMV is merely a random event. Nevertheless, the use of synchronized ventilation in the neonatal population was delayed as compared to adults, mainly because of technical reasons. Coordinating the infant's respiratory effort and the onset of mechanical ventilation (MV) in the neonatal population has requested high sensitivity instruments, able to detect minimal flows and tidal volumes (TVs).[2] Moreover, the almost unavoidable presence of consistent air leakage around the uncuffed endotracheal tube had to be considered to develop a functional system.

[a] Division of Neonatology, "V.Buzzi" Children's Hospital, ASST-FBF-Sacco, Via Castelvetro 32, Milan 20154, Italy; [b] Division of Neonatology, "F. Del Ponte" Hospital, Woman and Child Department, University of Insubria, Varese, Italy; [c] Department of Pediatrics, UC Davis Children's Hospital, Sacramento, CA, USA
* Corresponding author.
E-mail address: gianluca.lista@assti-fbf-sacco.it

Clin Perinatol 48 (2021) 813–824
https://doi.org/10.1016/j.clp.2021.07.008
0095-5108/21/© 2021 Elsevier Inc. All rights reserved.

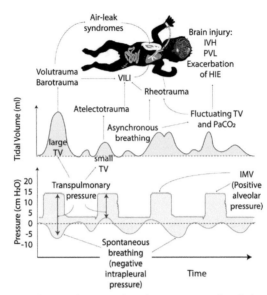

**Fig. 1.** IMV without synchrony. The green line (pressure waveform) shows positive alveolar pressure generated by the ventilator. The blue line is the negative intrapleural pressure generated by the neonate's spontaneous respiration. The light green color between these 2 lines indicates transpulmonary pressure. Fluctuating transpulmonary pressure leads to variable tidal volume (TV). Large TV is associated with volutrauma and barotrauma leading air-leak syndromes. Low TVs lead to atelectotrauma. Volutrauma, barotrauma, rheotrauma, and atelectotrauma contribute to ventilator-induced lung injury (VILI). Fluctuating TVs and Paco$_2$ can exacerbate brain injury in hypoxic-ischemic encephalopathy (HIE) or trigger intraventricular hemorrhage (IVH) and periventricular leukomalacia (PVL). (*Courtesy of* Satyan Lakshminrusimha.)

The need for neonatal-targeted synchronized ventilation finds its way in the multiple harmful effects, which may derive from asynchrony, from gas exchange impairment, air trapping, and air leak syndromes to central nervous system damage (see **Fig. 1**).[3–5] In contrast, with synchrony, adequate gas exchange can be achieved with lower inflating pressure with a subsequent lower risk for ventilator-induced lung injury (VILI). In fact, MV is known to be responsible for pulmonary injury.[6] Several types of damage can occur, and they are named according to the cause leading to them, which are as follows:

- Volutrauma, caused by over-distension and excessive stretch of tissues
- Barotrauma, when excessive pressure is delivered to the lung parenchyma
- Atelectotrauma, when TV is given in the presence of atelectasis with never re-cruited alveoli
- Biotrauma, when repetitive alveolar opening and closing of under-recruited al-veoli triggers a cascade of inflammatory mediators and cells causing biochemical and biophysical injury
- Rheotrauma, when inappropriate flow is delivered, either excessive or inadequate.[7]

Nowadays, the main goal for the neonatologist is to minimize VILI and reducing the work of breathing (WOB) by reducing the duration of ventilation, optimizing the use of ventilators, improving synchronized ventilatory strategies.

Until recently, asynchronous breathing was partially resolved with the use of pharmacologic agents, inducing muscle paralysis and deep sedation to prevent the baby from fighting the ventilator.

Currently, there are several ventilation techniques through which synchronization can be achieved, but there is still uncertainly on the optimal modality.[8] We hereby provide an overview of the commonly used synchronized ventilatory strategies among neonatal intensive care units (NICU), focusing on bedside application.

## MODES OF SYNCHRONIZED VENTILATION

Synchronized ventilatory modes are characterized by the delivery of a mechanical breath in response to a signal corresponding to the initiation of the patient's spontaneous breathing.

The most common modalities to provide synchronized MV to preterm infants are *synchronized intermittent mandatory ventilation (SIMV)*, *assist-control ventilation (A/C)*, otherwise known as *synchronized intermittent positive pressure ventilation (SIPPV)*, and *pressure support ventilation (PSV)* (**Fig. 4**). More recently, *neurally adjusted ventilatory assist (NAVA)* has been introduced, but it has not been incorporated yet into routine clinical practice in most NICUs.

### Signal Detection

A deep understanding of the interaction between the patient's effort and the ventilator's inflation is crucial to avoid suboptimal or excessive ventilation. The TV entering the lung is determined by the combination of the patient's inspiratory effort (negative intrapleural pressure) and the positive pressure generated by the ventilator, which together form the transpulmonary pressure (see **Fig. 1**). Preterm infant's breathing pattern is typically characterized by short inspiratory time and high respiratory rate (RR), especially when the degree of lung compliance is low, as it is during the acute phase of respiratory distress syndrome (RDS). Hence, the system response time (the so-called "trigger"), which refers to the interval between signal detection and the rise in pressure at the proximal airway, must be minimal (less than 50 ms) to detect the breaths producing minimal signals.

The respiratory effort's signal can be derived from different types of measurements, although only a few are in common clinically spread in NICUs (**Fig. 2**).

The first technique for synchronization was based on the pressure changes in the ventilator circuit, which depends on the infant making a sufficiently large inspiration to modify the circuit pressure (around 0.5 cmH$_2$O). However, this method is not accurate enough if the baby is very tiny or has a poor inspiratory effort.

Another option is the detection of abdominal movements. They are obtained through an applanation traducer, such as the so-called Graseby capsule, applied on the patient's abdominal wall. Although this method avoids the problem of increased dead space, the reliability depends on where the capsule is placed on the abdomen, since movement artifacts may lead to autocycling. More accuracy might be obtained through diaphragmatic electromyography, but the sensors are not so commonly available in most of the NICUs. Also, variations in the esophageal pressure have the advantage to avoid dead space interference, but peristalsis and cardiac movements may cause triggering artifacts.

Currently, in most of the ventilators in use, triggering is made through a hot wire flow sensor placed between the ventilator circuit and the endotracheal tube. Two tungsten wires heated to 400°C detect inspiratory gas flow, and when it reaches about 0.2 L/min, around 30 ms after the beginning of the inspiratory flow, a mechanical inflation

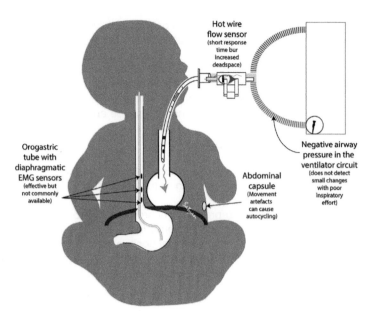

**Fig. 2.** Common modes of respiratory synchronization in neonates. Disadvantages or advantages associated with each mode are shown in small font. Negative airway pressure generated in the ventilatory circuit with spontaneous inspiration, abdominal wall movement, diaphragmatic electrical activity, and detection of flow with a hotwire sensor are 4 methods of synchronizing ventilator breaths with spontaneous breaths from the neonate. (*Courtesy of* Satyan Lakshminrusimha.)

is started. The delay time depends on the set trigger sensitivity on a scale ranging from 1 to 10 (1 is the most sensitive). This sensitivity should always be set to 1 so that the inflation occurs as close as possible to the onset of the baby's inspiration. A higher number will mean a longer delay between the beginning of inspiration and the start of inflation, resulting in nonsynchronous inflation. Accurate determination of exhaled tidal volume (eTV) is important especially when small TVs are delivered. To have an accurate eTV measurement, it is necessary to detect it at the patient airway. This is the reason why the flow sensor is placed between the T-piece and the endotracheal tube. Although this method allows measurement of TVs and minute ventilation, some clinicians are concerned about the additional dead space caused by the flow sensor, which may result in $Paco_2$ retention. However, the common use of uncuffed endotracheal tubes in the NICU is often associated with leaks around the tube. Even in the case of no leaks, the effect of a hotwire flow sensor on $Paco_2$ is moderate and not of clinical significance compared with the clinical gain. Nevertheless, to compensate for this dead space, in the most premature infants less than 1 kg, the TV set on the ventilator might be slightly increased (eg, 1 mL/kg plus the standard 5 mL/kg), in addition to a higher RR. Potential risks related to these modifications (eg, volutrauma) must be evaluated on an individual basis.

### Synchronized Intermittent Mandatory Ventilation

The SIMV is a form of patient-triggered ventilation characterized by a predetermined number of inflations (back up rate), which are synchronized with the onset of spontaneous infant's breath or delivered automatically if the infant's effort is inadequate or absent. It is pressure-limited and time-cycled. In SIMV, spontaneous breaths exceeding the predetermined number are not assisted and are supported only by the baseline positive end-expiratory pressure (PEEP) (**Figs. 3** and **4B**). SIMV can be combined with PSV (**Fig. 4C**). In this case, the ventilator delivers a determined number of inflations per minute. In between, the infant can take spontaneous breaths, and the ventilator provides pressure support (eg, 2–3 cmH$_2$O) above PEEP values, reducing WOB. In fact, using PSV, we can facilitate spontaneous breathing with a low back-up SIMV rate and maintain a background minute ventilation and lung volume.

Weaning from MV is probably the best application of SIMV, although some clinicians prefer to use it as an alternative mode to assist control (A/C).

Weaning from SIMV might be done by reducing peak pressure or TV before the ventilation rate, and extubation should be considered when the SIMV rate is low. In fact, decreasing the fixed rate to favor spontaneous breathing was previously considered a "pre-extubation training," but it has shown to be a useless respiratory effort, with an excessive WOB and ineffective minute ventilation, especially in the most premature infants.

### Assist-Control or Synchronized Intermittent Positive Pressure Ventilation

This technique (pressure-limited and time-cycled) is another form of patient-triggered ventilation. It supports any respiratory effort, either initiated by the patient ("assist") or by the ventilator ("control"), capable of overcoming the trigger threshold set by the neonatologist (**Fig. 4D**). It has been shown to be very useful in the acute phase of RDS, and it is a good ventilation strategy for virtually all patients. However, the various stages of RDS, corresponding to different lung compliances and shallow breathing,

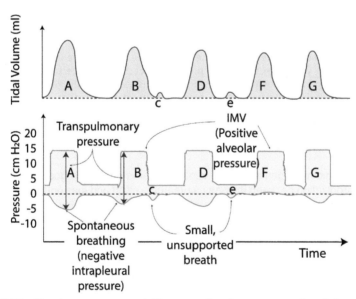

**Fig. 3.** SIMV without pressure support. The green line (pressure waveform) shows positive alveolar pressure generated by the ventilator. The blue line is the negative intrapleural pressure generated by the neonate's spontaneous respiration. The light green color between these 2 lines indicates transpulmonary pressure. Breaths A, B, D, and F are triggered by infant's spontaneous breaths. Breaths c and e are small breaths occurring soon after B and D, respectively, and do not trigger a mechanical inflation. Breath F is a mandatory breath without any triggering by the patient. (*Courtesy of* Satyan Lakshminrusimha.)

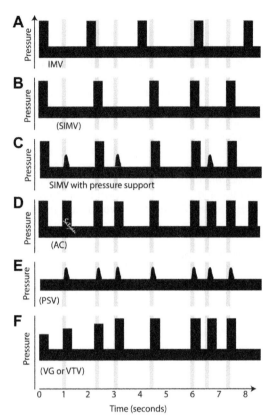

**Fig. 4.** Different modes of ventilation. The vertical gray bars indicate infant's own sponta-neous effort. The vertical axis refers to pressure in each mode. See text for details. The long, rectangular bars refer to full inflation breaths supported by PIP and time-cycled. The short, narrow inflation breaths are pressure support breaths that are flow-cycled. In mode F, the tidal volume is set up and the pressure is adjusted by the ventilator until the targeted volume is reached. VTV, volume-targeted ventilation. (*Courtesy* Satyan Lakshminrusimha.)

impose dynamic management of the ventilator parameters. The goal is to obtain the best synchronization between the baby's breathing effort and the ventilator, thus using lower ventilation pressures. Usually, a back-up rate slightly below the spontaneous rate (30–40 inflations/min) is set to provide a minimum rate in case of apnea. The TV should range 4 to 6 mL/kg, according to the RDS phase (acute/weaning), and pressure parameters should be set accordingly. During the weaning phase, the inspiratory peak is gradually lowered, keeping the RR initially unchanged. In this way, reducing the sup-port provided to each breath, the WOB for the infant increases gradually, as a compensation for the reduced volume supplied by the ventilator.

Especially in very preterm neonates, and infants with hypoxic-ischemic encepha-lopathy, the risk of hypocapnia warrants particular attention.

### Pressure Support Ventilation

PSV is a pressure-controlled mode that partially or fully supports every infant's breath, like A/C, but it is flow-cycled (**Fig. 4**E). This means that the patient initiates an inspiratory effort that results in an acceleration of airway flow. Once the breath is triggered, flow is delivered to the infant's airway and pressure rises rather quickly to the set pressure support. As long as the lung is filled, the inspiratory flow decreases its velocity and, when a threshold usually ranging 5% to 20% of the flow peak is reached, the support is terminated. This technique eliminates the pressure support for prolonged inspiration times and theoretically provides greater adherence to the ventilation synchronization. In fact, PSV allows the patient to determine the depth, length, flow, and rate of breathing. PSV reduces the need for sedatives and/or muscle relaxants. Further advantages may involve the reduction of intrathoracic and intracranial pressure fluctuations.[7]

This technique can be used alone with a backup frequency rate or, in some ventilators, in conjunction with SIMV. This "hybrid" mode tends to better support the spontaneous respiratory effort of the patient. A common mistake is using a high SIMV rate with PSV, as it compromised synchronization with the provision of unnecessary mandatory breaths. If there is a need for high SIMV rate, it is advisable to consider A/C until the baby is ready for PSV. PSV is designed primarily as weaning mode "to train" the neonate before extubation, but can be used also during the acute phase of RDS after improvement of lung compliance (eg, after surfactant) or in neonate mechanically ventilated after surgery but with normal lung compliance.

All these modalities of synchronized ventilation are pressure-limited, so they do not control the TV delivered to the patient, which can change according to lung compliance and airway resistance. This "TV variability" cannot reduce WOB and induce VILI (especially atelectrauma and volutrauma), therefore may predispose to bronchopulmonary dysplasia (BPD). This is the reason why in many NICUs all these modalities are often combined with a targeted-volume control of ventilation, that allows both synchronization and a more adequate lung volume. One of the most popular volume-targeted ventilation for the neonate is the volume-guarantee (VG). With the VG option, available in some neonatal ventilators, the operators set the target TV and the ventilator regulates the peak inspiratory pressure (PIP) using the eTV measurements (**Fig. 4**F). According to lung compliance and resistance, with an algorithm that compares the TV of the previous breath, the ventilator adjusts the ventilator operating PIP (working pressure) to achieve the target TV. The automatic reduction of the working pressure in response to the lung compliance improvement and increased patient effort makes VG a real self-weaning modality.[9,10]

### New Direction: Neurally Adjusted Ventilatory Assist

Recently, a new form of synchronization has been introduced, the so-called NAVA (**Fig. 5**). It allows the patient to control the initiation and the termination of each mechanical breath on a breath-by-breath basis. Using electrodes on a specialized nasogastric tube, it detects and analyzes the electrical activity of the diaphragm, triggering ventilator inflations in proportion and in synchrony with this signal. Synchrony is then improved not only in the initiation of breath but also for size and termination. NAVA reduces wrong triggering, even in the presence of large air leak, as it is frequent in the most premature infants.[11,12] These peculiarities lead to a significant reduction of asynchrony.[13]

NAVA is contraindicated in specific clinical conditions, which lead to a complete lack of respiratory drive or inability to place the NAVA sensor. This is the case of oversedation or paralysis, esophageal malformations, history of recent upper airways surgery, phrenic nerve lesion, and the clinical circumstances where the respiratory center in the brainstem is compromised (eg, severe hypoxic-ischemic encephalopathy, stroke).

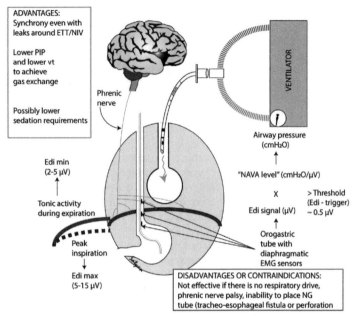

**Fig. 5.** The physiologic basis, advantages, and disadvantages of NAVA in neonates. The electrical activity of the diaphragm (Edi) is detected by sensors embedded in a specialized nasogastric tube. The Edi min value corresponds to the tonic activity of the diaphragm during expiration and the typical values in preterm infants are shown in parentheses. The Edi max indicates the peak generated during inspiration. When the Edi value exceeds a preset trigger value, a mechanical breath is initiated by the ventilator. The ventilator provides flow to generate a peak pressure above PEEP for the mechanical breath as determined by the product of (Edi max − Edi min) × NAVA level. EMG, electromyography; ETT, endotracheal tube; NIV, non-invasive ventilation; NG, nasogastric; Vt, tidal volume. (*Courtesy of* Satyan Lakshminrusimha.)

### Synchronization, short-term outcomes, and long-term sequelae

Although the use of synchronized mechanical ventilation in premature infants is currently widespread in various forms in worldwide NICUs, the superiority of one mode over another still requires further investigation.

Comparing A/C to SIMV, a few trials reported that the weaning duration tended to be shorter when A/C was used, while no differences were found with regard to weaning failure, extubation failure, and incidence of air leaks.[14,15] The meta-analysis conducted by Greenough and colleagues[8] showed no evidence of effect in any of these outcomes.

A/C and PSV have been compared in one study by Patel and coworkers, which reported no differences in terms of weaning from MV duration.[16]

The use of PSV compared to SIMV did not report statistical difference in terms of weaning duration, extubation failure, BPD, and air leaks.[17]

There is only one study analyzing the difference between the use of SIMV alone and SIMV with PSV and it showed no significant difference concerning death, BPD, IVH, and air leaks.[18]

The addition of VG to synchronized ventilation has shown interesting results, which encourage the clinician to increase its use. As shown by Duman and coworkers, the VG option in very premature infants, when combined with A/C (in the acute phase of RDS) and SIMV (in the weaning phase), reduced TV variability, and may have shortened the duration of ventilation. Overall mortality and BPD rates did not show a significant difference, although their combined outcome was significantly improved in infants treated with VG modes as compared to those treated with synchronized pressure-limited modes alone.[19] Liu and colleagues[10] compared the use of SIMV with PSV+VG. They showed superiority of PSV+VG regarding extubation failure and weaning duration. Similarly, Una and colleagues[20] showed that PSV+VG compared to SIMV+VG provided closer TVs to the set value and was not associated with overventilation or a difference in mortality or morbidity.

With regards to NAVA, predominantly short-term data are available. Although limited in number, the published studies showed promising findings.[21–24]

## BEDSIDE SUGGESTIONS

Given the wide variety of clinical conditions, types of ventilators, and modes of ventilation, standard recommendations are of limited utility, and should be customized on an individual basis. Although the SIMV we have previously described is for infants already recovered in NICU, it is of extreme importance that any ventilation management must be commenced early in the delivery room to be effective, using recruitment maneuvers for the optimization of lung volume.[25,26]

We provide a schematic summary of a potential approach to MV that we are used to following in our NICUs.

In preterm infants in the acute phase of RDS, start with AC+VG with the following initial parameters:

- RR 40 to 60 breaths per minute (bpm), adjusted to optimize the comfort of the baby during ventilation and according to $CO_2$ levels. If observing the flow curve on the ventilator screen, the expiration flow does not return completely to baseline before the following mechanical breath, it is important to increase the length of expiratory time or reduce the RR to avoid the risk of inadvertent PEEP.
- Inspiratory time (IT) 0.30 to 0.40 sec, changed several times in a day according to lung compliance, searching for the time constant (eg, adequate IT value is displayed when inspiratory flow curve comes back completely to baseline and immediately starts the expiratory flow)
- TV 5 to 7 mL/kg adjusted to reduce WOB, and according to the degree of lung inflation. In patients affected by BPD or ventilated for a prolonged time, it might be appropriate to increase TV up to 8 to 10 mL/kg to overcome the increased functional dead space and tracheal enlargement. TV might also be increased to 10 mL/kg when compensation of leaks is necessary. Avoid higher values because of the risk of rheotrauma.
- PEEP 5 cmH2O adjusted according to blood gases values (mainly $CO_2$), $Fio_2$ requirement, and lung inflation visible at chest X-ray. PEEP values higher than 8 cm $H_2O$ are rarely needed.

We use PSV + VG as a first-line treatment in very premature infants only if they dramatically respond to surfactant administration. PSV+VG is our preferred modality of ventilation in neonates affected by respiratory failure:

- Due to severe neurologic impairment
- Undergoing deep pharmacologic sedation
- During recovery of postabdominal surgery
- Due to heart diseases with ventilator dependence
- With normal lung compliance

Unless the baby is affected by BPD, during the weaning phase, we usually avoid changes in ventilation modality. We keep the patient on A/C, and we reduce RR (eg, 15–20 bpm), TV (not <4 mL/kg), and PEEP (not <4 cmH2O), trying for extubation when the PIP needed to reach the TV set is around 14 to 16 cmH2O and $Fio_2$ requirement is <0.30.

The use of SIMV+VG is usually limited to the weaning phase of very preterm infants, to avoid the risk of metabolic acidosis caused by the increase of WOB. However, if the WOB excessively increases using this modality, pressure support over PEEP (eg, 2–3 $cmH_2O$) is often associated. Of note, gradual weaning is recommended to avoid lung derecruitment.

Particular attention should be paid to autocycling and trigger failure. The most frequent cause for autocycling is the leakage around the endotracheal tube, which may be misinterpreted by the sensor, restarting the cycle. In some cases, the water bubbling in the ventilator circuit creates condensed flow which activates the trigger. To avoid trigger failure, setting the appropriate sensitivity is fundamental. If the trigger threshold is too low, artifacts may trigger inflations. If it is too high, the time until the infant reaches the threshold may be longer, causing a delay in the response time, or the infant may even not reach this threshold at all. The appropriate trigger response time should be the lowest possible, just above the level of observed artifacts, and 0.1 ms seems to be a reasonable choice.

## SUMMARY

Synchronized mechanical ventilation in preterm infants in any of the aforementioned modalities has been shown to be beneficial, compared to asynchronous conventional MV. Newly introduced modalities such as NAVA have shown intriguing results. However, there are still several aspects that need to be clarified, especially about how the different modalities can be tailored to specific neonatal populations and clinical circumstances. More large-scale clinical trials are required to better explore the long-term effects of synchronization in preterm infants.

## CLINICS CARE POINTS

- To synchronize the infant's breath with the mechanical breath, some methods are available in neonatal setting. These includes signal detection through pressure changes in the ventilator circuit, the detection of abdominal movements through the Graseby capsule, the use of a hot wire flow sensor to detect inspiratory and expiratory flow changes or the newest sensor to detect neuronal diaphragmatic activity. All of them have pros and cons, which should be considered in the clinical management.

- There are several ventilation techniques which can nowadays be used to synchronize mechanical ventilation in the neonatal population. These include SIMV, SIPPV, PSV, NAVA. There are various clinical indications for each of them, and their use should be tailored according to the patient's characteristics and ongoing clinical circumstances.

- In order to reduce the risk of early and long-term sequelae, synchronization must be associated to ventilatory strategies aiming to reduce VILI (e.g. volume and peak pressure control levels, tailored PEEP, inspiratory and expiratory time).

- Although synchronization has shown to be beneficial compared to asynchronous invasive ventilation, there is still lack of evidence regarding the best modalities to use in specific populations of infants and of clinical circumstances.

## BEST PRACTICES

- What is the current practice?
  - Neonatal ventilatory strategies have been improved significantly lately, and synchronization of ventilation has become part of routine clinical practice for neonatologists.

- What changes in current practice are likely to improve outcomes?
  - Synchronization has shown to improve neonatal clinical outcomes as compared to asynchronous modalities of ventilation. However, there is lack of evidence supporting the superiority of one technique over another. Tailoring the ventilation approach during the whole NICU stay is likely to improve both short term and long-term outcomes.

- Major recommendation
  - The use of synchronized modalities should be chosen as first line ventilation strategy in neonatal units
  - An accurate evaluation of the underlying clinical conditions should be made setting the ventilator's parameters to customize respiratory support on an individual basis
  - Appropriate tailoring of parameters according to the different phases of the lung development as well as the clinical conditions should be aimed. Excessive or insufficient delivery of pressure and volumes should be avoided to prevent lung trauma.

## CONFLICT OF INTEREST

None declared.

## REFERENCES

1. Owen LS, Manley BJ, Davis PG, et al. The evolution of modern respiratory care for preterm infants. Lancet 2017;389(10079):1649–59.
2. Donn SM, Sinha SK. Controversies in patient-triggered ventilation. Clin Perinatol 1998;25(1):49–61.
3. Lipscomb AP, Thorburn RJ, Reynolds EO, et al. Pneumothorax and cerebral haemorrhage in preterm infants. Lancet 1981;1(8217):414–6.
4. Rennie JM, South M, Morley CJ. Cerebral blood flow velocity variability in infants receiving assisted ventilation. Arch Dis Child 1987;62(12):1247–51.
5. Perlman JM, Goodman S, Kreusser KL, et al. Reduction in intraventricular hemorrhage by elimination of fluctuating cerebral blood-flow velocity in preterm infants with respiratory distress syndrome. N Engl J Med 1985;312(21):1353–7.
6. Attar MA, Donn SM. Mechanisms of ventilator-induced lung injury in premature infants. Semin Neonatol 2002;7(5):353–60.
7. Keszler M. Mechanical ventilation strategies. Semin Fetal Neonatal Med 2017; 22(4):267–74.
8. Greenough A, Rossor TE, Sundaresan A, et al. Synchronized mechanical ventilation for respiratory support in newborn infants. Cochrane Database Syst Rev Sep 2016;9:CD000456.
9. Scopesi F, Calevo MG, Rolfe P, et al. Volume targeted ventilation (volume guarantee) in the weaning phase of premature newborn infants. Pediatr Pulmonol 2007;42(10):864–70.
10. Liu WQ, Xu Y, Han AM, et al. [A comparative study of two ventilation modes in the weaning phase of preterm infants with respiratory distress syndrome]. Zhongguo Dang Dai Er Ke Za Zhi 2018;20(9):729–33.

11. Clement KC, Thurman TL, Holt SJ, et al. Neurally triggered breaths reduce trigger delay and improve ventilator response times in ventilated infants with bronchiolitis. Intensive Care Med 2011;37(11):1826–32.

12. Alander M, Peltoniemi O, Pokka T, et al. Comparison of pressure-, flow-, and NAVA-triggering in pediatric and neonatal ventilatory care. Pediatr Pulmonol 2012;47(1):76–83.

13. Bordessoule A, Emeriaud G, Morneau S, et al. Neurally adjusted ventilatory assist improves patient–ventilator interaction in infants as compared with conventional ventilation. Pediatr Res 2012;72(2):194–202.

14. Chan V, Greenough A. Comparison of weaning by patient triggered ventilation or synchronous intermittent mandatory ventilation in preterm infants. Acta Paediatr 1994;83(3):335–7.

15. Dimitriou G, Greenough A, Griffin F, et al. Synchronous intermittent mandatory ventilation modes compared with patient triggered ventilation during weaning. Arch Dis Child Fetal Neonatal Ed 1995;72(3):F188–90.

16. Shefali-Patel D, Murthy V, Hannam S, et al. Randomised weaning trial comparing assist control to pressure support ventilation. Arch Dis Child Fetal Neonatal Ed 2012;97(6):F429–33.

17. Erdemir A, Kahramaner Z, Turkoglu E, et al. Effects of synchronized intermittent mandatory ventilation versus pressure support plus volume guarantee ventilation in the weaning phase of preterm infants. Pediatr Crit Care Med 2014;15(3): 236–41.

18. Reyes ZC, Claure N, Tauscher MK, et al. Randomized, controlled trial comparing synchronized intermittent mandatory ventilation and synchronized intermittent mandatory ventilation plus pressure support in preterm infants. Pediatrics 2006;118(4):1409–17.

19. Duman N, Tuzun F, Sutcuoglu S, et al. Impact of volume guarantee on synchronized ventilation in preterm infants: a randomized controlled trial. Intensive Care Med 2012;38(8):1358–64.

20. Unal S, Ergenekon E, Aktas S, et al. Effects of volume Guaranteed ventilation combined with two different modes in preterm infants. Respir Care 2017; 62(12):1525–32.

21. de la Oliva P, Schüffelmann C, Gómez-Zamora A, et al. Asynchrony, neural drive, ventilatory variability and COMFORT: NAVA versus pressure support in pediatric patients. A non-randomized cross-over trial. *Intensive Care Med* May 2012;38(5): 838–46.

22. Stein H, Howard D. Neurally adjusted ventilatory assist in neonates weighing <1500 grams: a retrospective analysis. J Pediatr 2012;160(5):786–9.e1.

23. Kallio M, Peltoniemi O, Anttila E, et al. Neurally adjusted ventilatory assist (NAVA) in pediatric intensive care–a randomized controlled trial. Pediatr Pulmonol 2015; 50(1):55–62.

24. Shetty S, Hunt K, Peacock J, et al. Crossover study of assist control ventilation and neurally adjusted ventilatory assist. Eur J Pediatr 2017;176(4):509–13.

25. Lista G, Maturana A, Moya FR. Achieving and maintaining lung volume in the preterm infant: from the first breath to the NICU. Eur J Pediatr 2017. https://doi.org/10.1007/s00431-017-2984-y.

26. Lista G, Castoldi F, Cavigioli F, et al. Alveolar recruitment in the delivery room. J Matern Fetal Neonatal Med 2012;25(Suppl 1):39–40.

# Volume-Targeted Ventilation

Gusztav Belteki, MD, PhD, FRCPCH*, Colin J. Morley, MD, FRCPCH

## KEYWORDS

- Neonatology • Mechanical ventilation • Volume-targeted ventilation
- Volume guarantee • Neonatal lung injury

## KEY POINTS

- Evidence from animal experiments and clinical studies has demonstrated that excessive tidal volumes (VTs), rather than high inflating pressure, are responsible for ventilator-induced lung injury in infants.
- Volume-targeted ventilation (VTV), compared with pressure-limited ventilation, reduces the risk of hypocarbia and several neonatal complications including the combined outcome of death or bronchopulmonary dysplasia at 36 weeks of corrected gestation.
- VTV is an adaptive ventilation mode that uses the expired VT of the previous inflation to determine the inflating pressure used for the next inflation resulting in significant breath-to-breath variability of both the inflating pressure and the VT as a baby breathes.
- Modern ventilators have mechanisms built in their software to mitigate the effect of significant endotracheal tube leak and patient–ventilator interactions during VTV.
- VTV can be used with different triggered ventilator modes including assist control ventilation, synchronized intermittent mandatory ventilation, and pressure support ventilation.

## INTRODUCTION

The use of tidal volume-targeted ventilation (VTV), often called volume guarantee (VG), on neonatal intensive care units has increased significantly over the last decade.[1,2] This is due to wider availability of ventilators offering VTV, more awareness of the lung damage caused by excessive VTs, the clinical benefits VTV offers, and improvement in clinicians' understanding of this mode. Nonetheless, the apparent complexity of this adaptive ventilation mode still deters some neonatologists and they turn off volume targeting when the ventilator produces frequent alarms or shows "unusual" ventilator parameters or with an unexpectedly poor blood gas.

Neonatal Intensive Care Unit, The Rosie Hospital, Cambridge University Hospitals NHS Foundation Trust, Cambridge, UK
* Corresponding author. The Rosie Hospital, Box 402, Robinson Way, Cambridge CB2 0QQ, United Kingdom.
E-mail address: gbelteki@aol.com

Clin Perinatol 48 (2021) 825–841
https://doi.org/10.1016/j.clp.2021.08.001
0095-5108/21/© 2021 Elsevier Inc. All rights reserved.
perinatology.theclinics.com

The objective of this review is to further neonatal clinicians' understanding of VTV. First, we provide a background how neonatal ventilation has evolved. Next, we summarize the evidence from experimental models and clinical studies supporting the use of VTV. Finally, we discuss practicalities of VTV including the choice of target expired tidal volume (VTe), other ventilator parameters, and how to deal with frequent ventilator alarms and with situations such as large endotracheal tube (ETT) leaks or hyperventilating infants.

## VTV: THE HISTORY
### The Old Days

The purpose of mechanical ventilation of a baby with respiratory failure is to ensure satisfactory oxygenation and carbon dioxide clearance. The commonest reasons for neonatal ventilation are prematurity with respiratory distress syndrome (RDS), neonatal infections, hypoxic–ischemic encephalopathy (HIE), and congenital malformations affecting the airways, lungs, or heart.

Historically, neonatal ventilation was time cycled and pressure limited (PLV), where the ventilator delivered an inflation with a peak inflating pressure (PIP), flow rate, ventilator rate, inflation time, or I:E ratio and inspired oxygen concentration ($Fio_2$), all set by the clinical staff and delivered through an ETT.[3] These were the only parameters set, measured, and displayed. The PIP was used to push an unknown VT into the lungs. The PIP was chosen by protocol or experience and then adjusted after observation of chest wall movements, the infant's breathing effort, and measurement of arterial blood gases. It was not possible with the ventilators available at the time to measure VT or control it. Also, as the ETTs used in babies are usually uncuffed, an unknown amount of the VT leaked around the ETT depending on the ETT diameter, lung compliance, airway resistance, and the PIP and positive end expiratory pressure (PEEP).

Spontaneous breathing between inflations was not supported by PEEP in the early days but was used later. Continuous flow in the ventilator circuit enabled an infant to take breaths between ventilator inflations. Because infants were ventilated at a set rate, they usually breathed out of synchrony with the ventilator and were often considered to be "fighting the ventilator". In retrospect, it was the ventilator fighting the baby because its inflations were unsynchronized with baby's breaths. To control this, babies were commonly treated with muscle relaxants. This stopped them breathing, but without spontaneous breaths, higher PIP had to be used. Muscle relaxants led to babies becoming edematous and unresponsive and made it difficult to assess when they could be weaned from ventilation.

PLV was the only mode available for many years. With all its shortcomings, it was successful compared with giving only oxygen, sodium bicarbonate, and glucose, which were associated with a high mortality. PLV is still used in some places where only simple ventilators are available or during neonatal transport.

### Modern Neonatal Ventilators

With microprocessor technology and sensitive flow sensors at the outer end of the ETT, most modern neonatal ventilators are able to detect the onset of a baby's inspiration, accurately measure inspiratory and expiratory VTs and trigger synchronized inflations. If VTV is turned on, it enables delivery of a more stable VT by varying the PIP breath by breath depending on a baby's breathing effort, changes in lung mechanics, and varying ETT leak.

Different makes of neonatal ventilators deliver VTV in different ways, and it may not be obvious how they do it. Also, it can be difficult to understand the terminology used by different manufacturers.

## GAS EXCHANGE DURING MECHANICAL VENTILATION
### Carbon Dioxide Clearance

In a spontaneously breathing baby, $CO_2$ is controlled by altering the VT or respiratory rate. A high and rising $Paco_2$ is due to reduced gas exchange caused by either a slow respiratory rate, apnea, or a low VT because of incompliant lungs from lack of surfactant, pulmonary edema, a chest wall that retracts with inspiration, a disease with loss of lung volume, such as diaphragmatic hernia or tension pneumothorax, or exhaustion. In normal lungs $CO_2$ easily crosses the alveolar epithelium to the capillaries, but this is reduced if there is proteinaceous exudate, called hyaline membranes, on the alveolar surface and associated atelectasis.

In a ventilated baby, controlling $Paco_2$ requires adjusting VT and sometimes the ventilator rate. However, if a baby also breathes spontaneously, a set ventilator rate will be out of synchrony with the varying respiratory rate of the baby.[4] Even when the ventilator inflations are synchronized with a baby's inspirations, there is no set PIP that can deliver a known VT because it continually changes with the variable depth of spontaneous breaths, variable leak around the ETT, changes in lung compliance and resistance, or by a baby contracting the abdominal muscles and reducing the delivered VT.[5] When a set PIP is used, with a breathing baby, the delivered VT can vary from low to very high if a baby takes a large breath simultaneously with an inflation. This may damage the lungs.[6] The effect of a ventilator inflation and spontaneous breath augmenting the VT is usually unrecognized with PLV. This may cause increased clearance of $CO_2$ to low levels (<30 mm Hg) and may decrease cerebral blood flow and cause brain ischemia.[7,8]

### Oxygenation

Oxygenation can be improved by (1) increasing the $Fio_2$, (2) treating with surfactant if deficiency is suspected, and (3) increasing mean airway pressure (MAP), for example, by using continuous positive airway pressure (CPAP) or PEEP to improve the surface area for gas exchange and reduce atelectasis during expiration. In practice, increasing PEEP is probably the safest and most effective way to achieve an appropriate lung volume, in part because usually the longest part of a ventilation cycle is the expiratory phase.[9,10] Alveolar volume is normally supported by surfactant counteracting the surface tension of alveolar fluid and the elastic recoil of the tissues. In an infant with RDS, surfactant treatment increases the alveolar surface area and thereby oxygenation. However, without adequate surfactant and PEEP, with stiff lungs, a pliable chest wall retracts during inspiration and the lung cannot maintain an effective end expiratory volume. Unintubated babies help maintain lung volume by shortening their expiratory time or grunting using laryngeal expiratory braking.[11]

Ventilatory strategies for a baby with respiratory failure should include an "open lung strategy", avoidance of a high VT and $Fio_2$. An adequate pulmonary blood flow is essential for good gas exchange. Low pulmonary blood flow may be due to hypotension, persistent pulmonary hypertension of the newborn, or congenital cardiac anomalies. These need to be investigated by blood pressure recording, chest x-ray, and echocardiography and treated appropriately. It is important to appreciate that treating hypoxia is not simply about altering VT or ventilation rate.

## VTV: THE EVIDENCE

Ventilator-induced lung injury (VILI) has been known for many years. Sladen and colleagues[12] reported more than 50 years ago that patients ventilated for long periods suffered from deteriorating lung function with a fall in respiratory compliance and increased alveolar–arterial oxygen gradient. Initially, VILI was thought to be due to barotrauma caused by positive pressure ventilation. However, later experimental and clinical data pointed toward the importance of large VTs and excessive supplemental oxygen as the main causes in infants.[13,14]

### Laboratory Studies

A study in ventilated goats demonstrated that animals can be ventilated for 2 weeks without severe lung damage if low PIP and no extra oxygen were used.[15] In another study, using rats, higher PIP was associated with development of more rapid and more severe lung edema than lower PIP.[16] Although these studies in sedated and apneic animals demonstrated the significance of inflating pressures, they could not distinguish if the lung damage is caused directly by the high PIP or by the resultant large VTs.

To differentiate between these possibilities, Dreyfuss and colleagues[17] ventilated rats with large or small VTs using a PIP of 45 cmH$_2$O. Low VT ventilation with a high PIP was obtained by limiting thoracoabdominal movement by strapping the animal's chest. The rats subjected to high VTs and high PIP developed pulmonary edema with ultrastructural abnormalities. Strapped animals ventilated with a high PIP but a normal VT had no edema, and the ultrastructure of the lungs appeared normal. This suggested that high VT is responsible for ventilator-induced pulmonary edema and not the high PIP *per se*. Hernandez *and colleagues*[18] ventilated young rabbits at 15, 30, and 45 cmH$_2$O PIP and also at the same PIPs but with chest movement restricted. The capillary filtration coefficient of the lungs, removed after ventilation, was normal in animals ventilated at 15 cmH$_2$O, increased by 31% at 30 cmH$_2$O and by 430% at 45 cmH$_2$O in animals without VT restriction. Restricting chest movement stopped the increase in the filtration coefficient even at the highest PIP.[18] Adkins *and colleagues*[19] observed that the capillary infiltration coefficient increased more in young rabbits than adults probably because the lung and chest wall compliance of the younger animals was higher, allowing greater distension for the same PIP.

In summary, these studies suggest that, at least in normal lungs and in sedated animals, a large VT rather than a high PIP is crucial in the development of VILI.

### Clinical Studies

A major problem with studies comparing different modes of neonatal ventilation is that few of the studies have used exactly the same ventilator modes or criteria, and there have been various levels of bias. There were different criteria for setting PIP, PEEP and backup rate, different gestational age of recruited babies, different ventilators, lack of blinding, variable criteria for success or failure, and different and usually only short-term clinical outcomes in the trials. Also, many studies recruited small numbers of babies and so had little power to show significant differences even in short-term clinical outcomes.[20,21]

Most of our experience and detailed data are from studying and recording Dräger Babylog 8000 and VN500 ventilators, (Dräger, Lübeck, Germany), although we also have some data from Fabian ventilators (Vyaire, Mettawa, IL, United States)

There have been a number of studies and reviews of VTV compared with PLV. The latest review by Klingenberg *and colleagues*[22] in 2017 included 20 studies. Most were of moderate to low quality and none were blinded. The most important results from this review were based on data from 8 to 12 studies including 584 to 771 infants, depending on the outcome of interest, and because not all studies had the same outcomes or measured them in the same ways. There was no significant difference in the primary outcome, death before hospital discharge, between VTV modes and PLV modes (typical relative risk [RR]: 0.75, 95% confidence interval [CI] = 0.53 to 1.07;

low quality evidence). However, there was moderate quality evidence that the use of VTV modes resulted in a reduction in the primary outcome, death or BPD (bronchopulmonary dysplasia) at 36 weeks' gestation (typical RR: 0.73, 95% CI = 0.59–0.89; typical number needed to benefit (NNTB) 8, 95% CI = 5 to 20) and the following secondary outcomes: rates of pneumothorax (typical RR: 0.52, 95% CI = 0.31–0.87; typical NNTB: 20, 95% CI = 11–100), mean days of mechanical ventilation (mean difference: −1.35 days, 95% CI = -1.83 to −0.86), rates of hypocarbia (typical RR: 0.49, 95% CI = 0.33–0.72; typical NNTB: 3, 95% CI = 2–5), rates of grade 3 or 4 intraventricular hemorrhage (typical RR: 0.53, 95% CI = 0.37–0.77; typical NNTB: 11, 95% CI = 7–25), and the combined outcome of periventricular leukomalacia with or without grade 3 or 4 intraventricular hemorrhage (typical RR: 0.47, 95% CI = 0.27–0.80; typical NNTB: 11, 95% CI = 7–33). Importantly, VTV modes were not associated with any increased adverse outcomes.

VTV can also be used during neonatal transport, and it reduces VTs, their variability, and the inflating pressures.[23] It is not known if it improves clinical outcomes.

## VTV: THE PRACTICALITIES
### The Mechanism of Volume Targeting

VTV, also known as VG, is different from volume-controlled ventilation. During volume-controlled (volume limited) ventilation, constant inspiratory flow is used to deliver a set inspired tidal volume (VTi). On modern ventilators, VTi is calculated by integrating the flow data measured by the proximal flow sensor during inspiration. This works in adults and older children who are intubated with cuffed ETTs. However, babies are intubated with uncuffed tubes because of concerns about tracheal damage caused by cuffed tubes and increased work of breathing due to increased airway resistance of narrow ETTs.[24,25] Uncuffed tubes are associated with variable and sometimes large leaks, when the actual VT (the difference between the volume of gas in the lungs at the end of inspiration and at the end of expiration) is significantly lower than the delivered "VTi". This has made primary volume control in infants problematic, although more success has been reported with newer ventilators.[26]

In contrast to volume-controlled ventilation, VTV is pressure controlled (pressure limited) for each inflation, that is, at each inflation, gas flow ends when a PIP is reached that the ventilator has calculated is needed to deliver the set expired tidal volume (VTe). The ventilator's microprocessor determines the VTe and compares it to the set target VTe. If VTe is lower than the target, the PIP of the next inflation is increased and *vice versa*. There is a separate ventilator algorithm for triggered (synchronized) and untriggered inflations because the former uses lower PIPs due to the baby's contribution to the (**Fig. 1**). The clinician has no control over each PIP used in VTV mode, except setting a maximum PIP (Pmax), which cannot be exceeded, even if the target VTe cannot be delivered with lower PIP.

### Variability of Tidal Volume and Inflating Pressure

As the PIP used for an inflation is based on the PIP and the VTe of the previous inflation of the same type, triggered or untriggered, it is unlikely this PIP will deliver exactly the target VTe during the next inflation. Therefore, during VTV, there is significant breath-to-breath variability of VTe (**Fig. 2A**). This variability is primarily due to the breath-to-breath variability in a baby's own respiratory effort. For example, a baby can make a stronger breath than the previous one, resulting in a VTe above the target. Alternatively, the infant may splint the chest, resulting in delivery of very little VT. This variability is less in babies receiving sedatives or muscle relaxants than in babies

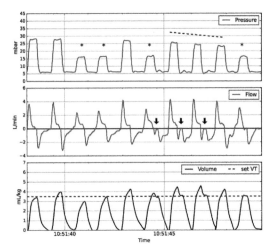

**Fig. 1.** This figure shows waves of pressure, flow and volume from a 14 s long recording of a term infant ventilated with AC-VG mode containing 10 inflations, 4 of them triggered (synchronized, marked with *asterisks*) and 6 untriggered (backup). The triggered inflations have PIPs ~17 mbar and the untriggered inflations PIPs ~28 mbar. During triggered inspirations, the infant has contributed to the VT with her own inhalations. The tidal volume was close to the targeted 3.5 mL/kg (dashed *line*) during both triggered and untriggered inflations. As the VTe of inflations 7 to 9 was above the target, the PIP was gradually reduced (marked with dashed *line*). Toward the end of the recording the baby takes small breaths, shown by the arrows, which interrupt the ventilator's expiratory flow (see **Fig. 5** for more details).

breathing normally. However, the average VTe is very close to the target VTe (**Fig. 2**B). Analyzing ventilator data downloaded with a high sampling rate, the average difference between the set and actual VTe was less than 1 mL/kg on several different neonatal ventilator models.[27–30] This stability of the VT is probably the reason for less variability in $Paco_2$ during VTV compared with PLV.[31]

Unlike stability of the VTe, the PIP varies significantly not only breath to breath but also in the longer term (**Fig. 2**C, D). Short-term variability of PIP is mostly due to patient–ventilator interactions. VTV algorithms usually do not allow PIP to change more than a few $cmH_2O$ from one inflation to the next, of the same type (triggered or untriggered), even if VTe deviates significantly from its target; this is to prevent sudden large changes in PIP. However, if VTe is repeatedly below the target, PIP may change significantly within 5 to 10 inflations. Also, if triggered and untriggered inflations alternate, there can be a large difference in the PIP of consecutive inflations due to the different algorithms the ventilator uses for them (see **Fig. 1**). Reducing the backup rate to below the spontaneous respiratory rate (to about 40/min) improves synchronization and reduces the variability in PIP if that was due to alternating triggered and untriggered inflations.[32]

Long-term variability of PIP reflects changes in the mechanics of the respiratory system, that is, increased or decreased compliance or airway resistance. This may be due to complications of mechanical ventilation (slippage or obstruction of the ETT, tension pneumothorax) or to progression or recovery of the lung disease.

### What Target Tidal Volumes Should Be Used

VTV targets VTe. VTe is used because if there is a leak around the ETT, some of the VTi is lost. Reviews usually suggest the use of VTe between 4 and 6 mL/kg for most

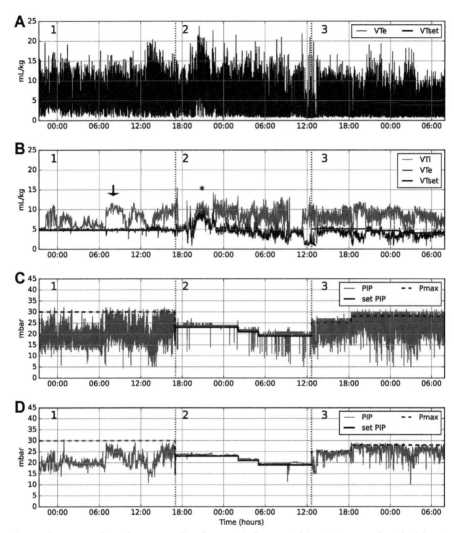

**Fig. 2.** This is a 34-hour-long recording from an infant weighing 690 g ventilated with AC-VG at the start and end sections but without VG in the middle section. VG was initially on (part 1) but turned off (part 2) because of large ETT leak. It was restarted for the last third (part 3) of the recording. When VG was on the set VTe (shown as horizontal black *line*) was 5 mL/kg, later gradually reduced to 4 mL/kg. (A) VTe of individual inflations (n = 210,870) show significant breath-to-breath variability, sometimes VTe is <1 mL/kg or greater than 10 mL/kg. This variability is due to the baby's own breathing and interaction with the ventilator inflations. (B). This graph shows the VTe of ventilator inflations averaged for each minute. During VG in part 1, the average VTe (blue *line*) was very close to the target value (black *line*), even when leak was ~50% (*arrow*). Because of the leak, the VTi (green *line*) is larger than the VTe, but very variable, as the ETT leak changes. When VG was turned off at part 2, the set PIP, about 23 mbar (see part C of this figure), was delivered for each inflation. The average VTe (blue *line*) became more variable, sometimes reaching 10 mL/kg when the leak was low (*asterisk*). When VG was turned back on, at part 3, the average VTe remained variable and below the target VT because the PIP continuously reached Pmax (see part C of this figure). (C). This shows the PIP of individual inflations over the same period. It shows significant variability during VG but not when the VG is turned off. The maximum allowed

babies.[33,34] Clinical studies of babies with different clinical conditions showed VTs in a similar range.[35–39] However, some of these studies were retrospective analyses, and the included patients received VTV, where clinicians setting the ventilators may have been influenced by similar recommendations. Moreover, VTs were measured in spontaneously breathing babies with a face mask or ETT and a flow sensor which may alter breathing patterns and add to the dead space. te Pas and colleagues,[40] investigated spontaneous breathing patterns of babies ≤32 weeks' gestation receiving CPAP of 8 cmH$_2$O at birth. There were five patterns. The mean (SD) VT for babies with a normal respiratory rate, not crying or panting, and unbraked expirations was 4.2 (1.5) mL/kg, and for those crying or grunting, it was 7.5 (4.2) mL/kg.

Infants with a large physiologic dead space (eg, meconium aspiration syndrome, BPD, or prolonged ventilation) may require larger VTs.[38,39,41] Interestingly, even in babies weighing less than 800 g, a VT of 5 to 6 mL/kg is enough to maintain normocapnia, which in their case is less than the instrumental dead space.[42] This suggests that other mechanisms of gas exchange rather than simple bulk gas flow need to be considered.[43]

Choosing the target VTe at the start of VTV is not an exact science. Initially, a set VTe around 5 mL/kg with an appropriate ventilator rate will suit most babies; blood gases need to be checked early to see if there is hypocarbia or hypercarbia because ventilation also depends on a baby's variable spontaneous breathing effort and rate. Weaning VT should be based on good blood gases, the stability of a baby's breathing pattern and VTs during a 30-s spontaneous breathing test.[44] There is no need to wean all babies to <5 mL/kg before extubation, as infants with severe BPD may have a larger physiologic dead space.[39,41]

### How to Set the Maximum Peak Inflating Pressure (Pmax) During VTV

With VTV, where the ventilator adjusts the PIP inflation by inflation to try and optimize VTe, the Pmax has to be set. This is a PIP which the ventilator cannot exceed. If it is too low, the set Pmax level may prevent the target VTe being delivered. It has been suggested that Pmax should be set 5 to 10 cmH$_2$O above the "working PIP" based on expert advice rather than evidence.[22,45] The difficulty is that due to the large variability of PIP during VTV, it is hard to define a working PIP (see **Fig. 2**C, D). We have shown that keeping Pmax 5 mbar (~5 cmH$_2$O) above the "usual" (most frequently occurring) PIP results in greater than 10% of inflations reaching Pmax, and the target VTe is not being delivered.[28] In our opinion, Pmax should be regarded as an alarm to notify the clinician about worsening lung function or complications of ventilation such as tube obstruction or pneumothorax. It is not a device to limit the VTe because that may cause underventilation. If there are concerns about the VTe being too high, a lower target VTe should be set if effective ventilation can be assured.

There is a trade-off between setting Pmax too low and limiting VTe delivery and setting it too high and risking late recognition of worsening lung disease or complications. The Pmax setting needs to be individualized; there is no default setting which is

---

inflating pressure (Pmax) is shown as a dashed black line. During part 1, PIP is close to Pmax when leak is large. During part 3, Pmax is set at a lower level and is constantly reached by PIP. This causes the VTe to be below the set VTe (see Part B of the figure). (D). This graph shows the average PIP for each minute. During part 1, the average PIP was 5 to 10 mbar below Pmax. During part 2 when VG was off, PIP was very close to the set PIP. During part 3 with the VG turned back on, the average PIP reached or was very close to Pmax.

good for all babies; but in our opinion, 10 mbar (~10 mmHg) above the mean PIP works for most babies. A very variable PIP (eg, in infants with BPD) may warrant a higher Pmax.

### The Effect of Leak Around the Endotracheal Tube

If there is no leak around the ETT, the VTi and VTe are equal. However, as uncuffed tubes are usually used during neonatal ventilation, there is often some leak of gas around the ETT.[46] With a leak, VTi is larger than VTe, as the gas escaping from the airways outside the ETT is not included in the VTe. In addition to the leak during inspiration, there is also some leak during expiration, as the pressure in the airways is always above atmospheric pressure during positive pressure ventilation when using PEEP. The actual VT will be lower than the measured VTi but higher than the VTe because the gas leaking during expiration was present in the lung at the end of inspiration and was part of the actual VT (**Fig. 3**).

During VTV, a large leak needs careful diagnosis and management. The ventilator will try to maintain the VTe at the set level by increasing the PIP until it reaches Pmax when a "low VT" alarm is triggered. This typically happens when the leak exceeds 50%.[29,47] Clinicians frequently respond by turning off VTV and using PLV with a set PIP. However, this can lead to excessive VTs and overventilation if the leak is variable or later decreases (see **Fig. 2**). An alternative is to upsize the ETT to ensure less leak. We note that many infants who tolerate a large leak can be successfully extubated unless they have an obstructed airway or inconsistent breathing effort.

The Dräger Babylog VN500 ventilator offers the opportunity to target "leak compensated" VT, which is the VTe plus the estimated leak during expiration. With this option, VT can be maintained at the target level even with a 90% leak (see **Fig. 3**).[47] Of note, this terminology is confusing because "leak compensation" is also used by manufacturers for ventilators automatically increasing their trigger threshold in case of a large leak because in this situation there is a continuous inward flow through the ETT between inflations which might otherwise cause autotriggering.

A large leak through an active chest drain represents a similar situation and causes similar challenges during VTV as a large leak around the ETT.

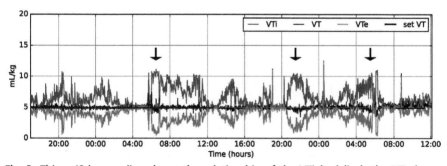

**Fig. 3.** This ~43-h recording shows the relationship of the VTi (red *line*), the VTe (green *line*), and now the leak-compensated expired tidal volume (VT) (blue *line*), which includes leak during expiration. When there is no leak, between the first 04:00 and 06:00, VTi, VT and VTe are very similar. With significant leak round the ETT, VT is less than VTi but more than VTe. VT can be maintained close to the target value even when the leak is ~80% (*arrows*). Importantly, VT is calculated by the ventilator as VTe plus an estimated leak during expiration because only VTi and VTe can be directly determined from the flow sensor data.

## Ventilator Interactions with an Infant's Breathing

During synchronized inflations, flow and VT are due to the combined work of (1) the ventilator generating a pressure gradient between the proximal airway and the alveoli and (2) the baby's inspiration generating a pressure gradient between the intrapleural space and the airway.[32] To ensure the target VTe is delivered, the ventilator needs to adapt to the strength of each breath. Because synchronized and backup inflations can follow each other, or alternate, VTV algorithms use a higher PIP for a backup inflation than for a synchronized one (see **Fig. 1**).

If a ventilated baby breathes hard but has normal work of breathing, the VTe can exceed the target VTe, and so the VTV algorithm will gradually reduce the PIP to near the PEEP level until the VTe matches its target (**Fig. 4**). Concerns have been raised that this is like giving endotracheal CPAP (ET-CPAP), which might cause exhaustion, hypercapnia, and acidosis.[31,34] However, no evidence has been presented to support this concern, and, in our experience, it does not happen during clinical practice. Firstly, this occurs only in babies who can generate the VT quickly and easily with large breaths and near normal lungs and are unlikely to get tired. Second, although this looks like ET-CPAP, it is fundamentally different because the ventilator analyzes the VTe after each inflation, determines whether the target VTe has been achieved, and, if not, it increases the PIP of the next inflations to deliver the set VTe. Nonetheless, the significance of this situation needs to be assessed in clinical studies. In our experience, when PIP less than 3 cmH$_2$O above PEEP, the SpO$_2$ and TcCO$_2$ are usually better than with higher PIP. If the baby continues to breathe regularly and the ETT is not required to overcome an upper airway obstruction, the infant can be extubated.

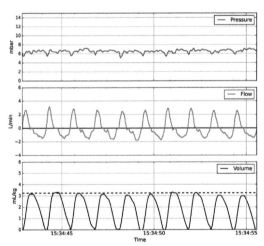

**Fig. 4.** This recording shows volume targeted ventilation in a term infant ventilated for hypoxic ischemic encephalopathy with SIMV-VG mode. The inflating pressure was low and similar to PEEP. This infant had normal lungs and was spontaneously hyperventilating to try to lower the Paco$_2$ as a response to the metabolic acidosis. The target VTe was at 3.25 mL/kg (dashed *line*). As the infant generated the set VTe alone, the VG algorithm has reduced the PIP of the triggered ventilator inflations to PEEP level. Please note that the set ventilator rate was 30/min. The infant's breathing rate here is ~60/min. Triggered SIMV inflations and spontaneous breaths cannot be distinguished from each other on the graph. The Paco$_2$ was in the normal range.

A safety mechanism to prevent large VTs during synchronized inflations is that the ventilator immediately stops an inflation when the VTi significantly (eg, >130%) exceeds the target VTe, provided there is no large leak. These inflations have a inspiratory time (Ti) shorter than the set Ti and a peaked appearance of the pressure waveform because the inflation has been stopped early (**Fig. 5**). Importantly, the ventilator does not prevent a baby taking a large breath because there is a continuous gas flow in the ventilator circuit. Therefore, breathing infants can have inflations with a VTe greater than 10 mL/kg even when the target VT is set at 5 mL/kg (see **Fig. 2A**).

Interrupted expirations, where a baby breathes in during ventilator expiration, can occur in some infants ventilated with VTV, particularly when the Ti of ventilator inflations is short (see **Fig. 5**). A study of 10 infants showed that interrupted expirations occurred in 2.2% of triggered and 3.3% of nontriggered inflations.[5] Expiratory flow is interrupted by a small, short inspiration within the 0.2 second refractory period of the ventilator, followed by the rest of expiration. The VG software interprets the small "interrupting" inspiration, early in expiration, as the end of expiration and the start of a new inflation. Because only a small proportion of expiratory flow has occurred by that time, an inappropriately small VTe is calculated for that inflation. Review of video recordings showed this was not due to hiccups, movement, handling, or crying. The causes have not been elucidated.

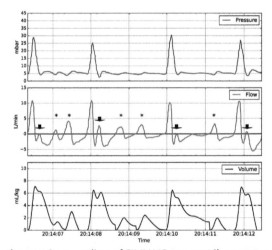

**Fig. 5.** This figure shows a 6-s recording of SIMV-VG at a ventilator rate of 30/min in a term infant ventilated for respiratory distress, sepsis, and hypoxic ischemic encephalopathy. It shows large tidal volumes, interrupted inspirations and expirations. The strong breathing effort of the baby was generating tidal volumes ~6 mL/kg, although the target VTe only 4 mL/kg (dashed *line*). The VG algorithm of the ventilator interrupts an inflation when the VTi exceeds 130% of the target VTe provided there is no large leak. It can be seen from the pressure recording that the ventilator inflations have been shortened (<0.3 seconds) and sharply peaked despite the set Ti being 0.4 seconds. The infant's inspirations continue beyond these short inflations and interrupt ventilator expirations (*arrows*), separating the expiratory flow into two parts. The effect of each inspiration can be seen as a small reduction in ventilator pressure. Please note that despite the large tidal volumes, the ventilator does not reduce the PIP of the following inflation because the VTV algorithm interprets the first part of the expiration as the main expiration with a lower VTe. Between ventilators, there are spontaneous breaths, shown by asterisks, which are not associated with any pressure rise above the PEEP level.

### Combination of VTV with Different Ventilator Modes

VTV only works with synchronized modes. A calibrated proximal flow sensor is required both for synchronized ventilation (to detect the infant's breathing effort) and for VTV (to calculate VTs from flow data). VTV can be used with synchronized intermittent mandatory ventilation (SIMV-VG), synchronized intermittent positive pressure ventilation (SIPPV-VG), also known as assist-control (AC-VG) or patient-triggered ventilation, and pressure support ventilation (PSV-VG). If an infant becomes apneic, the ventilator delivers volume-targeted mandatory inflations at the set backup rate.

SIMV-VG and SIPPV-VG are time cycled, that is, the inspiratory phase of the ventilator inflation ends when the set Ti finishes. If Ti is set too long, there is a period of inspiratory pressure hold with no gas flow until the end of the Ti (**Fig. 6**A). If Ti is set short, the VG algorithm can only deliver the target VTe by increasing the PIP; in this case, increasing the Ti will reduce the PIP while maintaining the MAP. When setting Ti, care should be taken to ensure enough time is available for expiration to avoid auto-PEEP, also known as dynamic hyperinflation.[48,49]

During SIMV-VG, only a set number of volume-targeted inflations are delivered. Between inflations, the baby can breathe from the continuous flow of the ventilator circuit

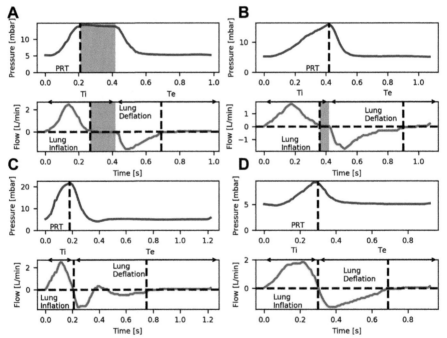

**Fig. 6.** This figure shows pairs of pressure and flow waves, with different pressure rise times (PRTs) during SIPPV-VG (*A-B*) and PSV-VG (*C-D*) modes. On the pressure waves, the end of each pressure rise is marked by a dashed vertical line, followed by a pressure plateau, if present, highlighted by shading. On the flow waves, the end of lung inflation and lung deflation are marked by dashed vertical lines; inspiratory hold, if present, is highlighted by shading. Inspiratory and expiratory times are showed by arrows above the flow waves. (*A*). SIPPV-VG with short (0.08 s) PRT. (*B*). SIPPV-VG with long (0.4 s) PRT; Ti was 0.4 s in both cases. (*C*). PSV-VG with short (0.08 s) PRT. (*D*). PSV-VG with long (0.4 s) PRT; Timax was 0.6 s in both cases. (*From* Chong D, Kayser S, Szakmar E, Morley CJ, Belteki G. Effect of pressure rise time on ventilator parameters and gas exchange during neonatal ventilation. Pediatr Pulmonol. 2020 May;55(5):1131-1138, with permission.)

(see **Fig. 5**). Spontaneous breaths can be optionally pressure supported with a pressure set by the clinicians. The VT and inspiratory time are not controlled by the ventilator. When using a low ventilator rate, spontaneous breaths between inflations contribute more to the minute ventilation during SIMV-VG than during SIMV without VG.[23,50] The clinical significance of this is unknown.

Unlike SIMV-VG, SIPPV-VG delivers inflations synchronized to each of a baby's inspirations as long as they reach the trigger threshold. The number of inflations may exceed the set ventilator rate. To avoid a very high ventilator rate, most manufacturers incorporate a "refractory period" after ventilator inflations, usually 0.1 to 0.2 seconds, during which another inflation cannot be triggered. Although it is commonly suggested that babies with respiratory distress syndrome (RDS) breathe about 60/min, it is common to see greater than 80/min in preterm infants with RDS and greater than 100/min in hyperventilating term babies with HIE and metabolic acidosis.

When assessing if enough expiratory time is available during SIPPV-VG, it is important to consider the actual ventilator rate, which can be significantly higher than the set backup rate. A fast rate is commonly driven by babies with lung disease specifically to shorten the expiratory time and stop the lung volume falling too low. In principle, it is possible to reduce the actual ventilator rate by increasing the trigger threshold; however, this can lead to a delay in triggering an inflation and patient–ventilator asynchrony. We suggest the most sensitive trigger threshold is always used, usually 0.1 to 0.2 L/min.

PSV-VG is flow cycled rather than time cycled, that is, ventilator inflation ends when flow drops to a fraction of the peak inspiratory flow, for example, 15%, which can be adjusted on some ventilators. The term "pressure support" can be confusing as it is also used for augmenting spontaneous breaths during SIMV (see above). During PSV-VG, Ti varies from breath to breath, but it is limited by a clinician set Timax. In babies with noncompliant lungs, the spontaneous Ti can be short (<0.3 seconds), particularly in infants with reduced lung compliance and a short time constant. Due to the logic of the mode, PIP holds and shortened expiratory time will not occur with PSV-VG, making this mode potentially useful for infants with increased airway resistance and a long time constant. Importantly, similar to SIPPV-VG, PSV-VG enables inflations synchronized to all breaths reaching the trigger threshold.

Mandatory minute ventilation (MMV) is a volume-targeted mode where the ventilator dynamically changes the rate of ventilator inflations to ensure a minute ventilation set by the clinician. MMV corresponds to SIMV-VG with a dynamic ventilator rate. If the baby has strong or frequent spontaneous breaths between ventilator inflations, the ventilator rate is reduced automatically, and the infant is responsible for most of the minute ventilation. Although MMV is potentially useful to prevent hypocapnia and as a weaning mode, there are few reports on its use in neonates, and they used older ventilator models than the ones available today.[51,52]

## Pressure Rise Time

A frequently overlooked set ventilator parameter during VTV is the pressure rise time (PRT, also known as slope time), which is the time from the beginning of pressure rise to when the PIP is reached. On older ventilators, the user sets the inspiratory flow rate (typically between 4–10 L/min) which implicitly defines the PRT. A long slope time or low circuit flow may be associated with insufficient inspiratory flow and "gas hunger" in large babies during deep breaths. There is also a concern that a high inspiratory flow rate associated with short PRT can cause airway damage due to stretching the airways and alveoli too quickly, called rheotrauma. However, this has only been demonstrated so far in animal studies using very high flow rates.[53]

PRT affects the characteristics of ventilator waveforms both during time-cycled and flow-cycled ventilation. During SIPPV-VG or SIMV-VG, a short slope time can result in a PIP hold and a higher MAP (see **Fig. 6**A). During PSV-VG, a longer PRT increases Ti and lowers the PIP (see **Fig. 6**B).[54] The clinical significance of using different PRTs in neonatal ventilation is unknown.

## 6: SUMMARY

VTV is available on most modern neonatal ventilators, and its use is supported by physiologic considerations and human trials showing improvement in several important clinical outcomes with no adverse effects compared with PLV. VTV should be the default neonatal ventilation mode. It can be used in most clinical situations including moderate leak or strong patient breathing effort. The comparison of different volume targeted modes (SIPPV, SIMV, PSV, MMV), the impact of spontaneous breathing, and ideal duration of pressure rise time warrant further investigations.

---

**Best Practices**

- Lung injury in ventilated infants is primarily due to excessive tidal volumes rather than high inflating pressures.
- Compared with pressure limited ventilation, volume-targeted ventilation improves several long-term clinical outcomes in preterm infants.
- During volume-targeted ventilation the expired tidal volume is maintained close to a target value set by the clinician.
- Although 4-6 mL/kg target tidal volume works for most babies, some infants require higher tidal volumes.
- There is always some variability in the expired tidal volume during volume-targeted ventilation, particularly in babies who are breathing and interacting with the ventilator.
- Hyperventilating infants can take breaths from the ventilator's circuit with much larger tidal volumes than the target VT.
- Most infants who tolerate a large leak around the endotracheal tube can be successfully extubated if they have consistent breathing effort and they do not have airway obstruction.

---

## DISCLOSURE

C.J. Morley is a consultant to Fisher and Paykel Healthcare, Auckland, New Zealand. Gusztav Belteki is a consultant to Vyaire, Mettawa, IL, United States, and Dräger Medical, Lübeck, Germany.

## ACKNOWLEDGMENTS

The authors thank to Thomas Krueger, Kreske Brunckhorst, and the engineers of Dräger Medical for help to export data from the ventilator. We thank to Roland Hotz, Rainer Kühner, and the engineers of Vyaire for their help to export data from the Fabian ventilator.

## REFERENCES

1. van Kaam AH, Rimensberger PC, Borensztajn D, et al, Neovent Study Group. Ventilation practices in the neonatal intensive care unit: a cross-sectional study. J Pediatr 2010;157(5):767–71.e3.

2. Gupta A, Keszler M. Survey of ventilation practices in the neonatal intensive care Units of the United States and Canada: use of volume-targeted ventilation and Barriers to its Use. Am J Perinatol 2019;36(5):484–9.

3. Ramsden CA, Reynolds EO. Ventilator settings for newborn infants. Arch Dis Child 1987;62(5):529–38.

4. Ramanathan R. Synchronized intermittent mandatory ventilation and pressure support: to sync or not to sync? Pressure support or no pressure support? J Perinatol 2005;25(Suppl 2):S23–7.

5. McCallion N, Lau R, Dargaville PA, et al. Volume guarantee ventilation, interrupted expiration, and expiratory braking. Arch Dis Child 2005;90(8):865–70.

6. Martherus T, Oberthuer A, Dekker J, et al. Supporting breathing of preterm infants at birth: a narrative review. Arch Dis Child Fetal Neonatal Ed 2019;104(1):F102–7.

7. Greisen G, Munck H, Lou H. Severe hypocarbia in preterm infants and neurodevelopmental deficit. Acta Paediatr Scand 1987;76(3):401–4.

8. Klinger G, Beyene J, Shah P, et al. Do hyperoxaemia and hypocapnia add to the risk of brain injury after intrapartum asphyxia? Arch Dis Child Fetal Neonatal Ed 2005;90(1):F49–52.

9. Monkman S, Kirpalani H. Peep - a "cheap" and effective lung protection. Paediatr Respir Rev 2003;4(1):15–20.

10. Probyn ME, Hooper SB, Dargaville PA, et al. Positive end expiratory pressure during resuscitation of premature lambs rapidly improves blood gases without adversely affecting arterial pressure. Pediatr Res 2004;56(2):198–204.

11. Kosch PC, Stark AR. Dynamic maintenance of end-expiratory lung volume in full-term infants. J Appl Physiol Respir Environ Exerc Physiol 1984;57(4):1126–33.

12. Sladen A, Laver MB, Pontoppidan H. Pulmonary complications and water retention in prolonged mechanical ventilation. N Engl J Med 1968;279(9):448–53.

13. Dreyfuss D, Saumon G. Ventilator-induced lung injury: lessons from experimental studies. Am J Respir Crit Care Med 1998;157(1):294–323.

14. Wispe JR, Roberts RJ. Molecular basis of pulmonary oxygen toxicity. Clin Perinatol 1987;14(3):651–66.

15. Nash G, Blennerhassett JB, Pontoppidan H. Pulmonary lesions associated with oxygen therapy and artifical ventilation. N Engl J Med 1967;276(7):368–74.

16. Webb HH, Tierney DF. Experimental pulmonary edema due to intermittent positive pressure ventilation with high inflation pressures. Protection by positive end-expiratory pressure. Am Rev Respir Dis 1974;110(5):556–65.

17. Dreyfuss D, Soler P, Basset G, et al. High inflation pressure pulmonary edema. Respective effects of high airway pressure, high tidal volume, and positive end-expiratory pressure. Am Rev Respir Dis 1988;137(5):1159–64.

18. Hernandez LA, Peevy KJ, Moise AA, et al. Chest wall restriction limits high airway pressure-induced lung injury in young rabbits. J Appl Physiol (1985) 1989;66(5):2364–8.

19. Adkins WK, Hernandez LA, Coker PJ, et al. Age effects susceptibility to pulmonary barotrauma in rabbits. Crit Care Med 1991;19(3):390–3.

20. Chowdhury O, Patel DS, Hannam S, et al. Randomised trial of volume-targeted ventilation versus pressure-limited ventilation in acute respiratory failure in prematurely born infants. Neonatology 2013;104:290–4.

21. Sinha SK, Donn SM, Gavey J, et al. Randomised trial of volume controlled versus time cycled, pressure limited ventilation in preterm infants with respiratory distress syndrome. Arch Dis Child Fetal Neonatal Ed 1997;77(3):F202–5.

22. Klingenberg C, Wheeler KI, McCallion N, et al. Volume-targeted versus pressure-limited ventilation in neonates. Cochrane Database Syst Rev 2017;10(10): CD003666.

23. Belteki G, Szell A, Lantos L, et al. Volume guaranteed ventilation during neonatal transport. Pediatr Crit Care Med 2019;20(12):1170–6.

24. Thomas RE, Rao SC, Minutillo C, et al. Cuffed endotracheal tubes in infants less than 3 kg: a retrospective cohort study. Paediatr Anaesth 2018;28(3):204–9.

25. Thomas J, Weiss M, Cannizzaro V, et al. Work of breathing for cuffed and uncuffed pediatric endotracheal tubes in an in vitro lung model setting. Paediatr Anaesth 2018;28(9):780–7.

26. Singh J, Sinha SK, Clarke P, et al. Mechanical ventilation of very low birth weight infants: is volume or pressure a better target variable? J Pediatr 2006;149(3): 308–13.

27. Farrell O, Perkins EJ, Black D, et al. Volume guaranteed? Accuracy of a volume-targeted ventilation mode in infants. Arch Dis Child Fetal Neonatal Ed 2018; 103(2):F120–5.

28. Szakmar E, Morley CJ, Belteki G. Analysis of peak inflating pressure and inflating pressure limit during neonatal volume guaranteed ventilation. J Perinatol 2019; 39(1):72–9.

29. Belteki G, Széll A, Lantos L, et al. Volume-targeted ventilation with a Fabian ventilator: maintenance of tidal volumes and blood $CO_2$. Arch Dis Child Fetal Neonatal Ed 2020;105(3):253–8.

30. Wong S, Wang H, Tepper R, et al. Expired tidal volume variation in extremely low birth weight and very low birth weight infants on volume-targeted ventilation. J Pediatr 2019;207:248–51.e1.

31. Keszler M, Abubakar K. Volume guarantee: stability of tidal volume and incidence of hypocarbia. Pediatr Pulmonol 2004;38(3):240–5.

32. McCallion N, Lau R, Morley CJ, et al. Neonatal volume guarantee ventilation: effects of spontaneous breathing, triggered and untriggered inflations. Arch Dis Child Fetal Neonatal Ed 2008;93(1):F36–9.

33. Sun Y, Zhang H. Ventilation strategies in transition from neonatal respiratory distress to chronic lung disease. Semin Fetal Neonatal Med 2019;24(5):101035.

34. Keszler M. Volume-targeted ventilation: one size does not fit all. Evidence-based recommendations for successful use. Arch Dis Child Fetal Neonatal Ed 2019; 104(1):F108–12.

35. Dawson C, Davies MW. Volume-targeted ventilation and arterial carbon dioxide in neonates. J Paediatr Child Health 2005;41(9–10):518–21.

36. Shah S, Kaul A. Volume targeted ventilation and arterial carbon dioxide in extremely preterm infants. J Neonatal Perinatal Med 2013;6(4):339–44.

37. Sharma S, Clark S, Abubakar K, et al. Tidal volume requirement in mechanically ventilated infants with meconium aspiration syndrome. Am J Perinatol 2015; 32(10):916–9.

38. Sharma S, Abubakar KM, Keszler M. Tidal volume in infants with congenital diaphragmatic hernia supported with conventional mechanical ventilation. Am J Perinatol 2015;32(6):577–82.

39. Keszler M, Nassabeh-Montazami S, Abubakar K. Evolution of tidal volume requirement during the first 3 weeks of life in infants <800 g ventilated with Volume Guarantee. Arch Dis Child Fetal Neonatal Ed 2009;94(4):F279–82.

40. te Pas AB, Davis PG, Kamlin CO, et al. Spontaneous breathing patterns of very preterm infants treated with continuous positive airway pressure at birth. Pediatr Res 2008;64(3):281–5.

41. Abman SH, Collaco JM, Shepherd EG, et al. Interdisciplinary care of children with severe bronchopulmonary dysplasia. J Pediatr 2017;18:12–28.e1.
42. Nassabeh-Montazami S, Abubakar KM, Keszler M. The impact of instrumental dead-space in volume-targeted ventilation of the extremely low birth weight (ELBW) infant. Pediatr Pulmonol 2009;44(2):128–33.
43. Hurley EH, Keszler M. Effect of inspiratory flow rate on the efficiency of carbon dioxide removal at tidal volumes below instrumental dead space. Arch Dis Child Fetal Neonatal Ed 2017;102(2):F126–30.
44. Kamlin CO, Davis PG, Argus B, et al. A trial of spontaneous breathing to determine the readiness for extubation in very low birth weight infants: a prospective evaluation. Arch Dis Child Fetal Neonatal Ed 2008;93(4):F305–6.
45. Keszler M, Abubakar KM. Volume guarantee ventilation. Clin Perinatol 2007; 34(1):107–vii.
46. Mahmoud RA, Proquitté H, Fawzy N, et al. Tracheal tube airleak in clinical practice and impact on tidal volume measurement in ventilated neonates. Pediatr Crit Care Med 2011;12(2):197–202.
47. Szakmar E, Morley CJ, Belteki G. Leak compensation during volume guarantee with the Dräger babylog VN500 neonatal ventilator. Pediatr Crit Care Med 2018;19(9):861–8.
48. Laghi F, Goyal A. Auto-PEEP in respiratory failure. Minerva Anestesiol 2012;78(2): 201–21.
49. Napolitano N, Jalal K, McDonough JM, et al. Identifying and treating intrinsic PEEP in infants with severe bronchopulmonary dysplasia. Pediatr Pulmonol 2019;54(7):1045–51.
50. Herrera CM, Gerhardt T, Claure N, et al. Effects of volume-guaranteed synchronized intermittent mandatory ventilation in preterm infants recovering from respiratory failure. Pediatrics 2002;110(3):529–33.
51. Claure N, Gerhardt T, Hummler H, et al. Computer-controlled minute ventilation in preterm infants undergoing mechanical ventilation. J Pediatr 1997;131(6):910–3.
52. Guthrie SO, Lynn C, Lafleur BJ, et al. A crossover analysis of mandatory minute ventilation compared to synchronized intermittent mandatory ventilation in neonates. J Perinatol 2005;25(10):643–6.
53. Bach KP, Kuschel CA, Hooper SB, et al. High bias gas flows increase lung injury in the ventilated preterm lamb. PLoS One 2012;7(10):e47044.
54. Chong D, Kayser S, Szakmar E, et al. Effect of pressure rise time on ventilator parameters and gas exchange during neonatal ventilation. Pediatr Pulmonol 2020; 55(5):1131–8.

# New Modes of Respiratory Support for the Premature Infant: Automated Control of Inspired Oxygen Concentration

Nelson Claure, MSc, PhD*, Eduardo Bancalari, MD

## KEYWORDS

- Premature infant • Intermittent hypoxemia • Hyperoxemia • Automated
- Supplemental oxygen

## KEY POINTS

- Owing to their respiratory instability premature infants show frequent episodes of intermittent hypoxemia. This, combined with limitations on staff availability, affects maintenance of $Spo_2$ within the target range.
- Tolerance of hyperoxemia in premature infants receiving supplemental oxygen is common.
- Automated $Fio_2$ control has been shown to be effective in reducing the more severe episodes of intermittent hypoxemia and the time spent in hyperoxemia, thereby improving the maintenance of $Spo_2$ within the target range compared with manual $Fio_2$ control.
- Randomized clinical trials will determine the beneficial effects or disadvantages of using automated $Fio_2$ control for longer periods on ophthalmic, respiratory, and neurodevelopmental outcomes in extremely premature infants.

Extremely premature infants present with persistent respiratory instability during the postnatal period and require oxygen supplementation to maintain adequate arterial oxygen saturation (oxygen saturation as measured by pulse oximetry [$Spo_2$]) levels. Supplemental oxygen is the most common form of respiratory support in this population and usually lasts for weeks or months. Caregivers target clinically recommended ranges of $Spo_2$ by manually adjusting the fraction of inspired oxygen ($Fio_2$), but consistent maintenance of $Spo_2$ within these ranges is not frequently achieved and premature infants on supplemental oxygen spend less than half of the time within the target range.[1,2]

Division of Neonatology, Department of Pediatrics, University of Miami Miller School of Medicine, Miami, FL, USA
* Corresponding author. PO Box 016960, R-131, Miami, FL 33101.
*E-mail address:* nclaure@miami.edu

Clin Perinatol 48 (2021) 843–853
https://doi.org/10.1016/j.clp.2021.08.002

## RESPIRATORY INSTABILITY AND SPONTANEOUS EPISODES OF INTERMITTENT HYPOXEMIA

The respiratory instability of the extreme premature infant typically manifests as spontaneous episodes of intermittent hypoxemia (IH). The frequency of these episodes increases over the first weeks after birth, and they are influenced by the severity of their underlying lung disease.[3–5] In mechanically ventilated infants episodes of IH are often associated with increased activity and forceful exhalations that lead to loss in lung volume and hypoventilation.[6–9] In spontaneously breathing infants, IH is often associated with apneic events,[10] but IH episodes triggered by forceful exhalations have also been observed.[11]

Exposure to episodic IH may have significant detrimental effects in this population. Recent data support the association between exposure to prolonged episodes of IH with the development of severe Retinopathy of Prematurity (ROP) and neurodevelopmental impairment.[12,13] There are also important hemodynamic consequences associated with low oxygen levels[14–18] and as shown in randomized trials, with increased mortality associated with exposure to lower $Spo_2$ ranges.[19,20]

## EXPOSURE TO HYPEROXEMIA DURING ROUTINE CARE

The frequency of IH episodes seems to be inversely related to the basal level $Spo_2$.[21,22] This relation is likely the reason why there exists considerable tolerance of high $Spo_2$ levels, which may be aimed at reducing the frequency of IH, due to limited staff availability or an excessive response to IH events.[1,23,24] Premature infants spend more than 30% of the time with $Spo_2$ greater than the target range,[1] which can exceed 50% of the time in the more chronic infants.[23,25] Limited caregiver availability often affects the maintenance of $Spo_2$ within the target range mainly because of increased hyperoxemia, which is more evident in the more stable convalescent preterm infants.[2,23] This prolonged exposure to hyperoxemia in extreme premature infants is primarily induced by an excessive $Fio_2$; this is of concern because hyperoxemia has been associated with eye, lung, and central nervous system damage.[26–30]

## RATIONALE FOR AUTOMATED CONTROL OF FRACTION OF INSPIRED OXYGEN

Maintenance of $Spo_2$ within the target range by limiting the severity of IH without increasing the exposure to hyperoxemia is essential to achieve the right balance and improved respiratory, ophthalmic, and neurodevelopmental outcomes in extremely premature infants. Under ideal conditions of staff availability, manual $Fio_2$ adjustment would be sufficient to keep $Spo_2$ within the target range. However, this is not usually the case under standard clinical conditions. For this reason, and because of the inherent respiratory instability of the preterm infant, automated control of $Fio_2$ has been proposed as a tool to improve $Spo_2$ targeting and reduce exposure to extreme high and low $Spo_2$ values, while minimizing exposure to supplemental oxygen.

## BASIC DESCRIPTION OF A SYSTEM FOR AUTOMATED CONTROL OF FRACTION OF INSPIRED OXYGEN

Systems for automated $Fio_2$ control in general consist of a respiratory gas delivery device (eg, ventilator, continuous airway positive pressure, or nasal cannula flow device), pulse oximeter, and the built-in algorithm that determines the $Fio_2$ adjustments. Although the exact manner in which these algorithms adjust $Fio_2$ varies, all of them increase or decrease $Fio_2$ in proportion to acute decline or increase in $Spo_2$ outside the target set by the clinician. These algorithms also adjust baseline $Fio_2$ following longer-term upward or downward trends in $Spo_2$. The response of these algorithms is also intended to provide an appropriate size change in $Fio_2$ to avoid an overshoot in $Spo_2$.

## AUTOMATED FRACTION OF INSPIRED OXYGEN CONTROL ON EPISODES OF INTERMITTENT HYPOXEMIA

In clinical studies automated $Fio_2$ control has not consistently reduced the frequency of episodes in which $Spo_2$ declines less than the target range (**Table 1**). This finding may seem counterintuitive; however, this is not unexpected because these automated systems were not designed to prevent IH episodes. The trigger for IH involves some form of ventilatory derangement that precedes the onset of hypoxemia. Keeping a high baseline $Spo_2$, which is often observed during routine care, may be the best effective strategy to prevent IH episodes by maintaining adequate oxygen reserves. However, this may come at a cost of exposure to a higher $Fio_2$ and $Pao_2$. This situation was frequently observed in some clinical studies in which tolerance of baseline $Spo_2$ values that exceeded the target was likely an attempt to prevent IH.

Although systems of automated $Fio_2$ control cannot achieve an immediate resolution of the hypoxemia, their responses have been shown to be quite effective in attenuating the duration and severity of the IH episodes. In clinical studies, automated $Fio_2$

| Table 1 Episodes of intermittent hypoxemia | | | |
|---|---|---|---|
| | Type of IH Episode (Range, Duration) | Number of IH Episodes/24 h | |
| | | Automated $Fio_2$ Control | Manual $Fio_2$ Control |
| Claure et al,[34] 2001 | $Spo_2$ <88%, >5 s | 386 | 360[a] |
| | $Spo_2$<85%, >5 s | 257 | 257[a] |
| | $Spo_2$ <75%, >5 s | 31 | 31[a] |
| Urschitz et al,[35] 2004 | $Spo_2$ <87%, >5 s | 223 | 305[a] |
| | | | 209[a] |
| Claure et al,[36] 2009 | $Spo_2$ <88%, ≥10 s | 552 | 360[a,b] |
| | $Spo_2$ <85%, >120 s | 15 | 33[a,b] |
| | $Spo_2$ <75%, >60 s | 12 | 23[a,b] |
| Claure et al,[38] 2011 | $Spo_2$ <87%, ≥10 s | 456 | 264[b] |
| | $Spo_2$ <85%, >120 s | 22 | 35[b] |
| | $Spo_2$ <75%, >60 s | 3 | 10[b] |
| Waitz et al,[43] 2015 | $Spo_2$ <88%, ≥10s | 586 | 588 |
| | $Spo_2$ <85%, >120 s | 54 | 115[b] |
| | $Spo_2$ <75%, >60 s | 2 | 13[b] |
| van Kaam et al,[41] 2015 | Target 89%–93%: | 4 | 15[b] |
| | $Spo_2$ <80%, >60 s | 4 | 13[b] |
| | Target 91%–95%: | | |
| | $Spo_2$ <80%, >60 s | | |
| Plottier et al,[44] 2017 | $Spo_2$ <85%, >60s | 0 | 11[a,b] |
| | $Spo_2$ <80%, >60s | 0 | 3.1[a,b] |
| Gajdos et al,[45] 2018 | $Spo_2$ <88%, >10 s | 526 | 597 |
| | $Spo_2$ <88%, >60 s | 35 | 91[b] |
| | $Spo_2$ <80%, >10 s | 405 | 457 |
| | $Spo_2$ <80%, >60 s | 43 | 75[b] |

[a] Extrapolated to 24 hours.
[b] Statistically significant.

control consistently achieved a reduction in the more severe IH episodes in which $Spo_2$ declined less than 80% for more than 1 minute. It is also important to note that the rates of overshoot into hyperoxemia after an episode of IH were negligible. **Fig. 1** shows a representative recording of automated $Fio_2$ control in an infant with multiple IH episodes during 4 hours. These findings suggest that automated $Fio_2$ control could ameliorate the damaging effects of the more severe IH episodes on the developing organs, specifically the eye and the brain.[4,12,13]

## AUTOMATED FRACTION OF INSPIRED OXYGEN CONTROL ON HYPEROXEMIA

In clinical studies, automated $Fio_2$ control has been consistently shown to be effective in reducing hyperoxemia (**Table 2**). As expected, the effect of the automated systems on the reduction of hyperoxemia was greater when manual $Fio_2$ control during routine care was suboptimal. Recently, the impact of introducing automated $Fio_2$ control for routine care in the neonatal intensive care unit has confirmed the observations reported from the clinical trials.[31]

## AUTOMATED FRACTION OF INSPIRED OXYGEN CONTROL ON THE MAINTENANCE OF A TARGET RANGE OF OXYGEN SATURATION AS MEASURED BY PULSE OXIMETRY

As a result of the combined reductions in hyperoxemia and IH in the clinical studies mentioned earlier, automated $Fio_2$ control has been shown to improve the maintenance of $Spo_2$ within the target range when compared with manual $Fio_2$ control during routine care and with a fully dedicated caregiver (**Table 3**).[31–45] The proportion of time $Spo_2$ was kept within the target range by manual or automated $Fio_2$ control varied considerably; this was likely due to different baseline oxygenation instability at study entry. Some of these studies included only infants with a high frequency of IH episodes to test the systems of automated $Fio_2$ control in a population that represents a significant challenge. Infants enrolled in some studies were receiving noninvasive respiratory support, which indicates a better lung function, whereas other studies enrolled mechanically ventilated infants. Regardless of these variabilities between studies, the improvement in the time $Spo_2$ was kept within the target range was significant and consistent.

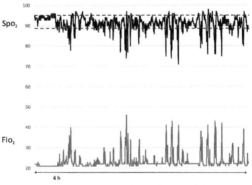

**Fig. 1.** The 4-hour recordings of $Spo_2$ (*top*) and $Fio_2$ (*bottom*) from an extremely premature infant during automated $Fio_2$ control. Increases in $Fio_2$ are in proportion with the severity of the IH episodes and only of duration necessary to bring $Spo_2$ to the target range (*dotted lines*).

**Table 2**
**Hyperoxemia**

| | Range | % Time in Range of Hyperoxemia | |
|---|---|---|---|
| | | Automated $Fio_2$ Control | Manual $Fio_2$ Control |
| Morozoff and Evans,[33] 1993 | $Spo_2$>95% | 23 | 39[c] |
| Claure et al,[34] 2001 | $Spo_2$>96% | 10 | 15 |
| Urschitz et al,[35] 2004 | $Spo_2$>96% | 1.3[b] | 4.9[b] |
| | | | 1.8[b] |
| Claure et al,[36] 2009 | $Spo_2$>95% | 9 | 31[c] |
| | $Spo_2$>97% | 3 | 16[c] |
| Claure et al,[38] 2011 | $Spo_2$>93%[a] | 21 | 37[c] |
| | $Spo_2$>98%[a] | 0.7 | 5.6[c] |
| Hallenberger et al,[39] 2014 | (4 centers [$Spo_2$ >95%, >92%, >93%, or >94%]) | 16 | 16 |
| Zapata et al,[40] 2014 | $Spo_2$ >95% | 27 | 55[c] |
| Waitz et al,[43] 2015 | $Spo_2$ >96% | 6.6 | 10[c] |
| Lal et al,[42] 2015 | $Spo_2$>95% | 4.8 | 10[c] |
| | $Spo_2$>97% | 0.08 | 1.7[c] |
| van Kaam et al,[41] 2015 | Target 89%–93%: | 21 | 25[c] |
| | $Spo_2$>93%[a] | 0.2 | 0.7[c] |
| | $Spo_2$>98%[a] | 22 | 19 |
| | Target 91%–95%: | 0.7 | 1.7[c] |
| | $Spo_2$>95%[a] | | |
| | $Spo_2$>98%[a] | | |
| Plottier et al,[44] 2017 | $Spo_2$>95%[a] | 5.1 | 25[c] |
| | $Spo_2$>98%[a] | 0 | 0.5[c] |
| Van Zanten et al,[31] 2017 | $Spo_2$>95% | 19 | 42[c] |
| | $Spo_2$>98% | 2 | 10[c] |
| Gajdos et al,[45] 2018 | $Spo_2$>96% | 4 | 6 |

[a] Excludes time with $Fio_2 = 0.21$.
[b] Estimated.
[c] Statistically significant.

## RELEVANT CONSIDERATIONS FOR THE USE OF AUTOMATED FRACTION OF INSPIRED OXYGEN CONTROL

Data from clinical studies indicate that there are large reductions in the need for manual adjustments to $Fio_2$ with automated $Fio_2$ control.[33–41,44] The lower frequency of manual adjustments also suggests a reduction in the time spent by caregivers who normally respond to an episode of IH and then remain at the bedside until the episodes resolve.

A potential risk of automated $Fio_2$ control is that it could potentially mask changes in respiratory status that would otherwise lead to low $Spo_2$ that would alert the caregiver. Although this risk has not been reported in clinical studies, most automated $Fio_2$ control systems should alert clinicians when there is an increase in basal $Fio_2$ to maintain adequate oxygenation. Still, when using these automated systems it is important to keep close continuous monitoring of the patient to detect any changes in clinical condition.

**Table 3**
Maintenance of a target range of $Spo_2$

| | $Spo_2$ Target Range | Proportion of Time in Target Range (%) | |
| --- | --- | --- | --- |
| | | Automated $Fio_2$ Control | Manual $Fio_2$ Control |
| Bhutani et al,[32] 1992 | 94%–96% | 81 | 54[b] |
| | | | 69 |
| Morozoff and Evans,[33] 1993 | 90%–95% | 50 | 39[b] |
| Claure et al,[34] 2001 | 88%–96% | 75 | 66 |
| Urschitz et al,[35] 2004 | 87%–96% | 91 | 82[b] |
| | | | 91[b] |
| Claure et al,[36] 2009 | 88%–95% | 58 | 42[b] |
| Morozoff,[37] 2009 | 90%–96% | 73 | 57 |
| Claure et al,[38] 2011 | 87%–93% | 47 | 39[b] |
| Hallenberger et al,[39] 2014 | All 4 centers | 72 | 61[b] |
| | 90%–95% | 71 | 63 |
| | 80%–92% | 69 | 64 |
| | 83%–93% | 66 | 43 |
| | 85%–94% | 84 | 65 |
| Zapata et al,[40] 2014 | 85%–93% | 58 | 34[b] |
| Waitz et al,[43] 2015 | 88%–96% | 76 | 69[b] |
| Lal et al,[42] 2015 | 90%–95% | 69 | 60[b] |
| van Kaam et al,[41] 2015 | 89%–93%[a] | 62 | 54[b] |
| | 91%–95%[a] | 62 | 58[b] |
| Plottier et al,[44] 2017 | 91%–95%[a] | 81 | 56[b] |
| Van Zanten et al,[31] 2017 | 90%–95%[a] | 62 | 48[b] |
| Gajdos et al,[45] 2018 | 88%–96% | 78 | 69[b] |

[a] Includes time with $Spo_2$ > target range, whereas $Fio_2$ = 0.21.
[b] Statistically significant.

One important consideration with the use of automated $Fio_2$ control systems is the selection of the target range of $Spo_2$ that will be used; this is because these systems will keep the target range more consistently than during routine care, which may uncover physiologic effects that would have not been observed otherwise. The contrast may be more evident in cases in which the staff maintains the baseline $Spo_2$ greater than the target range to reduce IH events, whereas bringing $Spo_2$ within the range by automated $Fio_2$ control may increase the number of events with $Spo_2$ declining less than the target range.

In summary, the respiratory instability of the extremely premature infants is associated with frequent episodes of IH. Clinically selected ranges of $Spo_2$ are not consistently kept, and excessive administration of supplemental oxygen that leads to hyperoxemia is common in this population. As exposure to high $Fio_2$, hyperoxemia, and prolonged episodes of IH have been associated with eye and lung injury as well as impaired neurodevelopment, several systems for automated $Fio_2$ control have been developed to improve $Spo_2$ targeting. Several clinical studies have documented the efficacy of automated $Fio_2$ control in reducing IH and hyperoxemia, thereby improving $Spo_2$ targeting. Future clinical trials should provide evidence on the benefits and limitations of automated $Fio_2$ control on long-term relevant clinical outcomes in these infants.[46]

## BEST PRACTICES

What is the current practice for targeting arterial oxygen saturation (SpO$_2$) in premature infants?

Currently, the fraction of inspired oxygen is manually adjusted to maintain the target range of SpO$_2$.

Best Practice/Guideline/Care Path Objective(s) Due to the respiratory instability of the premature infant and staff limitations, maintenance of the target range of SpO2 is not always possible. Periods of intermittent hypoxemia and hyperoxemia are frequently observed. Many practices have been implemented to improve SpO$_2$ targeting including the development of systems for automated control of inspired oxygen.

What changes in current practice are likely to improve outcomes?

Quality improvement initiatives that increase caregiver attentiveness to episodes of hypoxemia or hyperoxemia have been shown effective in improving SpO$_2$ targeting. Use of automated systems has also been shown effective in improving SpO$_2$ targeting.

Is there a Clinical Algorithm? If so, please include [either create your own, use from article or search from an Elsevier application] Major Recommendations

Continuous monitoring of SpO$_2$ with attentive response to attenuate the duration and severity of episodes of intermittent hypoxemia without inducing hyperoxemia. Use of automated systems for this purpose must be carefully implemented with particular attention to the selection of SpO$_2$ targets, continuous patient monitoring and maintenance of staff attentiveness.

Rating for the Strength of the Evidence Clinical studies have consistently provided strong evidence on improved SpO$_2$ targeting by quality improvement initiatives as well as by automated control of inspired oxygen.

Bibliographic Source(s): This is important list current sources relevant to evidence

Hagadorn JI, Furey AM, Nghiem TH, et al. Achieved versus intended pulse oximeter saturation in infants born less than 28 weeks' gestation: the AVIOx study.

Poets CF, Roberts RS, Schmidt B, et al. Association Between Intermittent Hypoxemia or Bradycardia and Late Death or Disability in Extremely Preterm Infants. Jama. 2015;314(6):595-603.

Di Fiore JM, Kaffashi F, Loparo K, et al. The relationship between patterns of intermittent hypoxia and retinopathy of prematurity in preterm infants. Pediatric research. 2012;72(6):606-612.

Sink DW, Hope SA, Hagadorn JI. Nurse:patient ratio and achievement of oxygen saturation goals in premature infants. Archives of disease in childhood Fetal and neonatal edition. 2011;96(2):F93-98.

van Zanten HA, Tan RN, Thio M, et al. The risk for hyperoxaemia after apnoea, bradycardia and hypoxaemia in preterm infants. Archives of disease in childhood Fetal and neonatal edition. 2014;99(4):F269-273.

Ford SP, Leick-Rude MK, Meinert KA, Anderson B, Sheehan MB, Haney BM, Leeks SR, Simon SD, Jackson JK. Overcoming barriers to oxygen saturation targeting. Pediatrics. 2006;118 Suppl 2:S177-86.

Claure N, Bancalari E, D'Ugard C, et al. Multicenter crossover study of automated control of inspired oxygen in ventilated preterm infants. Pediatrics. 2011;127(1):e76-83.

van Kaam AH, Hummler HD, Wilinska M, et al. Automated versus Manual Oxygen Control with Different Saturation Targets and Modes of Respiratory Support in Preterm Infants. The Journal of pediatrics. 2015;167(3):545-550 e541-542.

## CLINICS CARE POINTS

- Intermittent episodes of prolonged and severe hypoxemia have been associated with neurodevelopmental impairment in premature infants.

- Attentive response to these episodes is aimed at reducing their impact. A transient increase in the fraction of inspired oxygen in response to an episode of hypoxemia should be followed by a decrease to baseline when the episode resolves to avoid hyperoxemia.

- Systems of automated control of inspired oxygen that target a range of arterial oxygen saturation are effective in attenuating episodes of hypoxemia and in reducing exposure to hypoxemia.

- The range of arterial oxygenation to be targeted by automated systems must be carefully selected by the clinicians.

- Caregiver attentiveness and continuous monitoring of ventilation and general patient status should remain unchanged during use of automated systems for automated control of inspired oxygen. Particular attention should be given to warning of increased basal oxygen requirement to maintain a given target range of oxygen saturation.

## ACKNOWLEDGMENTS

The authors thank the University of Miami Project NewBorn for their continued support.

## CONFLICT OF INTEREST STATEMENT

Drs N. Claure and E. Bancalari developed and patented a system for automated control of inspired oxygen discussed in this article. The University of Miami, the assignee for this patent, has a licensing agreement with Vyaire Medical. Vyaire Medical supported some of the clinical studies to evaluate this system.

## REFERENCES

1. Hagadorn JI, Furey AM, Nghiem TH, et al. Achieved versus intended pulse oximeter saturation in infants born less than 28 weeks' gestation: the AVIOx study. Pediatrics 2006;118(4):1574–82.
2. Lim K, Wheeler KI, Gale TJ, et al. Oxygen saturation targeting in preterm infants receiving continuous positive airway pressure. J Pediatr 2014;164(4):730–6.e1.
3. Garg M, Kurzner SI, Bautista DB, et al. Clinically unsuspected hypoxia during sleep and feeding in infants with bronchopulmonary dysplasia. Pediatrics 1988;81(5):635–42.
4. Di Fiore JM, Bloom JN, Orge F, et al. A higher incidence of intermittent hypoxemic episodes is associated with severe retinopathy of prematurity. J Pediatr 2010; 157(1):69–73.
5. Raffay TM, Dylag AM, Sattar A, et al. Neonatal intermittent hypoxemia events are associated with diagnosis of bronchopulmonary dysplasia at 36 weeks postmenstrual age. Pediatr Res 2019;85(3):318–23.
6. Bolivar JM, Gerhardt T, Gonzalez A, et al. Mechanisms for episodes of hypoxemia in preterm infants undergoing mechanical ventilation. J Pediatr 1995;127(5):767–73.
7. Dimaguila MA, Di Fiore JM, Martin RJ, et al. Characteristics of hypoxemic episodes in very low birth weight infants on ventilatory support. J Pediatr 1997; 130(4):577–83.

8. Esquer C, Claure N, D'Ugard C, et al. Role of abdominal muscles activity on duration and severity of hypoxemia episodes in mechanically ventilated preterm infants. Neonatology 2007;92(3):182–6.

9. Lehtonen L, Johnson MW, Bakdash T, et al. Relation of sleep state to hypoxemic episodes in ventilated extremely-low-birth-weight infants. J Pediatr 2002;141(3):363–8.

10. Poets CF, Stebbens VA, Richard D, et al. Prolonged episodes of hypoxemia in preterm infants undetectable by cardiorespiratory monitors. Pediatrics 1995;95(6):860–3.

11. Esquer C, Claure N, D'Ugard C, et al. Mechanisms of hypoxemia episodes in spontaneously breathing preterm infants after mechanical ventilation. Neonatology 2008;94(2):100–4.

12. Poets CF, Roberts RS, Schmidt B, et al. Association between intermittent hypoxemia or bradycardia and late death or disability in extremely preterm infants. Jama 2015;314(6):595–603.

13. Di Fiore JM, Kaffashi F, Loparo K, et al. The relationship between patterns of intermittent hypoxia and retinopathy of prematurity in preterm infants. Pediatr Res 2012;72(6):606–12.

14. Tay-Uyboco JS, Kwiatkowski K, Cates DB, et al. Hypoxic airway constriction in infants of very low birth weight recovering from moderate to severe bronchopulmonary dysplasia. J Pediatr 1989;115(3):456–9.

15. Abman SH, Wolfe RR, Accurso FJ, et al. Pulmonary vascular response to oxygen in infants with severe bronchopulmonary dysplasia. Pediatrics 1985;75(1):80–4.

16. Skinner JR, Hunter S, Poets CF, et al. Haemodynamic effects of altering arterial oxygen saturation in preterm infants with respiratory failure. Arch Dis Child Fetal Neonatal Ed 1999;80(2):F81–7.

17. Noori S, Patel D, Friedlich P, et al. Effects of low oxygen saturation limits on the ductus arteriosus in extremely low birth weight infants. J Perinatol 2009;29(8):553–7.

18. Halliday HL, Dumpit FM, Brady JP. Effects of inspired oxygen on echocardiographic assessment of pulmonary vascular resistance and myocardial contractility in bronchopulmonary dysplasia. Pediatrics 1980;65(3):536–40.

19. Carlo WA, Finer NN, Walsh MC, et al. Target ranges of oxygen saturation in extremely preterm infants. N Engl J Med 2010;362(21):1959–69.

20. Stenson B, Brocklehurst P, Tarnow-Mordi W. Increased 36-week survival with high oxygen saturation target in extremely preterm infants. N Engl J Med 2011;364(17):1680–2.

21. McEvoy C, Durand M, Hewlett V. Episodes of spontaneous desaturations in infants with chronic lung disease at two different levels of oxygenation. Pediatr Pulmonol 1993;15(3):140–4.

22. Di Fiore JM, Walsh M, Wrage L, et al. Low oxygen saturation target range is associated with increased incidence of intermittent hypoxemia. J Pediatr 2012;161(6):1047–52.

23. Sink DW, Hope SA, Hagadorn JI. Nurse:patient ratio and achievement of oxygen saturation goals in premature infants. Arch Dis Child Fetal Neonatal Ed 2011;96(2):F93–8.

24. van Zanten HA, Tan RN, Thio M, et al. The risk for hyperoxaemia after apnoea, bradycardia and hypoxaemia in preterm infants. Arch Dis Child Fetal Neonatal Ed 2014;99(4):F269–73.

25. Durand M, McEvoy C, MacDonald K. Spontaneous desaturations in intubated very low birth weight infants with acute and chronic lung disease. Pediatr Pulmonol 1992;13(3):136–42.

26. Collins MP, Lorenz JM, Jetton JR, et al. Hypocapnia and other ventilation-related risk factors for cerebral palsy in low birth weight infants. Pediatr Res 2001;50(6): 712–9.

27. Back SA, Luo NL, Mallinson RA, et al. Selective vulnerability of preterm white matter to oxidative damage defined by F2-isoprostanes. Ann Neurol 2005;58(1): 108–20.

28. Haynes RL, Folkerth RD, Keefe RJ, et al. Nitrosative and oxidative injury to premyelinating oligodendrocytes in periventricular leukomalacia. J Neuropathol Exp Neurol 2003;62(5):441–50.

29. Supplemental Therapeutic oxygen for prethreshold retinopathy of prematurity (STOP-ROP), a randomized, controlled trial. I: primary outcomes. Pediatrics 2000;105(2):295–310.

30. Askie LM, Henderson-Smart DJ, Irwig L, et al. Oxygen-saturation targets and outcomes in extremely preterm infants. N Engl J Med 2003;349(10):959–67.

31. Van Zanten HA, Kuypers KL, Stenson BJ, et al. The effect of implementing an automated oxygen control on oxygen saturation in preterm infants. Arch Dis Child Fetal Neonatal Ed 2017;102(5):F395–9.

32. Bhutani VK, Taube JC, Antunes MJ, et al. Adaptive control of inspired oxygen delivery to the neonate. Pediatr Pulmonol 1992;14(2):110–7.

33. Morozoff PE, Evans RW. Closed-loop control of SaO2 in the neonate. Biomed Instrum Technol 1992;26(2):117–23.

34. Claure N, Gerhardt T, Everett R, et al. Closed-loop controlled inspired oxygen concentration for mechanically ventilated very low birth weight infants with frequent episodes of hypoxemia. Pediatrics 2001;107(5):1120–4.

35. Urschitz MS, Horn W, Seyfang A, et al. Automatic control of the inspired oxygen fraction in preterm infants: a randomized crossover trial. Am J Respir Crit Care Med 2004;170(10):1095–100.

36. Claure N, D'Ugard C, Bancalari E. Automated adjustment of inspired oxygen in preterm infants with frequent fluctuations in oxygenation: a pilot clinical trial. J Pediatr 2009;155(5):640–5, e641–2.

37. Morozoff EP, Smyth JA. Evaluation of three automatic oxygen therapy control algorithms on ventilated low birth weight neonates. Conf Proc IEEE Eng Med Biol Soc 2009;2009:3079–82.

38. Claure N, Bancalari E, D'Ugard C, et al. Multicenter crossover study of automated control of inspired oxygen in ventilated preterm infants. Pediatrics 2011;127(1): e76–83.

39. Hallenberger A, Poets CF, Horn W, et al. Closed-loop automatic oxygen control (CLAC) in preterm infants: a randomized controlled trial. Pediatrics 2014; 133(2):e379–85.

40. Zapata J, Gomez JJ, Araque Campo R, et al. A randomised controlled trial of an automated oxygen delivery algorithm for preterm neonates receiving supplemental oxygen without mechanical ventilation. Acta Paediatr 2014;103(9):928–33.

41. van Kaam AH, Hummler HD, Wilinska M, et al. Automated versus manual oxygen control with different saturation targets and modes of respiratory support in preterm infants. J Pediatr 2015;167(3):545–50, e541–2.

42. Lal M, Tin W, Sinha S. Automated control of inspired oxygen in ventilated preterm infants: crossover physiological study. Acta Paediatr 2015;104(11):1084–9.

43. Waitz M, Schmid MB, Fuchs H, et al. Effects of automated adjustment of the inspired oxygen on fluctuations of arterial and regional cerebral tissue oxygenation in preterm infants with frequent desaturations. J Pediatr 2015;166(2):240–4.e1.
44. Plottier GK, Wheeler KI, Ali SK, et al. Clinical evaluation of a novel adaptive algorithm for automated control of oxygen therapy in preterm infants on non-invasive respiratory support. Arch Dis Child Fetal Neonatal Ed 2017;102(1):F37–43.
45. Gajdos M, Waitz M, Mendler MR, et al. Effects of a new device for automated closed loop control of inspired oxygen concentration on fluctuations of arterial and different regional organ tissue oxygen saturations in preterm infants. Arch Dis Child Fetal Neonatal Ed 2019;104(4):F360–5.
46. Poets CF, Franz AR. Automated FiO2 control: nice to have, or an essential addition to neonatal intensive care? Arch Dis Child Fetal Neonatal Ed 2017; 102(1):F5–6.

# High-frequency Ventilation

Manuel Sánchez-Luna, MD, PhD[a],*,
Noelia González-Pacheco, MD, PhD[a], Martín Santos-González, DVM, PhD[b],
Francisco Tendillo-Cortijo, DVM, PhD[b]

## KEYWORDS

- High-frequency ventilation • Volume guarantee • Ventilation efficacy
- $CO_2$ elimination • Tidal volume

## KEY POINTS

- High-frequency ventilation (HFV) is an alternative to conventional mechanical ventilation (CMV) with less risk of ventilator-induced lung injury (VILI) and more effectivity in washout $CO_2$ from the lungs.
- Rescue high-frequency oscillatory ventilation (HFOV) has been used when severe respiratory distress syndrome needs aggressive CMV settings to prevent lung damage.
- HFOV is more effective to open atelectatic lungs but also has a role in air leak syndrome, meconium aspiration syndrome, and lung hypoplasia.
- Today it is possible to measure and to set directly high-frequency tidal volume (VThf), which can make it possible to decrease VThf to protect the immature lung from large tidal volumes and to decrease fluctuations in the VThf.
- This new strategy can be used in preterm infants with RDS using very low VThf and high frequencies to maintain ventilation and decrease the risk of VILI.

## INTRODUCTION

Very immature infants are at risk of lung damage soon after delivery due to exposure to oxygen and distension of the lung by breathing air. Knowledge that ventilator-induced lung injury (VILI) in premature newborn infants with respiratory failure can trigger bronchopulmonary dysplasia (BPD) recently led to modifications in the respiratory support applied to this population for a gentler and less invasive mechanical ventilation, and the combination of initial lung stabilization with early surfactant therapy has been shown to decrease the most severe forms of BPD.[1]

---

Conflict of interest: M. Sánchez-Luna has received advisory board consulting fees from Dräger. N. González-Pacheco, M. Santos-González, and F. Tendillo-Cortijo have no conflicts to declare.
[a] Neonatology Division, Instituto de Investigación Sanitaria Hospital General Universitario Gregorio Marañón, Complutense University of Madrid, Madrid, Spain; [b] Medical and Surgical Research Unit, Instituto de Investigación Sanitaria Puerta de Hierro–Segovia de Arana, Madrid, Spain
* Corresponding Author. Neonatology Department, C/ Dr. Esquerdo 46, E-28007 Madrid, Spain.
*E-mail address:* msluna@salud.madrid.org

But in some severe cases, using invasive mechanical ventilation still is needed. Most of the new ventilators can synchronize with the inspiratory effort using sophisticated trigger systems. Conventional mechanical ventilation (CMV), due to the need to use large tidal volume (TV) and high ventilator pressures, can damage the immature lung. High-frequency ventilation (HFV) emerged as an alternative to conventional ventilation in the 1970s, because this technique can be beneficial due to its efficacy in recruiting a collapsed lung and wash out more $CO_2$ with less lung trauma. Although HFV can reduce the incidence of VILI and BPD, the evidence of the potential benefits of its elective use is low, due to use of different ventilation protocols and devices and clinical situations,[2] so it has been considered a rescue therapy. Decades later, the use of a high lung-volume strategy and the possibility of measuring and controlling, in a very precise manner, high-frequency TV (VThf) during HFV with new ventilators[3] offer a new alternative to CMV, mostly in the more immature infants, to decrease the risk of lung damage during invasive ventilation.[4]

## THE HISTORY OF HIGH-FREQUENCY VENTILATION

HFV is defined as the use of a constant distension pressure to maintain a high-lung volume, normally over the functional residual capacity while transmitting energy to the airway by an oscillatory pressure amplitude ($\Delta P$) around the mean airway pressure (Paw) to produce TVs smaller than the dead space (VThf) delivered at supraphysiologic frequencies ($fr$).[5] This is possible when the lung is inflated to near its total lung capacity; then, the Paw can be reduced maintaining the lung volume and applying oscillatory pressure at the maximal curvature of the deflation limb of the pressure-volume relationship of the lung. This area is considered the safe area for ventilation.[6]

Although different types of HFV devices are in use, most experimental and clinical studies in neonates use high-frequency oscillatory ventilation (HFOV). Other devices, such as high-frequency flow interrupters (HFFIs) and high-frequency jet ventilators (HFJVs), are used less frequently in neonates and less information is available.

The HFJV delivers short pulses of pressurized gas directly into the upper airway through a narrow-bore cannula or jet injector, and exhalation is a result of passive lung recoil.[7]

With this modality, because exhalation is passive, a theoretical increase in the risk of gas trapping is possible, but no evidence of more gas trapping exists when comparing HFJV and HFOV in premature infants.[8]

HFFI ventilators create, over a continuous distending pressure, bursts of gas not directly into the airway but into the ventilator circuit at some distance back from the trachea and endotracheal tube, and exhalation also is passive.

HFOV works at frequencies between 3 Hz and 20 Hz (180–1200 cycles/min). Over a Paw, the ventilator produces small TV (VThf), smaller than the anatomic dead space, 2.4 mL/kg (range 1.0–3.6), that reach the airway by a piston or a membrane that create oscillatory pressure around the Paw; thus, the gas goes in and out to and from the airway actively, with an active exhalation unlike HFJV and HFFI.[9]

Explanations by which HFOV maintains normal gas exchange have been offered extensively, with multiple involved mechanisms to explain how the use of TVs smaller than the conducting airways volume can induce gas exchange. These mechanisms include convection (dependent on bulk flow), diffusion (spontaneous gas mixing due to brownian motion), and the combined effects of both mechanisms.[10]

In some instances, the VThf can gain alveolar areas and contribute to ventilation in a conventional way, with direct penetration of fresh gas into the alveolar space might being responsible in part for the improved gas exchange efficiency.[11]

HFOV is more effective than conventional ventilation for $CO_2$ removal,[12] because this is related to the square of VThf,[13,14] generated by variations on $\Delta P$[15] and transmitted distally into the airways. This transmission is easier when the airway is short and wide without reduction in the airway diameter. In adults, due to increased lung size and bronchial branching, DP is not well transmitted, $\Delta P$ is not well transmitted and the efficiency of the HFOV decreases,[16] making the HFOV more effective and probably less injurious in neonates compared with in adults.

The use of a high-volume strategy decreases the risk of neurologic lesions, described initially in some studies where this strategy was not used.

In the HIFI study, where no high-volume strategy was used, HFOV was associated with an increased incidence of pneumoperitoneum of pulmonary origin, grades 3 and 4 intracranial hemorrhage, and periventricular leukomalacia compared with CMV.[17]

In a meta-analysis of elective use of HFOV in preterm infants compared with CMV, the short-term neurologic morbidity with HFOV was found only in the subgroup of 2 trials not using a high-volume strategy with HFOV.[2]

## ELECTIVE USE OF HIGH-FREQUENCY VENTILATION

As evidenced in immature animal models,[18–20] small TVs and lung volume maintenance are able to prevent VILI in the preterm lung, and HFOV has been proposed as an ideal mode of ventilation to prevent damage of the immature lung; but, more than 40 years after the initial use of HFOV, there still is no consensus about the potential benefits of using electively HFOV in immature infants to prevent lung damage.

Earlier studies did not report measurement of VThf because most of the devices were not able to monitor TV or at all.

Although in some clinical studies, VThf as high as 3 mL/kg has been reported in neonates, exceeding the anatomic dead space and permitting some direct alveolar ventilation,[21] use of VThf of more than 2 mL/kg also is described, with these high TVs a possible explanation of why HFOV still put the infant lung at risk of damage during ventilation.[22]

More often, the frequency used and recommended by clinicians is 10 Hz, but, if there is $CO_2$ retention, then traditionally the frequency is reduced to less than 10 Hz to send a larger VThf,[23] because TV decreases when higher frequency is used.[24] A multicenter randomized controlled trial in 2002[25] demonstrated a higher rate of successfully extubation at 30 days, alive and weaned from all respiratory support at 36 weeks' postmenstrual age and less pulmonary hemorrhage in the HFOV group compared with the CMV group. In this study in premature infants of less than 1200 g, the ventilator device (SensorMedics) as in the original article only appears SensorMedics was a SensorMedics 3100A ventilator for HFOV, with an inspiratory to expiratory (I:E) ratio of 1:3, a frequency of 10 Hz to 15 Hz, and a lung recruitment strategy for an ideal lung inflation as expansion to 8 to 9.5 ribs on the chest radiography and compared with CMV using synchronized flow ventilation with expiratory TVs of 4 mL/kg to 7 mL/kg. No differences in other outcomes were found, demonstrating the safety of the HFOV when the lung recruitment strategy was used.

At the same time, a UK trial[26] randomized patients of less than 29 weeks' gestation to HFOV or CMV as the primary mode of ventilator support. In this study, different ventilators in different centers were used in the HFOV group with optimized lung volume, the Dräger Babylog 8000 (Dräger, Lübeck, Germany), the SensorMedics 3100A, or the SLE 2000 HFO (Specialised Laboratory Equipment Ltd, South Croydon, UK), with an I:E ratio of 1:1 in the Dräger and the SLE ventilators and 1:3 with the SensorMedics, and an initial frequency of 10 Hz modifying the $\Delta P$ to adjust $Paco_2$. No differences in the composite primary outcome of death or chronic lung disease (defined by a dependence on supplemental oxygen at 36 weeks' postmenstrual age) were found between the 2 groups. The effect of the type of ventilators was analyzed, and statistically differences in the frequency of the primary outcome between infants treated with the SensorMedics ventilator and those treated with either of the other 2 models were found, with a better result in the patients where these other ventilators.

These investigators followed the studied population, who at 11 years to 14 years of age demonstrated a superior lung function in the group who had undergone HFOV, compared with those who had received conventional ventilation, with no evidence of poorer functional outcomes.[27]

Some observational studies using a high-volume strategy described a higher survival rate at a mean of 2.6 years of follow-up in the HFOV group of premature infants, with a mean gestational age of 27 weeks, compared with CMV, but with no information about the HFOV settings.[28]

## HIGH-FREQUENCY OSCILLATORY VENTILATION AS A RESCUE THERAPY

Because the potential benefit of HFOV is to prevent lung damage related to volutrauma, RDS of premature infants is the most frequent indication. Although meta-analyses comparing rescue HFOV or HFJV therapy demonstrated no long-term benefits over CMV,[29–31] due to its efficacy in decreasing $CO_2$ and generating lung recruitment, there are other conditions that can be benefit from HFOV. The most frequent are[32]

- Air leak syndrome (ALS)
- Meconium aspiration syndrome (MAS)
- Lung hypoplasia (LH)
- Pulmonary hypertension of the newborn (PPHN)

## LUNG HYPOPLASIA

Congenital diaphragmatic hernia (CDH) represents a clinical situation where lung hypoplasia can be the limiting survival factor. The larger randomized controlled trial comparing the effect of HFOV as elective therapy to CMV failed to demonstrate any benefit and the trial was stopped early after an interim analysis.[33] In this international multicenter study, CDHs diagnosed prenatally were treated electively using CMV or HFOV; no statistically significant difference in the combined outcome of mortality or BPD between the 2 ventilation groups were found, and secondary outcomes favor the use of CMV. Probably, the use of HFOV in these conditions has to be individualized and apply when low TVs are preferred or $CO_2$ removal is a limiting factor.

## THERAPY FOR AIR-LEAK SYNDROME

Controlled trials demonstrated that the use of a short inspiratory time decreases the incidence of pulmonary interstitial emphysema, and, in animal neonatal models, the use of higher frequencies on HFOV decreases more the leakage than lower frequencies.[34]

Some mechanisms are described for the potential benefits of using HFOV in the ALS, as a decrease in the driving pressure of the gas through the site of the leak, or to decrease of the site size due to the short inspiratory time.

In some cases, HFOV can prevent the use of a thoracic tube to drain the air leak with a positive evolution.[35]

The HiFO study, a multicenter, prospective, no crossover, randomized trial to determine whether HFOV would decrease the development or progression of ALS in infants with severe RDS, using a frequency of 15 Hz, with a 1:2 I:E ratio and no background tidal breaths, demonstrated a significant lower risk to develop ALS but no effect in decreasing the worsening of the air leak when it was previously established.[36]

In the meta-analysis of elective HFOV in preterm infants,[2] however, ALS occurred more frequently in the HFOV group, but most of the studies used frequencies less than 15 Hz and no data about the I:E ratio were described.

## NEONATAL MECONIUM ASPIRATION SYNDROME

Although meconium staining of amniotic fluid occurs in up to 15% of all deliveries, meconium aspiration syndrome, described as respiratory distress in an infant born through meconium-stained amniotic fluid, appears in only 1.5% to 8% of those cases[37] but can be a life-threatening disorder in newborn infants. Coexistence of asphyxia and pulmonary hypertension are considered more important than the obstruction of the airways and/or damage to the lung produced by meconium. Although some experimental data suggest that HFOV can be superior to CMV,[38] and sometimes is recommended as a rescue therapy in severe MAS,[39] there are no clinical data demonstrating its potential benefit over CMV, so currently it is not recommended routinely.[40]

PPHN is a syndrome characterized by severe hypoxemia due to right-to-left shunting of desaturated blood through the foramen oval and/or the patent ductus arteriosus, not responding to supplemental oxygen. In some cases, this is due to parenchymal lung disease and recruitment of the lung with HFOV can improve its outcome.[41]

Also, the combined therapy of HFOV, surfactant, and inhaled nitric oxide can decrease the need of ECMO in the more severe forms. A better vehiculation of the inhaled nitric oxide by the HFOV can be achieved and a better respond sometimes is obtained, but cases need to be individualized.[42]

## VOLUME GUARANTEE COMBINED WITH HIGH-FREQUENCY OSCILLATORY VENTILATION—A NEW ERA

VThf is proportional to the $\Delta P$ generated in each cycle and the length of the inspiratory time and is inversely proportional to the oscillation frequency; thus, traditionally, an increase in $\Delta P$ or a decrease in frequency to finally increase VThf has been used to improve $CO_2$ clearance.[11,15] Also, the frequency has an important role in $CO_2$ removal[43] and has an independent effect on the distribution of the gas within the airways[44] and to changes in the volume when oscillating at or near the resonant frequency of the respiratory system.[45]

Measurement of the VThf gives an important advantage,[16] because there is a close correlation of the VThf and the $CO_2$ washout,[46] described as the diffusion coefficient of $CO_2$ ($DCO_2$) which is related to the $VThf^2$ and the frequency, as follows:

$$DCO_2 = VThf^2 \times fr^{15,47}$$

Traditionally, HFOV devices did not measured the VThf, so looking at the transmission of the oscillation to the thorax of the patient has been used to clinically control VThf. Today it is possible not only to measure but also to control and fix the VThf (volume guarantee [VG]) to maintain it as constant, similar to the VG described for conventional ventilation (**Fig. 1**), enabling an independent adjustment of the VThf and the

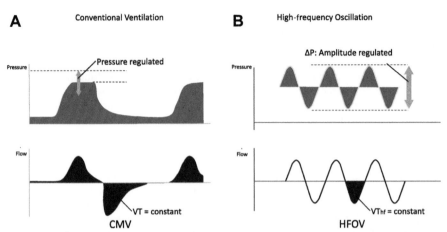

**Fig. 1.** Schematic representation of the VG modality, from the Dräger Babylog VN500. (*A*) Pressure regulation to control the TV set in CMV with the VG modality. (*B*) ΔP regulation to control the VThf set in HFOV with the VG modality.

frequency.[3] The ventilator, using this new technology, modifies ΔP to maintain the VThf at the setting value (**Fig. 2**).

When the VThf is fixed, any change in the frequency does not affect the VThf generated (**Fig. 3**) but directly modifies $DCO_2$ and $CO_2$ washout in the same direction as in conventional ventilation.[48]

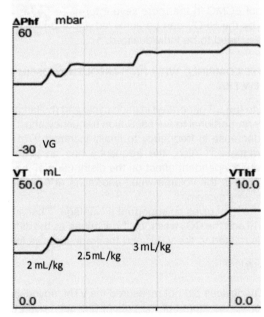

**Fig. 2.** Effect of increase in the VThf set on the ΔP of the ventilator during HFOV. Animal neonatal model with intact lung. Graphic obtained from the software of the Dräger Babylog VN500.

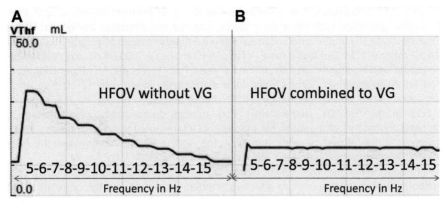

**Fig. 3.** (A) Effect of increase in the frequency during HFOV without VG. In this case, there is a drop in the VThf generated by the ventilator. (B) Effect of increase in the frequency during HFOV with VG. There is no change in the VThf generated by the ventilator because it is fixed. Graphic obtained from the software of the Dräger Babylog VN500, attached to a test lung.

To maintain a constant VThf, the ventilator increases the proximal ΔP when the frequency is increased, but this increase in the proximal ΔP is not transmitted into the distal airway,[16] so the lung is protected from ΔP, mostly because at lower frequencies pressure oscillations are "passed" from the airway opening to the alveolar spaces, while high-frequency pressure oscillations are heavily attenuated by resistive losses.[16,49] Also, the I:E ratio affects in a different manner if the VG is in use or not. When the HFOV does not use the VG modality, the longer the inspiratory time, the higher the VThf generated (I:E at 1:1), so more $CO_2$ washout is achieved at any frequency. But during HFOV combined to VG, a shorter inspiratory time (I:E at 1:2) is more effective to decrease $CO_2$ because the VThf is fixed and the only limitation is not having enough time to deliver the VThf set at very high frequencies.[50]

Some new generation devices can work with the VG modality, but differences in performance are described[51] as the capability of compensating the air leak around the endotracheal tube, making the VThf measured inaccurate,[52] so, it is important to use only devices that work with this leak compensation.[53]

## CLINICAL RESULTS WITH HIGH-FREQUENCY OSCILLATORY VENTILATION COMBINED WITH VOLUME GUARANTEE

Because it is possible to decrease VThf in HFOV and fix it with the VG modality, $DCO_2$ can be maintained as constant by increasing the frequency of the ventilator as the VThf is decreased. This effect recently was demonstrated in a neonatal animal model of RDS, where the use of an approach of very low VThf at high frequencies produced a lung protective effect, demonstrated by a lower histologic damage score.[54] This new strategy has been demonstrated to be feasible in newborn infants with respiratory failure, even extremely immature infants.[55] In very immature infants, it was possible to increase the standard $fr$ from 10 Hz to near 20 Hz maintaining similar $DCO_2$ and $P_{CO_2}$ with a very low VThf without side effects.

In a randomized crossover clinical trial, Iscan and colleagues[56] found lower fluctuations of the VThf and the $P_{CO_2}$, similar findings by Belteki and colleagues[57] in a single-center study.

Tuzun and colleagues,[58] in a retrospective study of preterm infants of less than 32 weeks' gestation with respiratory failure, studied the ventilator settings of HFOV combined with VG and showed a mean optimal airway pressure after lung recruitment of 10.2 mbar ± 1.7 mbar and a mean VThf of 1.61 mL/kg ± 0.25 mL/kg to provide normocapnia with no significant correlation between $Pco_2$ levels and VThf (per kilogram). VThf levels to maintain normocarbia were significantly lower with 12-Hz frequency compared with 10-Hz frequency (1.50 mL/kg ± 0.24 mL/kg vs 1.65 mL/kg ± 0.25 mL/kg; $P<.001$, respectively). The authors demonstrated this effect in a neonatal animal model, because the efficacy of $CO_2$ removal clearly increases with increments in the frequency more than expected, so the correlation between the $Pco_2$ and $DCO_2$ decreases if using the standard formula, $DCO_2 = VThf^2 \times fr$.

At frequencies higher than 15 Hz, similar $DCO_2$ measurements produce higher $CO_2$ washout, demonstrating a more effective alveolar ventilation; so, the correlation between $DCO_2$ and $Pco_2$ throughout increasing frequencies was not linear, showing a greater $CO_2$ elimination efficiency at higher frequencies, despite maintaining a constant $DCO_2$. To prevent this, the authors proposed a corrected formula of $DCO_2$ ($cDCO_2$) to be used at higher frequencies, which implies a better correlation of $DCO_2$ and $Pco_2$:

$$cDCO_2 = VThf^{1.78} \times fr^{1.15}\ [59]$$

This is probably due to modification of the gas flow behavior.[16] It has been suggested that the VThf during high-frequency oscillation steadily increases with increasing frequencies, reaching the maximum at the resonant frequency and subsequently decreasing again once that frequency is exceeded.[60]

The potential long-term benefits of this new modality remain to be demonstrated but there are some data showing this possibility.

Chen and colleagues[61] used HFOV combined with VG in 18 preterm infants as a rescue therapy and found a decrease in the combined outcome of BPD and death.

The authors compared a baseline period when HFOV was used without VG (2012–2013) against a period in which this strategy had been fully implemented (2016–2017). A total of 182 patients were exposed to invasive mechanical ventilation in the first 3 days after delivery, a higher proportion on HFOV at day 3 in the second period 79.5% (35) in 2016 to 2017 versus 55.4% (n 31) in 2012 to 2013. After adjusting for perinatal risk factors, the second period was associated with an increased rate of survival free of BPD (odds ratio [OR] 2.28; CI 95%, 1.072–4.878); this effect was more evident in neonates born at a gestational age of less than 29 weeks (OR 4.87; 95% CI, 1.9–12.48).[62]

A proposal of early rescue conventional ventilator settings to use HFOV combined to VG in premature infants is shown in **Table 1**, with the following initial setting of the HFOV combined with VG of the ventilator, always with a high-volume lung strategy (**Table 2**).

The lung high-volume strategy achieved using a lung recruitment protocol also is validated by other investigators.[56,63]

It is summarized as follows:

- Initial setting of the Paw 1 mbar to 2 mbar higher than that received during CMV (or similar for infants with ALS) and same fraction of inspired oxygen ($Fio_2$)
- Subsequently, slight increases in Paw (1–2 mbar every 2 min) until the critical lung opening pressure is reached, defined as an increase in oxygen saturation without signs of cardiocirculatory compromise
- $Fio_2$ then is decreased below 0.4 to 0.6, maintaining an oxygen transcutaneous saturation ($Spo_2$) of 90% to 95%.

**Table 1**
Proposed clinical criteria for switch to high-frequency oscillatory ventilation from conventional mechanical ventilation as a rescue therapy in severe respiratory failure in newborn infants

| | |
|---|---|
| Severe respiratory insufficiency refractory to CMV[a]:<br>Requirements of $Fio_2$ >50%[b]<br>and/or<br>$Paco_2$ >55–60 mm Hg that needs peak inspiratory pressure of ➡ | • >15 mbar in <1000 g<br>• >15–17 mbar between 1000 g and 1500 g<br>• >17 mbar between 1500 g and 2.000 g<br>• >20 mbar between 2000 g and 3000 g<br>• >25–30 mbar in >3000 g |
| ALS (interstitial emphysema, pneumothorax, or pneumomediastinum) | |
| PPHN wherein CMV fails | |
| Pulmonary atelectasis | |
| Pulmonary hypoplasia with $CO_2$ retention | |

[a] In preterm infants with RDS, failure of CMV is defined only after administering an initial dose of surfactant.
[b] In term infants, it is necessary to individualize and evaluate the cause of hypoxemia.

- After decreasing $Fio_2$, Paw is decreased by 1 mbar to 2 mbar every 2 min until $Spo_2$ less than 90%, defining the critical lung closing pressure.
- Paw then is increased again, to reopen the lung to the known critical lung opening pressure, and then decreased at 2 mbar above the critical lung closing pressure.
- Ideal lung inflation is defined as expansion to 8 ribs to 9 ribs (the top of the right hemidiaphragm relative to the posterior ribs on chest radiography at full inspiration).

Recently, the authors described a new clinical technique to effectively recruit the lung.

**Table 2**
Recommended initial settings of high-frequency oscillatory ventilation combined with volume guarantee

| | |
|---|---|
| $Fio_2$ | The same as in CMV |
| Paw | 1–2 mbar > Paw in CMV<br>Usual initial Paw for working in a safe zone:<br><1.000 g: 8–10 mbar<br>1000–1500 g: 10–12 mbar<br>1500–2000 g: 12–15 mbar<br>>2000 g: >15 mbar[a] |
| Frequency | 8–20 Hz:<br><2000 g: 14–20 Hz<br>>2000 g: 8–15 Hz |
| $\Delta P$ | 40–50 mbar |
| VThf | 1.5–2 mL/kg |
| Inspiratory time | I:E 1:2 (33%)<br>I:E 1:1 (50%) only when $fr$ >15 Hz |

[a] It is unusual to use Paw greater than 25 cm $H_2O$, although it may be necessary during lung volume recruit'ent maneuver. Always use a high-volume strategy after lung recruitment; for details of the lung recruitment scheme, see text.

In an ex vivo lung model, decreases in $\Delta P$ demonstrated the recruitment of the lung after increments in Paw. After reaching the recruitment of the lung, $\Delta P$ did not decrease more. This also was demonstrated in an in vivo animal lung study, where the decreases in $\Delta P$ also correlated with increases in $Pao_2$ until the recruitment of the lung was achieved; then, no further increases in $Pao_2$ or decrease in $\Delta P$ were observed. So, the changes in $\Delta P$, linked to a progressive increase in Paw, can be used to identify lung recruitment even earlier than oxygenation improvement.[64]

## BEST PRACTICES BOX

- Prevention of invasive mechanical ventilation and help to establish the functional residual capacity at delivery is the best respiratory support of immature infants at risk of developing respiratory failure.
- If invasive mechanical ventilation is needed, then prevent lung trauma using the lower tidal volume possible during ventilation.
- If a low compliance lung needs high respiratory pressures to maintain ventilation, the use of HFOV as a rescue therapy can be an effective and safe alternative to conventional ventilation.
- Monitoring and controlling of the tidal volume during HFOV improves its clinical use.
- Using the lower tidal volume at the higher respiratory rate in HFOV can reduce lung injury.

## CLINICS CARE POINTS

- Immature infants are at risk of lung injury and aggressive invasive ventilation must be prevented.
- Ventilator lung injury is mostly related to the use of large tidal volumes and can trigger chronic respiratory failure in premature infants.
- HFOV uses low tidal volumes and in several studies has demonstrated a protective effect compared with conventional ventilation.
- The use of HFV is effective as a rescue therapy in severe RDS in premature infants and it is safe as long term studies have demonstrated.
- Accurate measurement of the tidal volume and control of this volume by the use of VG combined to HFOV can be a new protective ventilator strategy to prevent lung trauma in the more immature infants with respiratory failure.

## DISCLOSURE

Dr Sánchez-Luna has received funding sources from National Grants (PI 14/00149-PI17/00838).

## REFERENCES

1. Rojas-Reyes MX, Morley CJ, Soll R. Prophylactic versus selective use of surfactant in preventing morbidity and mortality in preterm infants. Cochrane Database Syst Rev 2012;(3):CD000510.

2. Cools F, Henderson-Smart DJ, Offringa M, et al. Elective high frequency oscilla-tory ventilation versus conventional ventilation for acute pulmonary dysfunction in preterm infants. Cochrane Database Syst Rev 2015 Mar;19(3):CD000104.

3. Sánchez Luna M, Santos González M, Tendillo Cortijo F. High-frequency oscilla-tory ventilation combined with volume guarantee in a neonatal animal model of respiratory distress syndrome. Crit Care Res Pract 2013;2013:593915.

4. Sánchez-Luna M, González-Pacheco N, Belik J, et al. New ventilator strategies: high-frequency oscillatory ventilation combined with volume guarantee. Am J Perinatol 2018;35:545–8.

5. Slutsky A, Drazen F, Ingram RJ, et al. Effective pulmonary ventilation with small volume oscillations at high-frequency. Science 1980;209:609–71.

6. Rimensberger PC, Pristine G, Mullen BM, et al. Lung recruitment during small tidal volume ventilation allows minimal positive end-expiratory pressure without augmenting lung injury. Crit Care Med 1999;27:1940–5.

7. Weisberger SA, Carlo WA, Fouke JM, et al. Measurement of tidal volume during high-frequency jet ventilation. Pediatr Res 1986;20:45.

8. Ethawi YH, Abou Mehrem A, Minski J, et al. High frequency jet ventilation versus high frequency oscillatory ventilation for pulmonary dysfunction in preterm in-fants. Cochrane Database Syst Rev 2016;(5):CD010548.

9. Inwood S, Finley GA, Fitzhardinge PM. High-frequency oscillation: a new mode of ventilation for the neonate. Neonatal Netw 1986;4:53–8.

10. Slutsky AS, Drazen JM. Ventilation with small tidal volumes. N Engl J Med 2002; 29:630–1.

11. Isabey D, Harf A, Chang HK. Alveolar ventilation during high-frequency oscilla-tion: core dead space concept. J Appl Physiol Respir Environ Exerc Physiol 1984;56:700–7.

12. Froese AB, Bryan AC. High frequency ventilation. Am Rev Respir Dis 1987;135: 1363–74.

13. Rossing TH, Slutsky AS, Lehr JL, et al. Tidal volume and frequency dependence of carbon dioxide elimination by high-frequency ventilation. N Engl J Med 1981; 305:1375–9.

14. Jaeger MJ, Kurzweg UH, Banner MJ. Transport of gases in high-frequency venti-lation. Crit Care Med 1984;12:708–10.

15. Boynton BR, Hammond MD, Fredberg JJ, et al. Gas exchange in healthy rabbits during high frequency oscillatory ventilation. J Appl Physiol 1989;66:1343–51.

16. Herrmann J, Lilitwat W, Tawhai MH, et al. High-frequency oscillatory ventilation and ventilator-induced lung injury: size does matter. Crit Care Med 2020;48: e66–73.

17. High-frequency oscillatory ventilation compared with conventional mechanical ventilation in the treatment of respiratory failure in preterm infants. The HIFI Study Group. N Engl J Med 1989;12(320):88–93.

18. deLemos RA, Coalson JJ, deLemos JA, et al. Rescue ventilation with high fre-quency oscillation in premature baboons with hyaline membrane disease. Pediatr Pulmonol 1992;12:29–36.

19. Hamilton PP, Onayemi A, Smyth JA, et al. Comparison of conventional and high-frequency ventilation: oxygenation and lung pathology. J Appl Physiol 1983;55: 131–8.

20. Jobe AH, Kramer BW, Moss TJ, et al. Decreased indicators of lung injury with continuous positive expiratory pressure in preterm lambs. Pediatr Res 2002;52: 387–92.

21. Chan V, Greenough A, Milner AD. The effect of frequency and mean airway pressure on volume delivery during high frequency oscillation. Pediatr Pulmonol 1993; 15:183–6.
22. Dimitriou G, Greenough A, Kavvadia V, et al. Volume delivery during high frequency oscillation. Arch Dis Child Fetal Neonatal Ed 1998;78:F148–50.
23. Leipälä JA, Iwasaki S, Milner A, et al. Accuracy of the volume and pressure displays of high frequency oscillators. Arch Dis Child Fetal Neonatal Ed 2004;89: F174–6.
24. Laubscher B, Greenough A, Costeloe K. Performance of four neonatal high frequency oscillators. Br J Intens Care 1996;6:148–52.
25. Courtney SE, Durand DJ, Asselin JM, et al, Neonatal Ventilation Study Group. High-frequency oscillatory ventilation versus conventional mechanical ventilation for very-low-birth-weight infants. N Engl J Med 2002;347:643–52.
26. Johnson AH, Peacock JL, Greenough A, et al, United Kingdom Oscillation Study Group. High-frequency oscillatory ventilation for the prevention of chronic lung disease of prematurity. N Engl J Med 2002;347:633–42.
27. Zivanovic S, Peacock J, Alcazar-Paris M, et al. Late outcomes of a randomized trial of high-frequency oscillation in neonates. N Engl J Med 2014;370:1121–30.
28. Kessel I, Waisman D, Barnet-Grinnes O, et al. Benefits of high frequency oscillatory ventilation for premature infants. Isr Med Assoc J 2010;12:144–9.
29. Bhuta T, Henderson-Smart DJ. Rescue high-frequency oscillatory ventilation versus conventional ventilation for pulmonary dysfunction in preterm infants. Cochrane Database Syst Rev 2007;2:CD000438.
30. Joshi VH, Bhuta T. Rescue high frequency jet ventilation versus conventional ventilation for severe pulmonary dysfunction in preterm infants. Cochrane Database Syst Rev 2006;1:CD000437.
31. Henderson-Smart DJ, De Paoli AG, Clark RH, et al. High frequency oscillatory ventilation vs conventional ventilation for infants with severe pulmonary dysfunction born at or near term. Cochrane Database Syst Rev 2009;1:CD002974.
32. Meyers M, Rodrigues N, Ari A. High-frequency oscillatory ventilation: a narrative review. Can J Respir Ther 2019;55:40–6.
33. Snoek KG, Capolupo I, van Rosmalen J, et al, CDH EURO Consortium. Conventional mechanical ventilation versus high-frequency oscillatory ventilation for Congenital diaphragmatic Hernia: a randomized clinical trial (the VICI-trial). Ann Surg 2016;263:867–74.
34. Ellsbury DL, Klein JM, Segar JL. Optimization of high-frequency oscillatory ventilation for the treatment of experimental pneumothorax. Crit Care Med 2002;30: 1131–5.
35. Aurilia C, Ricci C, Tana M, et al. Management of pneumothorax in hemodynamically stable preterm infants using high frequency oscillatory ventilation: report of five cases. Ital J Pediatr 2017;43:114.
36. Randomized study of high-frequency oscillatory ventilation in infants with severe respiratory distress syndrome. HiFO Study Group. J Pediatr 1993;122:609–19.
37. Fanaroff AA. Meconium aspiration syndrome: historical aspects. J Perinatol 2008; 28:S3–7.
38. Calkovska A, Sun B, Curstedt T, et al. Combined effects of high-frequency ventilation and surfactant treatment in experimental meconium aspiration syndrome. Acta Anaesthesiol Scand 1999;43:135–45.
39. Dargaville PA, Copnell B. Australian and New Zealand Neonatal Network. The epidemiology of meconium aspiration syndrome: incidence, risk factors, therapies, and outcome. Pediatrics 2006;117:1712–21.

40. Vain NE, Szyld EG, Prudent LM, et al. What (not) to do at and after delivery? Prevention and management of meconium aspiration syndrome. Early Hum Dev 2009;85:621–6.

41. Kinsella JP. Inhaled nitric oxide in the term newborn. Early Hum Dev 2008;84:709–16.

42. Kinsella JP, Abman SH. Clinical approach to inhaled nitric oxide therapy in the newborn with hypoxemia. J Pediatr 2000;136:717–26.

43. Fredberg JJ, Glass GM, Boynton BR, et al. Factors influencing mechanical performance of neonatal high-frequency ventilators. J Appl Physiol (1985) 1987;62:2485–90.

44. Schuster DP, Karsch R, Cronin KP. Gas transport during different modes of high-frequency ventilation. Crit Care Med 1986;14:5–11.

45. Lee S, Alexander J, Blowes R, et al. Determination of resonance frequency of the respiratory system in respiratory distress syndrome. Arch Dis Child Fetal Neonatal Ed 1999;80:F198–202.

46. Zimová-Herknerová M, Plavka R. Expired tidal volumes measured by hot-wire anemometer during high-frequency oscillation in preterm infants. Pediatr Pulmonol 2006;41:428–33.

47. Weinmann GG, Mitzner W, Permutt S. Physiological dead space during high-frequency ventilation in dogs. J Appl Physiol 1984;57:881–7.

48. Mukerji A, Belik J, Sanchez-Luna M. Bringing back the old: time to reevaluate the high-frequency ventilation strategy. J Perinatol 2014;34:464–7.

49. Zannin E, Dellaca RL, Dognini G, et al. Effect of frequency on pressure cost of ventilation and gas exchange in newborns receiving high-frequency oscillatory ventilation. Pediatr Res 2017;82:994–9.

50. Sánchez-Luna M, González-Pacheco N, Santos M, et al. Effect of the I/E ratio on $CO_2$ removal during high-frequency oscillatory ventilation with volume guarantee in a neonatal animal model of RDS. Eur J Pediatr 2016;175:1343–51.

51. Grazioli S, Karam O, Rimensberger PC. New generation neonatal high frequency ventilators: effect of oscillatory frequency and working principles on performance. Respir Care 2015;60:363–70.

52. Szakmar E, Morley CJ, Belteki G. Leak compensation during volume guarantee with the dräger Babylog VN500 neonatal ventilator. Pediatr Crit Care Med 2018;19:861–8.

53. Belteki G, Széll A, Lantos L, et al. Volume-targeted ventilation with a Fabian ventilator: maintenance of tidal volumes and blood $CO_2$. Arch Dis Child Fetal Neonatal Ed 2020;105:253–8.

54. González-Pacheco N, Sánchez-Luna M, Chimenti-Camacho P, et al. Use of very low tidal volumes during high-frequency ventilation reduces ventilator lung injury. J Perinatol 2019;39:730–6.

55. González-Pacheco N, Sánchez-Luna M, Ramos-Navarro C, et al. Using very high frequencies with very low lung volumes during high-frequency oscillatory ventilation to protect the immature lung. A pilot study. J Perinatol 2016;36:306–10.

56. Iscan B, Duman N, Tuzun F, et al. Impact of volume guarantee on high-frequency oscillatory ventilation in preterm infants: a randomized crossover clinical trial. Neonatology 2015;108:277–82.

57. Belteki G, Morley CJ. High-frequency oscillatory ventilation with volume guarantee: a single-centre experience. Arch Dis Child Fetal Neonatal Ed 2019;104:F384–9.

58. Tuzun F, Deliloglu B, Cengiz MM, et al. Volume guarantee high-frequency oscillatory ventilation in preterm infants with RDS: tidal volume and DCO2Levels for optimal ventilation using open-lung strategies. Front Pediatr 2020;8:105.

59. González-Pacheco N, Sánchez-Luna M, Arribas-Sánchez C, et al. DCO2/PaCO2 correlation on high-frequency oscillatory ventilation combined with volume guarantee using increasing frequencies in an animal model. Eur J Pediatr 2020;179:499–506.

60. Lee S, Alexander J, Blowes R, et al. Determination of resonance frequency of the respiratory system inrespiratory distress syndrome. Arch Dis Child Fetal Neonatal Ed 1999;80:F198–202.

61. Chen LJ, Chen JY. Effect of high-frequency oscillatory ventilation combined with volume guarantee on preterm infants with hypoxic respiratory failure. J Chin Med Assoc 2019;82:861–4.

62. Ramos-Navarro C, González-Pacheco N, Rodríguez-Sánchez de la Blanca A, et al. Effect of a new respiratory care bundle on bronchopulmonary dysplasia in preterm neonates. Eur J Pediatr 2020;179:1833–42.

63. De Jaegere A, van Veenendaal MB, Michiels A, et al. Lung recruitment using oxygenation during open lung high-frequency ventilation in preterm infants. Am J Respir Crit Care Med 2006;174:639–45.

64. Rodríguez Sánchez de la Blanca A, Sánchez Luna M, González Pacheco N, et al. New indicators for optimal lung recruitment during high frequency oscillator ventilation. Pediatr Pulmonol 2020;55:3525–31.

# Lung Protection During Mechanical Ventilation in the Premature Infant

Emma E. Williams, MBBS[a], Anne Greenough, MD[a,b,c],*

## KEYWORDS

- Lung injury • Atelectrauma • Oxygen toxicity • Volutrauma • Open lung ventilation
- PEEP • Respiratory function monitoring

## KEY POINTS

- Lung injury is caused by atelectrauma, oxygen toxicity, and volutrauma.
- Optimum approaches of positive end-expiratory pressure delivery aimed at facilitating initial lung aeration after birth in preterm infants and during mechanical ventilation have yet to be determined.
- Volume-targeted ventilation is superior to pressure-limited ventilation in preterm infants for decreasing the incidence of death or bronchopulmonary dysplasia at 36 weeks postmenstrual age. It is important that appropriate tidal volumes are used.
- Respiratory function monitoring, such as capnography and ventilator graphics, provides clinicians with continuous real-time information that could aid in the optimization of lung-protective ventilatory strategies.
- Further research is needed to assess which lung-protective strategies result in a decrease in long-term respiratory morbidity.

## BACKGROUND

Mechanical ventilation can be life-saving for the premature infant, but is often injurious to immature and underdeveloped lungs. As a consequence, affected infants develop bronchopulmonary dysplasia (BPD), diagnosed by chronic oxygen dependency, which is the most common complication of very premature birth. Infants born very prematurely, even those without BPD, can suffer chronic respiratory morbidity, with troublesome symptoms, lung function abnormalities, and exercise intolerance into adulthood. It is, therefore, important to identify lung protection strategies and to do

[a] NICU, 4th floor Golden Jubilee Wing, King's College Hospital NHS Foundation Trust, Denmark Hill, London, SE5 9RS, UK; [b] Asthma UK Centre for Allergic Mechanisms in Asthma, London, SE9 0RT, UK; [c] NIHR Biomedical Research Centre Based at Guy's and St Thomas' NHS Foundation Trust and King's College London, London, SE9 0RT, UK
* Corresponding author. Professor Anne Greenough, NICU, 4th floor Golden Jubilee Wing, King's College Hospital NHS Foundation Trust, Denmark Hill, London, SE5 9RS, UK.
*E-mail address:* anne.greenough@kcl.ac.uk

Clin Perinatol 48 (2021) 869–880
https://doi.org/10.1016/j.clp.2021.08.006
0095-5108/21/© 2021 Elsevier Inc. All rights reserved.

so it is essential to understand the mechanisms by which lung injury is caused. In this article, we first discuss lung injury mechanisms, the efficacy of possible lung protection strategies during mechanical ventilation, and the relevance of respiratory function monitoring.

## LUNG INJURY MECHANISMS
### Atelectrauma

Atelectrauma is lung injury caused by cyclic atelectasis or repeated alveolar expansion and collapse. The injury is caused by shearing forces as alveoli next to each other collapse and reexpand. Unstable alveoli are susceptible to shear stress forces and exhibit vulnerability to the adverse effects of ventilator-induced injury, often independent of neutrophil-mediated inflammatory lung damage.[1]

### Oxygen Toxicity

Hyperoxia can lead to increased levels of reactive oxygen species and the subsequent development of BPD.[2] Low levels of reactive oxygen species are important in homeostasis and cell signaling.[3] The overproduction of reactive oxygen species, however, can lead to oxidative stress, which can be harmful and lead to chronic inflammatory damage.[4] Prematurely born infants have a decreased antioxidant defense system[5] and are also prone to infection, which leads to further activation of reactive oxygen species by inflammatory cells.[5] Oxidative stress affects the regulation of fibrotic pathways, with the overproduction of reactive oxygen species disrupting the extracellular matrix, with resulting airway remodeling and the triggering of fibrosis and development of chronic lung disease.[6] Hyperoxia, even at resuscitation, can be detrimental. Among preterm infants born at less than 28 completed weeks of gestation, infants receiving a fraction of inspired oxygen ($Fio_2$) of 0.9 had higher levels of markers of oxidative stress (eg, IL-8 and tumor necrosis factor alpha) than infants resuscitated with an $Fio_2$ of 0.3; the latter group had lower levels of BPD at 36 weeks postmenstrual age (15.4% vs 31.7%; $P<.05$).[7] Bronchoalveolar lavage samples from preterm infants with respiratory disease demonstrated that infants exposed to higher levels of oxidative stress to have increased expression of type IV collagenase, which resulted in disruption of the alveolar basement membrane.[6] The effects of hyperoxia on lung growth and development have been described in a baboon BPD model.[8] Baboons who received a high $Fio_2$ for the first 2 weeks after birth, regardless of ventilatory pressures and volumes, had larger airspaces ($P = .0003$), a decrease in the number of alveolar cells ($P = .004$), and a decreased internal alveolar surface area ($P = .05$).[8] Maintaining a narrow range of oxygen saturations using new technologies such as automated control[9] may be beneficial to preterm infants[9] (as discussed elsewhere in this article).

### Volutrauma

The delivery of excessive tidal volumes can lead to ventilator-induced lung injury. Volutrauma has adverse effects on the developing lung by increasing inflammation, edema, and ventilation–perfusion mismatching, inhibiting optimal gas exchange at the alveolar–capillary interface.[10] Lung inflation and overdistension have been association with increased expression of cytokines and interleukins. In a study of preterm lambs, inflammatory mediators were increased in response to resuscitation with high tidal volumes.[11] Furthermore, preterm lambs manually ventilated with high volumes before surfactant administration exhibited not only greater lung injury, but also a diminished response to surfactant compared with the low tidal volume group.[12]

Treatment with surfactant before tidal volume delivery decreased the severity of lung injury.[13] The delivery of "normal" physiologic tidal volumes to derecruited alveoli is often redistributed to "open" alveolar lung units and the resulting overdistension can cause damage to healthy alveoli.[14] Preterm infants with surfactant-depleted lungs have areas of atelectasis unavailable to gas exchange and, therefore, injury occurs to the open lung areas because the whole tidal volume is preferentially delivered to only the healthy lung units.[15] Furthermore, lung overinflation from mechanical ventilation can lead to alveolar edema as tidal volumes increase, and the damage is further affected by extremes of positive end-expiratory pressure (PEEP) levels.[16,17]

Preterm infants are susceptible to volutrauma, owing to factors such as exposure to inflammatory mediators in utero, surfactant deficiency, decreased chest wall compliance, and a decreased antioxidant defense system.[15] An increase in tracheal aspirate proinflammatory cytokines within the first week after birth has been found in preterm infants with respiratory distress syndrome (RDS) who were ventilated with small rather than larger tidal volumes (3 mL/kg vs 5 mL/kg).[18] Furthermore, the low tidal volume group also required a longer duration of invasive mechanical ventilation (16.8 days vs 9.2 days; $P = .005$).[18] The impact of high-frequency ventilation with both low and high targeted tidal volumes was examined in a piglet model.[19] Inflammatory infiltrates and areas of parenchymal consolidation were found more often where high-frequency oscillation ventilation (HFOV) was used with high tidal volumes, with significantly lower lung histology scores for inflammation ($P = .043$) and emphysema ($P = .027$) in the piglets supported by low tidal volume HFOV.[19]

## LUNG PROTECTION STRATEGIES
### Resuscitation Strategies

#### Lung recruitment
The lungs of new born infants are susceptible to injury as they transition from in utero to postnatal life. Aeration of the lungs occurs as fluid is expelled and the functional residual capacity is established.[20,21] To minimize damage to the immature lung during this transition, gradual aeration and recruitment of the alveoli should be homogenous to ensure the tidal volume is distributed evenly throughout the lung units, thereby avoiding regional differences in lung inflation.[22,23] Lung injury during the initial resuscitation of preterm lambs was assessed by comparing 2 lung recruitment maneuvers. The first was a sustained inflation to achieve rapid clearance of lung fluids and the second made use of PEEP followed by gradual aeration to prevent outward flow of lung fluid. Both methods were superior to tidal ventilation with no active recruitment maneuvers.[24] Resuscitation using sustained inflation maneuvers with the primary aim of rapidly aerating the lungs at birth, however, was associated with nonuniform lung aeration in an animal model.[25] Furthermore, the results of a systematic review comparing standard lung inflations with sustained lung inflations during resuscitation of newborn infants at birth found sustained lung inflations not to be superior.[26]

#### Open lung ventilation and positive end-expiratory pressure
In a randomised trial of preterm lamb resuscitation, the efficacy of different ventilatory techniques with regard to lung inflation, establishment of end-expiratory lung volume, and spatiotemporal aeration of the lungs at birth was assessed.[23] More uniform and homogenous distribution of tidal volume occurred after open lung ventilation with transient escalation and deescalation of PEEP levels to aid in recruitment of alveoli; there were also beneficial effects regarding oxygenation, surfactant response, compliance, ventilatory requirements, and lung mechanics.[23] The optimal approaches of PEEP

delivery aimed at facilitating initial lung aeration after birth in preterm infants have yet to be determined; however, results from recent animal studies suggest this is a promising field to explore.[23,25]

### Volume-targeted resuscitation

The development of volume-targeted rather than pressure-driven resuscitation devices have been assessed during mask and endotracheal resuscitation simulation scenarios using a neonatal mannikin.[27,28] During mask resuscitation with standard pressure devices (such as the self-inflating bag or t-piece), the tidal volume delivery was consistently higher than when the volume-controlled prototype device was used when using high compliant test lungs (10.0 mL/kg vs 4.9 mL/kg; $P<.001$). Using a low compliant test lung, however, the volume-controlled device underdelivered the set tidal volume.[27] The volume-controlled resuscitator device delivered the most consistent tidal volume, regardless of compliance of the test lung.[28] The results from this prototype device should encourage further research.

## Mechanical Ventilation Strategies in the Neonatal Intensive Care Unit

### Lung recruitment and maintenance of lung volumes

A systematic review demonstrated that lung recruitment maneuvers guided by changes in oxygenation decreased the duration of invasive ventilatory support (95% confidence interval [CI], −1.85 to −0.26).[29] There was, however, low evidence that oxygen-guided lung recruitment maneuvers decrease mortality (relative risk [RR], 1.0; 95% CI, 0.17–5.77) or BPD (RR, 0.25; 95% CI, 0.03–2.07) compared with routine care.[30,31]

### Positive end-expiratory pressure

Lung recruitment can be achieved by the application of PEEP. Optimal levels of PEEP are required to maintain lung volume, prevent atelectasis, and avoid overdistension. PEEP protects the alveoli from repeated opening and collapse, which in turn can cause damage to the immature lung.[32] The application of PEEP prevents total collapse of alveoli at the end of expiration, microatelectasis, and the ensuing instability of alveoli. Specimens of surfactant deactivated lung tissue in an in vivo study demonstrated that the application of PEEP to unstable alveoli decreased the histopathologic features of thickened walls and intra-alveolar edema.[1] A systematic review of studies of PEEP levels in mechanically ventilated preterm infants with RDS found insufficient evidence to determine global PEEP levels and recommended an individualized infant-by-infant approach.[29] No randomised trials have investigated optimal levels of PEEP during invasive mechanical ventilation in infants with established BPD.[29]

### Volume-targeted ventilation

A systematic review highlighted that volume-targeted ventilation was superior to pressure-limited ventilation in preterm infants with regard to decreasing the incidence of death or BPD at 36 weeks postmenstrual age (RR, 0.73, 95% CI, 0.59–0.89), the duration of mechanical ventilation (95% CI, −1.83 to −0.86), and the pneumothorax rate (RR, 0.52, 95% CI, 0.31–0.87).[33] It is important, however, that appropriate tidal volumes are used. Low tidal volumes increase the work of breathing in infants with RDS; targeting tidal volumes of at least 5 mL/kg decreased the work of breathing.[34] Preterm infants with evolving BPD who were still ventilator dependent beyond 1 week of age had a decrease in the work of breathing when higher volumes of 7 mL/kg were targeted,[35] likely reflecting the greater physiologic dead space of infants with evolving BPD compared with those with RDS.

### Short inspiratory times
Spontaneously breathing, preterm newborns with RDS have previously been shown to have inspiratory times of between 0.26 and 0.34 seconds.[32] The use of short inspiratory times (0.2 seconds) has been examined in a 2-unit lung model with regard to improving the balance between preventing alveolar collapse and avoiding overinflation of lung units with differing compliance levels. An improvement in ventilation homogeneity was seen with a more equal distribution of tidal volume between compartments with different compliances when short inspiratory times were used ($P<.001$).[36] Adjustment of the inspiratory time might confer benefit in extremely preterm infants with inhomogeneous lungs.

### High-frequency oscillation ventilation
Animal studies have shown HFOV to be superior to conventional modes of invasive mechanical ventilation in improving the stability of alveoli.[37] An in vitro study assessing the inflammatory response at different amounts of cyclical strain designed to mimic what occurs during conventional ventilation or HFOV demonstrated lower levels of IL-6 release in the HFOV exposed alveolar cell analogues.[38] The United Kingdom Oscillation Study (UKOS) reported no difference in the primary outcome of mortality or BPD at 36 weeks postmenstrual age in extremely preterm infants randomised to conventional ventilation or HFOV within the first hour after birth (RR, 0.98; 95% CI, 0.89–1.08),[39] yet those supported by HFOV had superior lung function at 11 to 14 years of follow-up.[40] In that trial,[39] a high-volume strategy was used, during which the mean airway pressure (MAP) is increased to improve oxygenation. In an observational study, during which the MAP was increased until the maximum oxygenation was achieved (optimal MAP), the optimal MAP had an inverse correlation with the function residual capacity before starting high-flow oxygenation and the change in MAP also correlated negatively with the baseline function residual capacity.[41] Noninvasive techniques of measuring lung volumes by electrical impedance tomography have been described.[42] Using such a technique, a stepwise recruitment maneuver in preterm infants with RDS who were receiving HFOV resulted in homogenous increases in end-expiratory lung volumes.[43]

### Surfactant

Surfactant has many benefits regarding decreasing mortality and morbidity in preterm infants. It has been shown in animal models to beneficially modify regional lung ventilation and tidal volume distribution.[44] Additionally, surfactant can be used to recruit alveoli, with an increase in lung compliance and both total and residual lung volumes[45]; indeed, 1 study showed a mean increase in lung volume of 61% after surfactant administration.[45] Furthermore, the combined effect of PEEP with postnatal surfactant has been associated with an increase in functional residual capacity in preterm infants with RDS.[46]

### Decrease in Oxygen Toxicity

#### Antioxidants
Various antioxidants have been investigated with regard to decreasing BPD. Meta-analysis of randomised controlled trials has demonstrated that supplementation with vitamin A decreased BPD, but did not improve long-term outcomes, further emphasizing that BPD is not an appropriate outcome for randomised controlled trials assessing agents to prevent the chronic respiratory morbidity of prematurely born infants. Potentially interesting results have been demonstrated with the antioxidant, recombinant superoxide dismutase, but these finding have not encouraged other

studies, perhaps because multiple doses of superoxide dismutase had to be given via the trachea. In animal models, augmentation of the endogenous anti-inflammatory pathway with a recombinant analogue of Clara cell secretory protein, rhCC10, has yielded promising results, but these data have not yet been translated into important clinical outcomes. Azithromycin, a macrolide used to treat *Ureaplasma* infection, also has anti-inflammatory properties and has been shown to decrease BPD. It has, however, been linked to the development of hypertrophic pyloric stenosis, although the results were from a retrospective study. Pentoxifylline is a synthetic methylxanthine derivative that has anti-inflammatory, antifibrotic, and immunomodulatory properties. In an initial study, it was shown to decrease BPD, but this finding was not conformed subsequently. There is less robust evidence for other antioxidants. Appropriately powered studies with long-term outcomes are required to assess the efficacy of antioxidants.[47]

### Automated closed loop oxygen delivery

Closed loop automated oxygen control systems automate the adjustment of the inspired oxygen concentrations according to peripheral oxygen saturation levels. In a systematic review,[9] 18 studies in neonates were identified. Overall, closed loop automated oxygen control was associated with an increased percentage of time spent within the target oxygen saturation range and there were fewer manual adjustments to the inspired oxygen concentration when compared with manual oxygen control. The systems were effective in infants on noninvasive respiratory support or mechanically ventilated, but no study included term-born infants. No long-term data are available to determine if the complications of oxygen toxicity were decreased.

### Monitoring Techniques

### Respiratory function monitoring

Respiratory function monitoring provides clinicians with continuous real-time information and could act as an adjunct to optimize lung protective ventilatory strategies. An early evaluation of neonatal resuscitation monitoring use and how practitioners interpreted the respiratory function data, however, revealed that many did not use the data to inform acute changes and indeed often wrongly interpreted the data.[48,49] More recently, eye tracking demonstrated that, during simulated resuscitation of a neonatal mannikin, clinicians spent more time looking at the exhaled tidal volume waveform than any other waveform on the respiratory function monitor.[50] In a cohort of preterm infants requiring noninvasive positive pressure ventilation during resuscitation, the use of a respiratory function monitor was associated with a decrease in high tidal volume delivery (5.8 mL/kg vs 7 mL/kg; $P = .001$); however, the use of monitoring did not decrease the need for intubation with the first 72 hours after birth.[51] Furthermore, the use of respiratory function monitoring in newborn infants has been evaluated during anesthetic care.[52] During anesthesia, a significant decrease in the delivery of tidal volumes of greater than 10 mL/kg was observed when respiratory function monitoring was used (RR, 0.61; 95% CI, 0.42–0.89) with a trend in decreasing tidal volumes inflations of lower than 4 mL/kg in the unblinded group (9.8% vs 6.5%).[52]

### Capnography

Capnography is used to measure exhaled carbon dioxide; a continuous waveform together and the maximal value at the end of each expired breath are displayed. Exhaled carbon dioxide levels during the resuscitation of newborn rabbit pups have been used to indicate initial lung aeration.[53] The establishment of the functional residual capacity and lung aeration correlated with an increase in the exhaled carbon dioxide levels. Those results have been replicated in a study of preterm infants; the increase in tidal volume immediately after birth correlated with increases in exhaled carbon dioxide levels.[54] The shape of the volumetric capnogram can provide data to calculate the homogeneity of alveolar ventilation, dead space ventilation, and the degree of ventilation perfusion matching.[55,56]

The slope gradients of the different phases of the capnogram have been assessed in preterm infants. The phase III slope has been shown to be steeper in ventilated preterm infants who have high ventilatory requirements in comparison with term infants,[57] and furthermore in a cohort of preterm infants with BPD a steeper phase III slope was present in those receiving supplemental oxygen, suggestive of greater ventilation perfusion mismatching.[58] Specific lung-protective ventilatory strategies involving carbon dioxide are those of permissive hypercapnia in an attempt to avoid volutrauma to the immature lung. A multicenter randomised trial of permissive hypercapnia in low birth weight infants found infants exposed to higher levels of carbon dioxide did not have decreased levels of pulmonary inflammatory mediators.[59] There was, however, no significant difference in the incidence of BPD between the permissive hypercapnic group and the controls.[60]

The use of end-tidal capnography on the neonatal intensive care unit can be used to assess gas exchange, with increasing discrepancy of expired end-tidal carbon dioxide levels relative to arterial carbon dioxide levels, indicating a worsening of lung pathology in preterm infants.[61] Interpretation of the volumetric capnogram can be used additionally to calculate dead space, the part of tidal volume that does not partake in gas exchange. Alveolar dead space has been shown to be increased significantly in preterm infants who had a greater duration of mechanical ventilation[62]; this finding might be explained by progressive alveolar distension and ventilator-induced lung injury together with a greater severity of lung disease.[63] The use of capnography on the neonatal unit and quantification of the dead space may, therefore, be able to guide optimal ventilatory strategies and targeting of appropriate tidal volume delivery.

### Ventilatory graphics

Pressure–volume curves can provide valuable information regarding lung compliance, alveolar recruitment, and distension of the lung.[64] The ascending inflation limb of the curve gives a lower inflection point, the opening pressure at which lung recruitment occurs, together with an upper inflection point, the pressure above which volutrauma can occur.

Maintaining functional residual capacity and ventilation within a 'safe zone' requires a balance to exist between alveolar decruitment and overdistension. Using the relationship between the pressure and the volume on the ventilator graphics curve has been suggested as an alternative method to guide different lung recruitment approaches, but this is not uniformly agreed on.[65] Setting the PEEP level relative to the lower inflection point has been described in a cohort of preterm infants with the lower inflection point signifying the onset of alveolar recruitment.[66] Using the upper curvature point on the deflation limb, as is used in high-frequency ventilation,[67] might confer greater oxygenation benefits, because this upper curvature signifies the level of alveolar recruitment, but may result in overdistension.[68] Lung recruitment in preterm infants with acute RDS receiving volume guarantee ventilation has been described using incremental increases in PEEP, followed by a stepwise decrease in PEEP with the lung volume being set on the deflation limb of the pressure–volume curve.[30] The group exposed to lung recruitment maneuvers exhibited a decreased time to achieve the lowest $Fio_2$ (94 minutes vs 435 minutes; $P<.001$) and had a shorter duration of oxygen dependency (29 days vs 12 days, $P = .04$).[30] Furthermore, in an animal study assessing the effects of open lung ventilation with small tidal volumes, optimal compliance during ventilation was achieved after an initial recruitment maneuver followed by subsequent PEEP levels, which were less than the inflation pressures, yet higher than the closing pressures.[69] Airway pressure release ventilation is a mode of time cycled–pressure limited ventilation that uses the inflection points from the pressure volume curve to deliver respiratory support in a more physiologic manner.[70] A high distending pressure for a prolonged time is used to achieve alveolar recruitment and followed by a short time spent at a lower pressure; this modality aims to achieve oxygenation while minimizing ventilator-induced lung injury.[71]

In a neonatal lamb model of acute lung injury, airway pressure release ventilation augmented alveolar ventilation and was associated with a decrease in peak airway pressure compared with conventional pressure ventilation (19.7 cm $H_2O$ vs 36.4 cm $H_2O$; $P<.05$), while maintaining the same oxygenation and carbon dioxide clearance.[72] Evidence is limited, however, and randomised clinical trials are required to determine whether this mode of ventilation supported by ventilator graphics may improve neonatal outcomes.

## SUMMARY

During mechanical ventilation, it is vital that there is a balance between achieving adequate gas exchange and minimizing damage to the pulmonary system. Open lung ventilation may avoid atelectasis and volutrauma while decreasing excessive oxygen toxicity by using lung recruitment maneuvers to improve oxygenation. Novel modes and monitoring devices may facilitate the appropriate delivery of ventilation during both resuscitation and on the neonatal intensive care unit. The display of visual parameters in real time may further aid clinicians to optimally deliver lung protective ventilation to preterm infants. Further research is needed to assess which lung-protective strategies result in a decrease in long-term respiratory morbidity.

## GOALS

- Prevention of atelectasis and maintenance of lung recruitment.
- Minimization of volutrauma and oxidative stress.
- Avoidance of regional lung injury and pulmonary inflammation.
- Accomplishment of optimal alveolar capillary gas exchange.
- A decrease in adverse long-term pulmonary outcomes, which are more appropriate end-points than the binary outcome of BPD, when assessing a decrease in lung damage.

## CLINICS CARE POINTS

- Lung damage may arise at resuscitation.
- Importance of optimizing ventilatory strategies to improve long-term outcomes.
- Individualized approach based on infant lung pathology.
- An appropriate evidence base for novel modes and monitoring techniques to further promote lung protection before they are used in routine care.

## DISCLOSURE

Professor A. Greenough has held grants from various manufacturers (Abbot Laboratories, MedImmune) and ventilator manufacturers (SLE). Professor A. Greenough has received honoraria for giving lectures and advising various manufacturers (Abbot Laboratories, MedImmune) and ventilator manufacturers (SLE). Professor A. Greenough is currently receiving a nonconditional educational grant from SLE.

## REFERENCES

1. Steinberg JM, Schiller HJ, Halter JM, et al. Alveolar instability causes early ventilator-induced lung injury independent of neutrophils. Am J Respir Crit Care Med 2004;169:57–63.
2. Perrone S, Bracciali C, Di Virgilio N, et al. Oxygen use in neonatal care: a two-edged sword. Front Pediatr 2016;4:143.
3. D'Autreaux B, Toledano MB. ROS as signalling molecules: mechanisms that generate specificity in ROS homeostasis. Nat Rev Mol Cell Biol 2007;8:813–24.
4. Rosanna DP, Salvatore C. Reactive oxygen species, inflammation, and lung diseases. Curr Pharm Des 2012;18:3889–900.
5. Saugstad OD. Bronchopulmonary dysplasia-oxidative stress and antioxidants. Semin Neonatol 2003;8:39–49.
6. Schock BC, Sweet DG, Ennis M, et al. Oxidative stress and increased type-IV collagenase levels in bronchoalveolar lavage fluid from newborn babies. Pediatr Res 2001;50:29–33.
7. Vento M, Moro M, Escrig R, et al. Preterm resuscitation with low oxygen causes less oxidative stress, inflammation, and chronic lung disease. Pediatrics 2009; 124:e439–49.
8. Coalson JJ, Winter V, deLemos RA. Decreased alveolarization in baboon survivors with bronchopulmonary dysplasia. Am J Respir Crit Care Med 1995;152: 640–6.
9. Sturrock S, Williams E, Dassios T, et al. Closed loop automated oxygen control in neonates-A review. Acta Paediatr 2020;109:914–22.
10. Attar MA, Donn SM. Mechanisms of ventilator-induced lung injury in premature infants. Semin Neonatol 2002;7:353–60.
11. Polglase GR, Miller SL, Barton SK, et al. Initiation of resuscitation with high tidal volumes causes cerebral hemodynamic disturbance, brain inflammation and injury in preterm lambs. PLoS One 2012;7:e39535.
12. Bjorklund LJ, Ingimarsson J, Curstedt T, et al. Manual ventilation with a few large breaths at birth compromises the therapeutic effect of subsequent surfactant replacement in immature lambs. Pediatr Res 1997;42:348–55.
13. Wada K, Jobe AH, Ikegami M. Tidal volume effects on surfactant treatment responses with the initiation of ventilation in preterm lambs. J Appl Physiol 1997; 83:1054–61.
14. Berger TM, Fontana M, Stocker M. The journey towards lung protective respiratory support in preterm neonates. Neonatology 2013;104:265–74.
15. Clark RH, Gerstmann DR, Jobe AH, et al. Lung injury in neonates: causes, strategies for prevention, and long-term consequences. J Pediatr 2001;139:478–86.
16. Dreyfuss D, Saumon G. Barotrauma is volutrauma, but which volume is the one responsible? Intensive Care Med 1992;18:139–41.
17. Dreyfuss D, Saumon G. Ventilator-induced lung injury: lessons from experimental studies. Am J Respir Crit Care Med 1998;157:294–323.
18. Lista G, Castoldi F, Fontana P, et al. Lung inflammation in preterm infants with respiratory distress syndrome: effects of ventilation with different tidal volumes. Pediatr Pulmonol 2006;41:357–63.

19. Gonzalez-Pacheco N, Sanchez-Luna M, Chimenti-Camacho P, et al. Use of very low tidal volumes during high-frequency ventilation reduces ventilator lung injury. J Perinatol 2019;39:730–6.

20. Schmolzer GM, Te Pas AB, Davis PG, et al. Reducing lung injury during neonatal resuscitation of preterm infants. J Pediatr 2008;153:741–5.

21. Hooper SB, Kitchen MJ, Wallace MJ, et al. Imaging lung aeration and lung liquid clearance at birth. FASEB J 2007;21:3329–37.

22. Krause MF, Jakel C, Haberstroh J, et al. Alveolar recruitment promotes homogeneous surfactant distribution in a piglet model of lung injury. Pediatr Res 2001;50: 34–43.

23. Tingay DG, Rajapaksa A, Zonneveld CE, et al. Spatiotemporal aeration and lung injury patterns are influenced by the first inflation strategy at birth. Am J Respir Cell Mol Biol 2016;54:263–72.

24. Tingay DG, Rajapaksa A, Zannin E, et al. Effectiveness of individualized lung recruitment strategies at birth: an experimental study in preterm lambs. Am J Physiol Lung Cell Mol Physiol 2017;312:L32–41.

25. Tingay DG, Togo A, Pereira-Fantini PM, et al. Aeration strategy at birth influences the physiological response to surfactant in preterm lambs. Arch Dis Child Fetal Neonatal Ed 2019;104:F587–93.

26. Bruschettini M, O'Donnell CP, Davis PG, et al. Sustained versus standard inflations during neonatal resuscitation to prevent mortality and improve respiratory outcomes. Cochrane Database Syst Rev 2020;3:CD004953.

27. Solevag AL, Haemmerle E, van Os S, et al. A novel prototype neonatal resuscitator that controls tidal volume and ventilation rate: a comparative study of mask ventilation in a newborn manikin. Front Pediatr 2016;4:129.

28. Solevag AL, Haemmerle E, van Os S, et al. Comparison of positive pressure ventilation devices in a newborn manikin. J Matern Fetal Neonatal Med 2017;30: 595–9.

29. Bamat N, Fierro J, Wang Y, et al. Positive end-expiratory pressure for preterm infants requiring conventional mechanical ventilation for respiratory distress syndrome or bronchopulmonary dysplasia. Cochrane Database Syst Rev 2019;2: CD004500.

30. Castoldi F, Daniele I, Fontana P, et al. Lung recruitment maneuver during volume guarantee ventilation of preterm infants with acute respiratory distress syndrome. Am J Perinatol 2011;28:521–8.

31. Wu R, Li SB, Tian ZF, et al. Lung recruitment maneuver during proportional assist ventilation of preterm infants with acute respiratory distress syndrome. J Perinatol 2014;34:524–7.

32. Ahluwalia JS, Morley CJ, Mockridge JN. Computerised determination of spontaneous inspiratory and expiratory times in premature neonates during intermittent positive pressure ventilation. II: results from 20 babies. Arch Dis Child Fetal Neonatal Ed 1994;71:F161–4.

33. Zivanovic S, Peacock J, Alcazar-Paris M, et al. Late outcomes of a randomized trial of high-frequency oscillation in neonates. N Engl J Med 2014;370:1121–30.

34. Dimitriou G, Greenough A. Measurement of lung volume and optimal oxygenation during high frequency oscillation. Arch Dis Child Fetal Neonatal Ed 1995;72: F180–3.

35. van der Burg PS, Miedema M, de Jongh FH, et al. Cross-sectional changes in lung volume measured by electrical impedance tomography are representative for the whole lung in ventilated preterm infants. Crit Care Med 2014;42:1524–30.

36. Baumgartner J, Klotz D, Schneider H, et al. Ultrashort inspiratory times homogenize ventilation distribution in an inhomogeneous two-compartment model of the neonatal lung. Pediatr Pulmonol 2021;56(2):418–23.

37. Miedema M, de Jongh FH, Frerichs I, et al. Changes in lung volume and ventilation during lung recruitment in high-frequency ventilated preterm infants with respiratory distress syndrome. J Pediatr 2011;159:199–205.

38. Gommers D, Vilstrup C, Bos JA, et al. Exogenous surfactant therapy increases static lung compliance, and cannot be assessed by measurements of dynamic compliance alone. Crit Care Med 1993;21:567–74.

39. Frerichs I, Dargaville PA, van Genderingen H, et al. Lung volume recruitment after surfactant administration modifies spatial distribution of ventilation. Am J Respir Crit Care Med 2006;174:772–9.

40. Goldsmith LS, Greenspan JS, Rubenstein SD, et al. Immediate improvement in lung volume after exogenous surfactant: alveolar recruitment versus increased distention. J Pediatr 1991;119:424–8.

41. da Silva WJ, Abbasi S, Pereira G, et al. Role of positive end-expiratory pressure changes on functional residual capacity in surfactant treated preterm infants. Pediatr Pulmonol 1994;18:89–92.

42. Klingenberg C, Wheeler KI, McCallion N, et al. Volume-targeted versus pressure-limited ventilation in neonates. Cochrane Database Syst Rev 2017;10:CD003666.

43. Patel DS, Rafferty GF, Lee S, et al. Work of breathing and volume targeted ventilation in respiratory distress. Arch Dis Child Fetal Neonatal Ed 2010;95:F443–6.

44. Carney D, DiRocco J, Nieman G. Dynamic alveolar mechanics and ventilator-induced lung injury. Crit Care Med 2005;33:S122–8.

45. Harris C, Thorpe SD, Rushwan S, et al. An in vitro investigation of the inflammatory response to the strain amplitudes which occur during high frequency oscillation ventilation and conventional mechanical ventilation. J Biomech 2019;88: 186–9.

46. Johnson AH, Peacock JL, Greenough A, et al. High-frequency oscillatory ventilation for the prevention of chronic lung disease of prematurity. N Engl J Med 2002; 347:633–42.

47. Ling R, Greenough A. Advances in emerging treatment options to prevent bronchopulmonary dysplasia. Expert Opin Orphan Drugs 2017;5:229–39.

48. Milner A, Murthy V, Bhat P, et al. Evaluation of respiratory function monitoring at the resuscitation of prematurely born infants. Eur J Pediatr 2015;174:205–8.

49. Schilleman K, Siew ML, Lopriore E, et al. Auditing resuscitation of preterm infants at birth by recording video and physiological parameters. Resuscitation 2012;83: 1135–9.

50. Katz TA, Weinberg DD, Fishman CE, et al. Visual attention on a respiratory function monitor during simulated neonatal resuscitation: an eye-tracking study. Arch Dis Child Fetal Neonatal Ed 2019;104:F259–64.

51. Sarrato GZ, Luna MS, Sarrato SZ, et al. New strategies of pulmonary protection of preterm infants in the delivery room with the respiratory function monitoring. Am J Perinat 2019;36:1368–76.

52. Atkins WK, McDougall R, Perkins EJ, et al. A dedicated respiratory function monitor to improve tidal volume delivery during neonatal anesthesia. Pediatr Anesth 2019;29:920–6.

53. Hooper SB, Fouras A, Siew ML, et al. Expired $CO_2$ levels indicate degree of lung aeration at birth. PLoS One 2013;8:e70895.

54. Murthy V, O'Rourke-Potocki A, Dattani N, et al. End tidal carbon dioxide levels during the resuscitation of prematurely born infants. Early Hum Dev 2012;88: 783–7.

55. Stromberg NO, Gustafsson PM. Ventilation inhomogeneity assessed by nitrogen washout and ventilation-perfusion mismatch by capnography in stable and induced airway obstruction. Pediatr Pulmonol 2000;29:94–102.

56. Ream RS, Schreiner MS, Neff JD, et al. Volumetric capnography in children. Influence of growth on the alveolar plateau slope. Anesthesiology 1995;82:64–73.

57. Dassios T, Dixon P, Williams E, et al. Volumetric capnography slopes in ventilated term and preterm infants. Physiol Meas 2020;41:055001.

58. Fouzas S, Hacki C, Latzin P, et al. Volumetric capnography in infants with bronchopulmonary dysplasia. J Pediatr 2014;164:283–8.

59. Gentner S, Laube M, Uhlig U, et al. Inflammatory mediators in tracheal aspirates of preterm infants participating in a randomized trial of permissive hypercapnia. Front Pediatr 2017;5:246.

60. Thome UH, Genzel-Boroviczeny O, Bohnhorst B, et al. Permissive hypercapnia in extremely low birthweight infants (PHELBI): a randomised controlled multicentre trial. Lancet Respir Med 2015;3:534–43.

61. Williams E, Dassios T, Greenough A. Assessment of sidestream end-tidal capnography in ventilated infants on the neonatal unit. Pediatr Pulmonol 2020;55: 1468–73.

62. Dassios T, Dixon P, Hickey A, et al. Physiological and anatomical dead space in mechanically ventilated newborn infants. Pediatr Pulmonol 2018;53:57–63.

63. Jobe AH, Ikegami M. Mechanisms initiating lung injury in the preterm. Early Hum Dev 1998;53:81–94.

64. Hickling KG. The pressure-volume curve is greatly modified by recruitment. A mathematical model of ARDS lungs. Am J Respir Crit Care Med 1998;158: 194–202.

65. Dargaville PA, Tingay DG. Lung protective ventilation in extremely preterm infants. J Paediatr Child Health 2012;48:740–6.

66. Mathe JC, Clement A, Chevalier JY, et al. Use of total inspiratory pressure-volume curves for determination of appropriate positive end-expiratory pressure in newborns with hyaline membrane disease. Intensive Care Med 1987;13:332–6.

67. Tingay DG, Mills JF, Morley CJ, et al. The deflation limb of the pressure-volume relationship in infants during high-frequency ventilation. Am J Respir Crit Care Med 2006;173:414–20.

68. Albaiceta GM, Luyando LH, Parra D, et al. Inspiratory vs. expiratory pressure-volume curves to set end-expiratory pressure in acute lung injury. Intensive Care Med 2005;31:1370–8.

69. Rimensberger PC, Cox PN, Frndova H, et al. The open lung during small tidal volume ventilation: concepts of recruitment and "optimal" positive end-expiratory pressure. Crit Care Med 1999;27:1946–52.

70. Daoud EG. Airway pressure release ventilation. Ann Thorac Med 2007;2:176–9.

71. van Kaam AH, De Luca D, Hentschel R, et al. Modes and strategies for providing conventional mechanical ventilation in neonates. Pediatr Res 2019. [Epub ahead of print].

72. Martin LD, Wetzel RC, Bilenki AL. Airway pressure release ventilation in a neonatal lamb model of acute lung injury. Crit Care Med 1991;19:373–8.

# Mechanical Ventilation During Chronic Lung Disease

Christopher D. Baker, MD

## KEYWORDS

- Preterm infants • Chronic ventilation • Tracheostomy

## KEY POINTS

- Infants with severe bronchopulmonary dysplasia (BPD) and other neonatal respiratory disorders can go on to develop chronic respiratory failure.
- When weaning of mechanical ventilation fails, chronic ventilation via tracheostomy may be considered.
- Strategies for chronic ventilation differ dramatically from those used in the acute period of respiratory distress. Rather than aiming to avoid lung injury, chronic ventilation aims to optimally support infants with established chronic lung disease.
- Family-centered care by an interdisciplinary team is essential for the successful management of infants who require mechanical ventilator for severe chronic lung disease.

## INTRODUCTION

Chronic lung disease (CLD) can develop after a wide-range of respiratory disorders in both preterm and full-term infants.[1] The most common and well-recognized is bronchopulmonary dysplasia (BPD), the severe CLD associated with preterm birth.[2] Many preterm infants who fail to meet criteria for BPD, however, nevertheless suffer from postprematurity respiratory disease and are at risk for respiratory complications later in life.[3,4] Moreover, neonatal respiratory disorders not due to prematurity, such as congenital diaphragmatic hernia (CDH), giant omphalocele, and other conditions associated with pulmonary hypoplasia also can result in CLD.[1,5,6] Disrupted lung growth and postnatal injury lead to impaired gas exchange and, in the most severe cases of CLD, chronic respiratory failure.[7,8] When chronic respiratory failure fails to improve during the first weeks of life, mechanical ventilation may be considered.[9] The number of infants receiving tracheostomies after prolonged mechanical ventilation has been increasing in recent years.[10] This article outlines approaches to invasive and noninvasive chronic ventilation for infants with severe CLD in the neonatal intensive care unit (NICU) and at home.

Disclosure statement: The author has nothing to disclose.
Section of Pulmonary and Sleep Medicine, Department of Pediatrics, University of Colorado School of Medicine, 13123 East 16th Avenue Box B-395, Aurora, CO 80045, USA
E-mail address: Christopher.Baker@CUAnschutz.edu

## IDENTIFYING CHRONIC RESPIRATORY FAILURE IN INFANTS WITH CHRONIC LUNG DISEASE

Both preterm and full-term neonates may develop respiratory distress syndrome (RDS) soon after birth. Some infants with RDS do not require intubation for invasive ventilation or stabilize rapidly, leading to timely extubation and ventilator liberation. Meanwhile, others experience severe and sustained respiratory failure that precludes ventilator weaning and extubation.[11] Identification of those infants who go on to require prolonged mechanical ventilation is difficult during early postnatal life. In addition to low birthweight and gestational age, the degree of ventilator support (higher tidal volume, peak inspiratory pressure, or minute ventilation) during the first day of life in preterm infants born before 32 weeks postmenstrual age is associated with persistent ventilator dependence on day 28.[12] This suggests that early ventilator-induced lung injury may contribute to the subsequent development of CLD. Some investigators have shown that an increase in mean airway pressure during the first weeks of life as well as tracheobronchomalacia may predict which babies require chronic ventilation via tracheostomy.[13,14]

The 2 groups, discussed previously, those with severe RDS who improve promptly to tolerate decreased support and those with severe persistent respiratory failure, are straightforward to identify. There also is an intermediate group of patients, however, who tolerate extubation but remain dependent on significant noninvasive support (eg, bilevel positive airway pressure, continuous positive airway pressure [CPAP], oxygen via heated humidified high-flow nasal cannula [HHHFNC], or other modalities).[15] Clinically, it then must be decided whether to continue weaning support or to consider chronic ventilation and, potentially, place a tracheostomy.

Importantly, infants with CLD who decompensate when CPAP or HHHFNC is interrupted are not stable for discharge. **Fig. 1** outlines how decision making may progress when caring for these infants. It is essential that an infant remain stable from both respiratory and developmental perspectives for weaning of support to be considered successful. Weaning that leads to increased respiratory distress (hypoxemia, tachypnea, increased work of breathing, or air hunger), impaired growth, or interruptions in developmental progress should be considered unsuccessful.[16]

This subacute form of chronic respiratory failure (inability to wean noninvasive support) can lead to marked hypercapnia with metabolic compensation (compensated respiratory acidosis). Some infants are given more time before weaning support is attempted again whereas others may be candidates for tracheostomy placement. This decision can be challenging for families.[17] Although debate remains, there is a growing understanding of the role of chronic ventilation via tracheostomy for infants with severe CLD.[18–20]

## ACUTE VERSUS CHRONIC VENTILATION: DIFFERENT GOALS

In the early postnatal period, ventilation strategies are aimed primarily at avoiding lung injury before CLD is established.[21] These acute strategies emphasize weaning whenever possible. As **Fig. 1** outlines, an infant may be weaned from invasive ventilation to progressively lower levels of noninvasive support. When a baby is stable with a safe amount of oxygen via low-flow nasal cannula or potentially room air, discharge can be considered. Home oxygen therapy is recommended for infants with chronic hypoxemia.[22]

Some neonates become unstable, however, when respiratory support is reduced and warrant consideration for chronic ventilation. The impression of whether or not an infant is tolerating reduced support is highly subjective. Nevertheless, as discussed

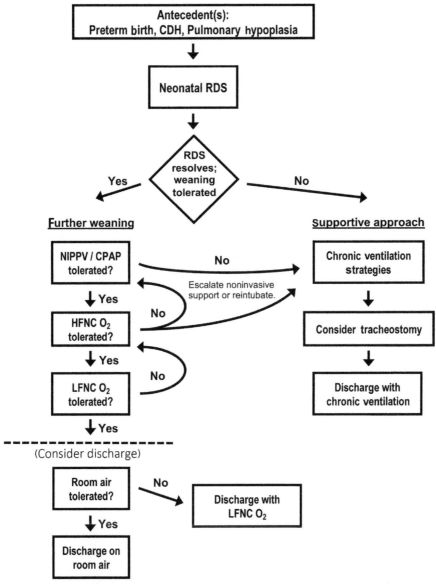

**Fig. 1.** Flowchart for attempting weaning in an infant with RDS, at risk for chronic respiratory failure. If weaning is tolerated, the baby should continue to grow and develop with respiratory stability and minimal distress. The speed of progression is at the discretion of the treating clinician. NIPPV, noninvasive positive pressure ventilation. HFNC, high-flow nasal cannula; LFNC, low-flow nasal cannula (<2 L/min).

previously, successful weaning should include consideration for all aspects of a child's stability. When weaning leads to compromises in these other areas, the baby likely benefits from returning to the higher level of support.

As the clinical course progresses and a child develops evidence of CLD, the goal of ventilation changes from preventing lung injury to supporting the child's breathing.

Once lung injury is established, larger volumes and higher pressures from the ventilator may be required. Moving forward, the priority shifts to providing optimal respiratory stability such that the child with CLD can grow, thrive, and participate in developmental therapy while minimizing life-threatening events.

## SPECIFIC CHRONIC STRATEGIES FOR INVASIVE VENTILATION

Abman and Nelin[11] first described strategies for chronic ventilation in 2011. Unlike protective ventilation, when the goal of ventilation is to optimally support the infant's breathing, a different approach to ventilation is required.[16,21] Chronic strategies are intended to optimally ventilate heterogeneously diseased lungs (interspersed areas of fibrosis/atelectasis and marked hyperinflation), as is common in infants with severe BPD (**Fig. 2**A).[23,24] Although the pathophysiology of CDH differs significantly from BPD, the most severe cases also have regionally heterogeneous lung disease, which is exaggerated further by the distinct structural differences between the ipsilateral and contralateral lung to the side of the diaphragm defect (**Fig. 2**B).[5] Although some forms of pulmonary hypoplasia consist of more homogeneous alveolar simplification and impaired microvascular growth, infants with severe hypoplasia also develop heterogeneous lung disease over time as CLD progresses (**Fig. 2**C).

Appropriate ventilator strategies for established CLD account for the observed pathophysiology. Large, slow breaths (10–12 mL/kg tidal volume with an inspiratory time of 0.6 seconds or longer) distribute air more evenly throughout the heterogeneously diseased lungs. A volume-targeted ventilator mode increases the likelihood that large breaths will continue to be given when resistance or compliance change (as occurs with illness or acutely when airways are occluded by mucus or secretions). Air trapping can be reduced by decreasing the respiratory rate to 10 breaths per minute to 14 breaths per minute, providing more time for exhalation. Sufficient positive end-expiratory pressure (PEEP) is essential for overcoming dynamic collapse of the airways or tracheobronchomalacia. In many cases, a clinician reduces the PEEP after observing hyperinflation on a chest radiograph only to find that hyperinflation worsens. Counterintuitively, when hyperinflation is due to tracheobronchomalacia (in large or small airways), increasing PEEP reduces hyperinflation by stenting open airways during exhalation and allowing the hyperinflated lung to degas. Implementation of these

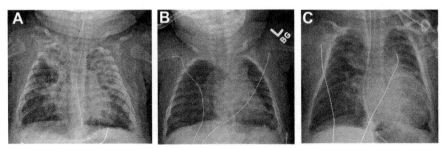

**Fig. 2.** Chest radiographs from 3 infants with severe heterogeneous lung disease of different etiologies. (*A*) A 3-month-old, 24-week preterm infant with severe BPD and lung disease characterized by severe upper lobe atelectasis and lower lobe hyperinflation. (*B*) A 4-month-old, full-term infant with left-sided CDH, right lung hyperinflation, and marked atelectasis in the lower left lung fields. (*C*) A 3-month-old, full-term infant with a repaired giant omphalocele, associated pulmonary hypoplasia, and regional hyperinflation and atelectasis.

chronic ventilation strategies often leads to a dramatic respiratory stabilization of babies with severe CLD.[11,25] Airways malacia also may occur in the small airways, distal to the trachea and large bronchi, which cannot be visualized by bronchoscopy. Babies with small airways malacia also may benefit from higher PEEP, which matches the intrinsic PEEP (or auto-PEEP) that the child must generate to open the collapsing airways.[26] Gibbs and colleagues[27] recently demonstrated how PEEP can be optimized to reduce airways resistance and respiratory system compliance. Additional breaths (those in excess of the set ventilator rate) should be treated with a pressure support, which does not exceed the peak inspiratory pressure delivered during the synchronized rated breaths.[9] Some centers use pressure-targeted ventilator modes with a similar ventilation strategy. In this case, a peak inspiratory pressure is chosen that results in delivery of an appropriately large tidal volume, as described previously.

## TIMING THE TRANSITION FROM ACUTE TO CHRONIC VENTILATION

Just as it is challenging to know whether and when to wean respiratory support in infants with severe CLD, it also is difficult to know when to transition from acute protective strategies to chronic supportive ventilation. The neonatologist must make this decision for each infant as the child's clinical course evolves during the first weeks of life. If an infant shows signs of improvement, weaning can be attempted, potentially aided by short courses of low-dose dexamethasone.[28] Chronic ventilation is indicated when a neonate develops the signs and symptoms of CLD (worsening hypoxemia, acute hypoxemic events, chronic hypoventilation, patchy atelectasis, and hyperinflation on chest radiograph).[2,29] In preterm infants, the change to chronic ventilation strategies can be made as soon as established heterogeneous lung disease is identified.[27]

Although some infants may tolerate only small changes in ventilation at any given moment, others dramatically improve when significant changes are made to the ventilator settings. For example, a preterm infant with established CLD, severe decompensation spells, hypercapnia, and marked hypoxemia who currently is ventilated with small tidal volumes (5–6 mL/kg) and a fast rate (25–30 breaths per minute) can improve dramatically when the tidal volume is increased to 10 mL/kg and the rate reduced to 14 breaths per minute Clinical stabilization can be observed immediately, the fraction of inspired oxygen needed to maintain normal saturation quickly decreases, and improvements in the chest radiograph may follow several days after the change in ventilation strategy. The individual components of this strategy work in tandem with each other; increasing the tidal volume and inspiratory time without lowering the rate can worsen hyperinflation or cause pneumothoraces. Failing to treat with sufficient PEEP also can be detrimental for the reasons previously described.

Full-term infants with CDH or other forms of pulmonary hypoplasia and established heterogeneous CLD also can benefit from the supportive ventilation strategies, discussed previously. The clinical course of these infants is highly variable, however, from those who require support by extracorporeal membrane oxygenation (ECMO) early in life and are unable to be liberated from the ventilator after ECMO is discontinued to those who do not require ECMO, intubation, or mechanical ventilation at all and no longer are hypoxemic after 30 days of life.[30]

## TO TRACH OR NOT TO TRACH

When infants with CLD and chronic respiratory failure are stabilized with chronic ventilation, consideration of tracheostomy is warranted. An interdisciplinary team should utilize shared decision making with the infant's family to determine the best way to proceed.[17,31] When the ultimate neurodevelopmental potential of the child is poor or uncertain, the decision to place a tracheostomy for chronic mechanical ventilation can be ethically challenging. The family's social situation also should be considered, not as a reason for denying tracheostomy but to make sure the family is fully informed as to how dramatically their lives will change when they begin to care for a chronically ventilated child at home.[32,33] Before the tracheotomy procedure occurs, it is essential that family caregivers understand how this will have an impact on their child for the remainder of the hospital stay and during the years to follow.

If a baby shows signs of improvement, additional time to grow and stabilize may be warranted. If subsequent attempts to wean support are not tolerated or if the current respiratory support modality is interfering with the child's ability to make developmental progress, however, tracheostomy may be considered. In most centers, tracheostomy placement for chronic ventilation in severe BPD does not occur before a preterm neonate reaches 40 weeks' postmenstrual age.[34,35] At this point, when there is a high risk of delaying development, a tracheostomy may be placed. Families must understand that their child likely will be 2 years to 3 years old when mechanical ventilation no longer is needed and the tracheostomy can be removed safely.[36] Some children even are liberated from the ventilator sooner than this, but a small number require mechanical ventilation for years longer. Early predictors of long-term outcomes remain unclear for chronically ventilated infants with severe CLD.

After the tracheotomy procedure, close monitoring in an NICU is essential while the tracheostomy stoma heals and becomes epithelialized. This may require increased sedation, and potentially medical paralysis, to facilitate healing. Typically, on postoperative day 5 to day 7, the tracheostomy tube is changed for the first time by the surgical team. When the stoma is healed and the infant is stable, sedation and paralysis may be discontinued cautiously. Prompt involvement of occupational and physical therapists and speech language pathologists is critical when the child is sufficiently stable and alert to tolerate therapies. Even in somewhat unstable children, trained developmental therapists may collaborate with the medical team to optimize state regulation, aid in managing agitation, cautiously begin passive range of motion therapy, and even work on important prefeeding skills to avoid oral aversion.

## SEVERE AGITATION AND PATIENT-VENTILATOR DYSSYNCHRONY

The strategies for chronic ventilation, discussed previously, enable a majority of infants with CLD to stabilize. After the child has recovered from tracheostomy placement, sedation can be weaned in most cases. One of the goals of chronic ventilation via tracheostomy is to facilitate sedation weaning so that the child can devote attention to growing and developing. A small number of the most severe infants remain unstable after tracheostomy and decompensate acutely whenever sedation is weaned. The severity of lung disease can limit an infant's ability to pneumatically trigger the ventilator to deliver a breath. As discussed previously, an insufficient PEEP requires additional patient effort to keep airways open, which are prone to dynamic collapse.[27] Some clinicians may elect to provide prolonged sedation (and medical paralysis if needed) for a period of time to appropriately ventilate the infant, followed by very slow weaning of sedation in hope of better tolerating chronic ventilation with improved synchrony. Certain centers offer neurally adjusted ventilatory assist (NAVA) ventilation, which has been shown to improve patient-ventilator synchrony, reduce cyanotic events, and facilitate sedation weaning.[37,38] NAVA ventilation requires a nasogastric catheter, which monitors the electrical signal from the phrenic nerve to the diaphragm to determine when the child is attempting to take a breath. The timing and strength of this signal direct the ventilator to deliver an appropriately sized breath, effectively eliminating patient-ventilator dyssynchrony. NAVA ventilation requires an intact respiratory drive, however, and does not ensure that a chronic ventilation strategy (larger, longer, and less frequent breaths, as described previously) is followed. Finally, even if NAVA is effective, the infant eventually needs to be transitioned back to conventional ventilation because NAVA ventilation can be delivered only in an intensive care unit (ICU).

## NONINVASIVE CHRONIC VENTILATION

If a decision is made to not place a tracheostomy tube, noninvasive ventilation likely is required because an infant with severe CLD cannot remain intubated and mechanically ventilated indefinitely in the NICU. Several noninvasive modalities exist to either provide ventilation or support the baby's own ventilation. Many devices and patient interfaces are available for noninvasive support. These include masks (nasal and full face), nasal pillows, and firmer cannulas that are capable of delivering positive pressure ventilation.[39] Noninvasive support may be an excellent option for infants who require mechanical ventilation intermittently (eg, only with sleep). In cases of an infant with severe CLD who cannot tolerate periods of time without ventilation, noninvasive support may be more dangerous in that the interface may become dislodged more easily than a properly secured tracheostomy tube. Continuous noninvasive ventilation also interferes with oral skills (feeding, swallowing, and speech) and increases the risk of skin breakdown where the interface comes into contact with the face.[40]

## MECHANICALLY VENTILATING INFANTS WITH CHRONIC LUNG DISEASE AT HOME

For infants who are stable with chronic ventilation via tracheostomy, the transition from ICU ventilator to home ventilator may be attempted. When treating the most severe forms of CLD, this transition may be challenging. An attempt should be made to replicate the settings from the ICU ventilator on the home device to the degree that it is possible. Some home ventilators limit how long the inspiratory time can be set for synchronized rated breaths, which can make the transition to home ventilator challenging for smaller infants. Although there currently is no standard of care pertaining to this transition, Willis and colleagues[41] implemented a standardized protocol for the home ventilator transition and observed that successful transition to the home ventilator occurred sooner than before their process was standardized. Some infants fail transition to the home ventilator initially and must remain in the ICU for future attempts when they have grown and become more stable. Typically, clinical teams allow 1 or more weeks to pass before attempting the transition again. A detailed description of a failed trial can be informative for subsequent attempts. In the author's center, families can become discouraged by failed attempts given their strong desire to keep making progress toward home discharge. It is emphasized that, during these key developmental periods, remaining stable to continue growing and tolerating developmental therapies is most important.

Once stable on a home ventilator, care coordination and discharge readiness become the focus of care.[42] The key elements of discharge preparation are

- Confirming that the infant with severe CLD is medically stable for discharge
- Completing comprehensive family education—caregivers must demonstrate competence in providing both routine cares and emergency interventions **(Table 1)**.[42–50]
- Obtaining durable medical equipment with accessible technical support
- Recruiting sufficient in-home private duty nursing

**Table 1**
Family caregivers (at least 2 per family) must receive comprehensive education (emphasis placed on competence and demonstration of skills). The format of education may vary but typically includes a combination of didactic instruction, hands-on practice, printed materials, videos (readily available online if possible), and emergent scenarios.[42–50]

| Education of Family Caregivers for Home Ventilation Via Tracheostomy | |
| --- | --- |
| **Category** | **Specific Topics to Cover** |
| Knowing their child | Normal respiratory system anatomy, specific anatomic and pathologic understanding of the child's disease (in lay persons' terms), indication(s) for tracheostomy and chronic ventilation, need for prolonged hospitalization, discharge process, impact on family and life at home |
| Tracheostomy tube | Suctioning (open or in-line), daily cares (cleaning stoma, changing tracheostomy ties), assessing the tracheostomy stoma, primary tracheostomy tube size and characteristics, back-up tracheostomy tube size, routine tracheostomy changes (2 people), emergency tracheostomy changes (1–2 people), bag-tracheostomy ventilation, bagging/suctioning with saline, emergencies (plugged tracheostomy, decannulation) |
| Home ventilator | Ventilator set-up, ventilator settings, circuit changes, portable/back-up ventilator set-up (if applicable), humidification set-up and troubleshooting, ventilator alarms, emergencies (ventilator malfunction and circuit disconnect) |
| Additional equipment | Pulse oximetry monitoring and device use, home oxygen (concentrator, tanks, regulators, and connecting to circuit/patient), nebulized/inhaled medications, using gastrostomy tube and feeding pump |
| Transportation | Transferring patient to the portable ventilator; go bag (emergency equipment to be with the child at all times: suction machine/supplies and extra and back-up tracheostomy tubes); heat moisture exchanger to trap humidity; car ride, where (at a minimum) family practices loading and unloading patient and equipment into their vehicle under supervision |
| Cardiopulmonary resuscitation training | Cardiopulmonary resuscitation training with focus on ventilation with advanced airway (tracheostomyeostomy tube) in place |
| Simulation training | High-fidelity simulation for rehearsing emergent scenarios (not available in all centers) |
| Independent stays | Two or more 12+-hour periods completed before discharge (often 1 day shift and 1 night shift or 1 24-h shift; each trained family caregiver must individually demonstrate competence to provide all routine cares; medical team remains available if caregiver needs help and for emergencies). The goal is to identify knowledge gaps and ensure caregiver competence. |

The format of education may vary but typically includes a combination of didactic instruction, hands-on practice, printed materials, videos (readily available online if possible), and emergent scenarios.

For most families, home nursing support is necessary to ensure that the chronically ventilated child remains in the presence of an awake, trained caregiver at all times.[50] Home ventilators and pulse oximeters may fail to alarm, endangering the infant, and thus are no substitute for an awake, trained caregiver.[51] Most families cannot provide continuous care without home professionals providing some degree of respite. Home nursing shortages, however, often result in discharge delays.[52–54]

Infants who require mechanical ventilation for CLD are in the hospital for many months.[42] Standardizing the discharge process (while still customizing it for each patient) is essential for ensuring the safety of the child, limiting the distress of the family, and delivering cost-effective care. The discharge process can be improved by formalizing a team with dedicated care coordinators and by tracking progress in the electronic medical record.[55–57]

Once the infant and family are finally home, life changes dramatically. Although many families report joyful feelings and a sensation of returning to normalcy after an extremely prolonged hospitalization, family caregivers of children with home ventilation also describe experiencing fatigue, depression, anxiety, and a reduced quality of life.[58–61] Improved access to quality home nursing resources may help alleviate parental anxiety and may reduce hospital readmissions.[62] New technologies, such as telemedicine and remote monitoring, also may increase safety at home.[63–65] This is important because mortality for severe BPD remains approximately 15% to 20%, often due to preventable complications rather than disease progression.[36,66,67] The mortality rate for CDH after tracheostomy is higher than for BPD (33%), but this is similar to the mortality rate of patients with CDH who do not receive tracheostomies (29%).[30]

In time, it can be expected that most infants with CLD will improve and the need for mechanical ventilation will resolve. Although the likelihood of developmental delay remains, a long-term survival of 81% was reported by Cristea and colleagues,[36] who noted that most survivors were liberated from the ventilator (83%) and decannulated (72%).

Given the likelihood of ventilator liberation and tracheostomy decannulation, chronic ventilation should not be considered a failure. If a supportive approach to ventilation can enable an infant with CLD to breathe comfortably, wean sedation, and make developmental progress, then tracheostomy for chronic ventilation may be the most appropriate intervention. Chronic mechanical ventilation may be warranted for all infants with chronic respiratory failure, rather than reserved for only the sickest infants who are unlikely to survive.[31] There is a strong need for studies examining the impact of chronic ventilation on long-term neurodevelopmental outcomes in this very high-risk infant population.

## SUMMARY

- Many preterm and full-term infants with severe CLD can benefit from chronic ventilation via tracheostomy.
- The overall goals of care and the specific ventilation strategies are uniquely different for treating acute and chronic respiratory failure.
- Eventual survival with liberation from mechanical ventilation and tracheostomy decannulation during early childhood is the most likely outcome for infants who require chronic ventilation for CLD.
- Further study is needed to determine how chronic ventilation during infancy affects respiratory and neurodevelopmental outcomes later in life.

## DISCLOSURE

A. Guarantor of the article: C.D. Baker.
  B. Any potential competing conflicts of interest: none.
  C. Statement of financial support: none.

## BEST PRACTICES BOX

---

- When a neonate with chronic lung disease fails to tolerate weaning from invasive or noninvasive ventilation, chronic ventilation should be considered.

For infants who warrant chronic ventilation, tracheostomy may be considered.

The majority of infants who are chronically ventilated via tracheostomy will be liberated from mechanical ventilation and undergo tracheostomy decannulation during early childhood.

Comprehensive training of family caregivers and a plan for observation by an awake trained caregiver at all times is critical to each child's safety at home.

---

## REFERENCES

1. Jobe AH, Bancalari E. Bronchopulmonary dysplasia. Am J Respir Crit Care Med 2001;163(7):1723–9.
2. Northway WH, Rosan RC, Porter DY. Pulmonary disease following respirator therapy of hyaline-membrane disease. Bronchopulmonary dysplasia. N Engl J Med 1967;276(7):357–68.
3. Keller RL, Feng R, Demauro SB, et al. Bronchopulmonary dysplasia and perinatal characteristics predict 1-year respiratory outcomes in newborns born at extremely low gestational age: a prospective Cohort study. J Pediatr 2017;187:89–97.e3.
4. Doyle LW, Andersson S, Bush A, et al. Expiratory airflow in late adolescence and early adulthood in individuals born very preterm or with very low birthweight compared with controls born at term or with normal birthweight: a meta-analysis of individual participant data. Lancet Respir Med 2019;7(8):677–86.
5. Hislop A, Reid L. Persistent hypoplasia of the lung after repair of congenital diaphragmatic hernia. Thorax 1976;31(4):450–5.
6. Argyle JC. Pulmonary hypoplasia in infants with giant abdominal wall defects. Pediatr Pathol 1989;9(1):43–55.
7. Jobe AJ. The new BPD: an arrest of lung development. Pediatr Res 1999;46(6):641–3.
8. Albertine KH, Jones GP, Starcher BC, et al. Chronic lung injury in preterm lambs. Disordered respiratory tract development. Am J Respir Crit Care Med 1999;159(3):945–58.
9. Baker CD. Long-term ventilation for children with chronic lung disease of infancy. Curr Opin Pediatr 2019;31(3):357–66.
10. Overman AE, Liu M, Kurachek SC, et al. Tracheostomy for infants requiring prolonged mechanical ventilation: 10 years' experience. Pediatrics 2013;131(5):e1491–6.
11. Abman SH, Nelin LD. Management of the infant with severe bronchopulmonary dysplasia. In: Bancalari E, editor. The newborn lung: neonatology questions and controversies, 2012 2011;. p. 407–25.
12. Ali K, Kagalwalla S, Cockar I, et al. Prediction of prolonged ventilator dependence in preterm infants. Eur J Pediatr 2019;178(7):1063–8.

13. Hysinger EB, Friedman NL, Padula MA, et al. Tracheobronchomalacia is associated with increased morbidity in bronchopulmonary dysplasia. Ann Am Thorac Soc 2017;14(9):1428–35.

14. Wai KC, Keller RL, Lusk LA, et al. Characteristics of extremely low gestational age newborns undergoing tracheotomy. JAMA Otolaryngol Head Neck Surg 2017; 143(1):13–7.

15. Wilkinson D, Andersen C, O'Donnell CP, et al. High flow nasal cannula for respiratory support in preterm infants. Cochrane Database Syst Rev 2016;2: CD006405.

16. Gien J, Abman SH, Baker CD. Interdisciplinary care for ventilator-dependent infants with chronic lung disease. J Pediatr 2014;165(6):1274–5.

17. Edwards JD, Panitch HB, Nelson JE, et al. Decisions for long-term ventilation for children. Perspectives of family members. Ann Am Thorac Soc 2020;17(1):72–80.

18. Barbato A, Bottecchia L, Snijders D. Tracheostomy in children: an ancient procedure still under debate. Eur Respir J 2012;40(6):1322–3.

19. Chotirmall SH, Flynn MG, Donegan CF, et al. Extubation versus tracheostomy in withdrawal of treatment-ethical, clinical, and legal perspectives. J Crit Care 2010; 25(2):360.e1–8.

20. Edwards JD, Morris MC, Nelson JE, et al. Decisions around long-term ventilation for children. Perspectives of directors of pediatric home ventilation programs. Ann Am Thorac Soc 2017;14(10):1539–47.

21. Abman SH, Collaco JM, Shepherd EG, et al. Interdisciplinary care of children with severe bronchopulmonary dysplasia. J Pediatr 2017;181:12–28.e1.

22. Hayes D Jr, Wilson KC, Krivchenia K, et al. Home oxygen therapy for children. An Official American Thoracic Society Clinical Practice guideline. Am J Respir Crit Care Med 2019;199(3):e5–23.

23. Coalson JJ. Pathology of new bronchopulmonary dysplasia. Semin Neonatal 2003;8(1):73–81.

24. Castile RG, Nelin LD. Lung function, structure and the physiologic basis for mechanical ventilation of infants with established BPD. In: Abman SH, editor. Bronchopulmonary dysplasia. New York, NY: Informa Healthcare; 2010. p. 328–46.

25. Hysinger EB, Panitch HB. Paediatric tracheomalacia. Paediatr Respir Rev 2016; 17:9–15.

26. Napolitano N, Jalal K, McDonough JM, et al. Identifying and treating intrinsic PEEP in infants with severe bronchopulmonary dysplasia. Pediatr Pulmonol 2019;54(7):1045–51.

27. Gibbs K, Jensen EA, Alexiou S, et al. Ventilation strategies in severe bronchopulmonary dysplasia. Neoreviews 2020;21(4):e226–37.

28. Doyle LW, Davis PG, Morley CJ, et al. Low-dose dexamethasone facilitates extubation among chronically ventilator-dependent infants: a multicenter, international, randomized, controlled trial. Pediatrics 2006;117(1):75–83.

29. Bolivar JM, Gerhardt T, Gonzalez A, et al. Mechanisms for episodes of hypoxemia in preterm infants undergoing mechanical ventilation. J Pediatr 1995;127(5): 767–73.

30. Al Baroudi S, Collaco JM, Lally PA, et al. Clinical features and outcomes associated with tracheostomy in congenital diaphragmatic hernia. Pediatr Pulmonol 2020;55(1):90–101.

31. Gien J, Kinsella J, Thrasher J, et al. Retrospective analysis of an interdisciplinary ventilator care program intervention on survival of infants with ventilator-dependent bronchopulmonary dysplasia. Am J Perinatol 2017;34(2):155–63.

32. Amar-Dolan LG, Horn MH, O'Connell B, et al. "This is how hard it is": family experience of hospital-to-home transition with a tracheostomy. Ann Am Thorac Soc 2020;17(7):860–8.

33. Baker CD. Take me home to the place I belong: discharging the tracheostomy-dependent child. Ann Am Thorac Soc 2020;17(7):809–10.

34. Mandy G, Malkar M, Welty SE, et al. Tracheostomy placement in infants with bronchopulmonary dysplasia: safety and outcomes. Pediatr Pulmonol 2013;48(3):245–9.

35. Rane S, Bathula S, Thomas RL, et al. Outcomes of tracheostomy in the neonatal intensive care unit: is there an optimal time? J Matern Fetal Neonatal Med 2014;27(12):1257–61.

36. Cristea AI, Carroll AE, Davis SD, et al. Outcomes of children with severe bronchopulmonary dysplasia who were ventilator dependent at home. Pediatrics 2013;132(3):e727–34.

37. Lee J, Kim HS, Jung YH, et al. Neurally adjusted ventilatory assist for infants under prolonged ventilation. Pediatr Int 2017;59(5):540–4.

38. McKinney RL, Keszler M, Truog WE, et al. Multicenter experience with neurally adjusted ventilatory assist in infants with severe bronchopulmonary dysplasia. Am J Perinatol 2020;28(S01):e162–6.

39. De Jesus Rojas W, Samuels CL, Gonzales TR, et al. Use of nasal non-invasive ventilation with a RAM cannula in the outpatient home setting. Open Respir Med J 2017;11:41–6.

40. Fedor KL. Noninvasive respiratory support in infants and children. Respir Care 2017;62(6):699–717.

41. Willis LD, Lowe G, Pearce P, et al. Transition from an ICU ventilator to a portable home ventilator in children. Respir Care 2020;65(12):1791–9.

42. Baker CD, Martin S, Thrasher J, et al. A standardized discharge process decreases length of stay for ventilator-dependent children. Pediatrics 2016;137(4):e20150637.

43. Amin R, Parshuram C, Kelso J, et al. Caregiver knowledge and skills to safely care for pediatric tracheostomy ventilation at home. Pediatr Pulmonol 2017;52(12):1610–5.

44. Amin R, Zabih W, Syed F, et al. What families have in the emergency tracheostomy kits: identifying gaps to improve patient safety. Pediatr Pulmonol 2017;52(12):1605–9.

45. Graf JM, Montagnino BA, Hueckel R, et al. Children with new tracheostomies: planning for family education and common impediments to discharge. Pediatr Pulmonol 2008;43(8):788–94.

46. Tolomeo CT, Bazzy-Asaad A. Utilization of a second caregiver in the care of a child with a tracheostomy in the homecare setting. Pediatr Pulmonology 2010;45(7):656–60.

47. Agarwal A, Marks N, Wessel V, et al. Improving knowledge, technical skills, and confidence among pediatric health care providers in the management of chronic tracheostomy using a simulation model. Pediatr Pulmonoly 2016;51(7):696–704.

48. Thrasher J, Baker J, Ventre KM, et al. Hospital to home: a quality improvement initiative to implement high-fidelity simulation training for caregivers of children requiring long-term mechanical ventilation. J Pediatr Nurs 2017;38:114–21.

49. Tofil NM, Rutledge C, Zinkan JL, et al. Ventilator caregiver education through the use of high-fidelity pediatric simulators: a pilot study. Clin Pediatr 2013;52(11):1038–43.

50. Sterni LM, Collaco JM, Baker CD, et al. An Official American Thoracic Society Clinical Practice Guideline: pediatric chronic home invasive ventilation. Am J Respir Crit Care Med 2016;193(8):e16–35.
51. Kun SS, Nakamura CT, Ripka JF, et al. Home ventilator low-pressure alarms fail to detect accidental decannulation with pediatric tracheostomy tubes. Chest 2001; 119(2):562–4.
52. Sobotka SA, Hird-McCorry LP, Goodman DM. Identification of fail points for discharging pediatric patients with new tracheostomy and ventilator. Hosp Pediatr 2016;6(9):552–7.
53. Sobotka SA, Gaur DS, Goodman DM, et al. Pediatric patients with home mechanical ventilation: the health services landscape. Pediatr Pulmonol 2019;54(1):40–6.
54. Sobotka SA, Dholakia A, Berry JG, et al. Home nursing for children with home mechanical ventilation in the United States: key informant perspectives. Pediatr Pulmonol 2020;55(12):3465–76.
55. Tearl DK, Cox TJ, Hertzog JH. Hospital discharge of respiratory-technology-dependent children: role of a dedicated respiratory care discharge coordinator. Respir Care 2006;51(7):744–9.
56. Rowan CM, Cristea AI, Hamilton JC, et al. Nurse practitioner coverage is associated with a decrease in length of stay in a pediatric chronic ventilator dependent unit. World J Clin Pediatr 2016;5(2):191–7.
57. Hanks J, Carrico CA. Evaluating the use of a stability guideline for long-term ventilator-dependent children discharging to home: a quality improvement project. J Pediatr Health Care 2017;31(6):648–53.
58. Carnevale FA, Alexander E, Davis M, et al. Daily living with distress and enrichment: the moral experience of families with ventilator-assisted children at home. Pediatrics 2006;117(1):e48–60.
59. Meltzer LJ, Boroughs DS, Downes JJ. The relationship between home nursing coverage, sleep, and daytime functioning in parents of ventilator-assisted children. J Pediatr Nurs 2010;25(4):250–7.
60. Seear M, Kapur A, Wensley D, et al. The quality of life of home-ventilated children and their primary caregivers plus the associated social and economic burdens: a prospective study. Arch Dis Child 2016;101(7):620–7.
61. Graham RJ, Rodday AM, Weidner RA, et al. The impact on family of pediatric chronic respiratory failure in the home. J Pediatr 2016;175:40–6.
62. Sobotka SA, Lynch E, Peek ME, et al. Readmission drivers for children with medical complexity: home nursing shortages cause health crises. Pediatr Pulmonol 2020;55(6):1474–80.
63. Battista L. A new system for continuous and remote monitoring of patients receiving home mechanical ventilation. Rev Sci Instrum 2016;87(9):095105.
64. Casavant DW, McManus ML, Parsons SK, et al. Trial of telemedicine for patients on home ventilator support: feasibility, confidence in clinical management and use in medical decision-making. J Telemed Telecare 2014;20(8):441–9.
65. Vitacca M, Guerra A, Assoni G, et al. Weaning from mechanical ventilation followed at home with the aid of a telemedicine program. Telemed J E Health 2007;13(4):445–50.
66. Boroughs D, Dougherty JA. Decreasing accidental mortality of ventilator-dependent children at home: a call to action. Home Healthc Nurse 2012;30(2):103–11, quiz 112-103.
67. Edwards JD, Kun SS, Keens TG. Outcomes and causes of death in children on home mechanical ventilation via tracheostomy: an institutional and literature review. J Pediatr 2010;157(6):955–9.e2.

# Weaning from the Ventilator in Bronchopulmonary Dysplasia

Giovanni Vento, MD*, Chiara Tirone, MD, Angela Paladini, MD,
Claudia Aurilia, MD, Alessandra Lio, MD, Milena Tana, MD

## KEYWORDS

- Bronchopulmonary dysplasia • Chronic ventilation • Prematurity
- Mechanical ventilation weaning • Noninvasive ventilation weaning • Tracheostomy

## KEY POINTS

- To facilitate weaning from mechanical ventilation in infants with severe form of bronchopulmonary dysplasia (sBPD) one of the main concept to be considered is that the respiratory stability (ie, no retractions, no tachypnea, no recurrent cyanotic or bradycardic episodes), better reflect successful strategies than traditional metrics of $PaCO_2$;
- In patients with sBPD in whom mechanical ventilation provides adequate gas exchange and reduces work of breathing by promoting the growth and healing of the injured lungs with the other therapies, there is a slow but steady decrease in the amount of oxygen needed to provide stable saturation;
- The focus should be to slowly and daily reduce the oxygen concentration achieving $SpO_2$ targets.

## INTRODUCTION

Bronchopulmonary dysplasia (BPD) is a debilitating lung disease that occurs in premature infants, resulting from an abnormal reparative response to both prenatal and postnatal damage of the developing lung.[1] Many diagnostic criteria have been developed over the years. In 2001 Jobe and Bancalari published the first severity-based definition of BPD.[2] This classification scheme categorizes BPD as mild, moderate, or severe according to the respiratory support provided at 36 weeks postmenstrual age (PMA) among very preterm infants treated with supplemental oxygen for at least 28 days. A significant center-to-center variability in oxygen use was noted. To decrease this variability Walsh and colleagues proposed in 2003 a standardized oxygen reduction

Dipartimento Universitario Scienze della Vita e Sanità Pubblica, Unità Operativa Complessa di Neonatologia, Fondazione Policlinico Universitario A. Gemelli IRCCS, Università Cattolica del Sacro Cuore, Largo Agostino Gemelli 8, Rome 00168, Italy
* Corresponding author.
*E-mail address:* giovanni.vento@unicatt.it

Clin Perinatol 48 (2021) 895–906
https://doi.org/10.1016/j.clp.2021.08.005
0095-5108/21/© 2021 Elsevier Inc. All rights reserved.
**perinatology.theclinics.com**

test to determine supplemental oxygen dependency among infants receiving 30% or less supplemental oxygen.[3] Later studies showed that although this "physiologic definition" decreases intercenter variability in BPD rates, it may not improve outcome prognostication among infants who qualify for testing.[4] Different strategies for oxygen supplementation can influence the diagnosis of the severity of BPD that is made clinically. As a consequence, it is extremely necessary to identify the minimum noninvasive respiratory assistance and $Fio_2$ necessary to guarantee adequate respiratory support for the infant. With this aim in a previous study our group suggested a modified physiologic test for BPD that can be used as a clinical tool.[5]

Unfortunately, additional limitations to the 2001 definition emerged over time. In recent years, several systems that administer heated and humidified "high-flow" nasal cannula have been introduced into clinical practice. In 2017, the multicenter BPD Collaborative proposed that infants treated with "high-flow" nasal cannula at 36 weeks PMA (along with those receiving other forms of noninvasive positive airway pressure) be defined as having type 1 severe BPD. They further recommended that infants receiving invasive mechanical ventilation at 36 weeks PMA be classified as a new type 2 severe BPD[6]. The proposed definition maintains a categorical, severity-based structure, but a grade I to III scale replaces the mild, moderate, and severe terminology.[4] The 2018 NICHD workshop definition proposed a grade IIIA BPD for infants with early death between 14 days postnatal age and 36 weeks PMA from persistent parenchymal lung disease and respiratory failure that is not attributable to other neonatal morbidities.[4] In 2019 Jensen and colleagues suggested a modified definition of BPD severity at 36 weeks PMA, based on type of respiratory support, instead of $O_2$ supplementation, as best predictor of respiratory outcomes.[7]

Our institutional practice is to proceed with a weaning protocol according to the type of respiratory support delivered at 36 weeks PMA.

## DISCUSSION
### Weaning from Invasive Mechanical Ventilation in Infants with Severe Bronchopulmonary Dysplasia

For the newborns needing invasive respiratory support at 36 weeks PMA, regardless of the type of ventilation used, it will be necessary to take into account the mechanics properties of both airways and lungs affected by severe BPD (sBPD), in particular increased airway resistances, decreased lung compliance, and reduced functional residual capacity in lungs containing regional heterogeneity in the severity of their disease.[6–9]

For all these reasons ventilator strategies, settings, and weaning must change dramatically after sBPD is established, but to date there is almost no high-quality evidence base supporting a specific approach to guide the optimal ventilator management and weaning in patients with sBPD.

Identifying phenotypical presentation of sBPD and its underlying lung pathology may therefore be the first important step in determining the appropriate individual management strategy, because both ventilator strategies and weaning should be selected on the lung physiology and pathologic changes of each patient.[7]

Although during acute lung disease the mechanical ventilation (MV) strategies provide a fast rate, low tidal volume (VT) and short inspiratory time (Ti) with a rapid weaning from MV to avoid lung injury, the goals of MV in the ventilated infants with sBPD are to reach adequate gas exchange, minimize ventilation/perfusion (V/Q) mismatch, provide relatively stable respiratory support reducing the work of breathing and respiratory distress (no retractions, no tachypnea, no recurrent cyanotic or bradycardic episodes), reducing the need for chronic sedation, preventing the development or progression of pulmonary hypertension (PH), and promoting optimal growth (both somatic and alveolar/vascular growth).[6,9]

To date clinical experience and current understanding of the pathophysiology of sBPD validate the strategy of slow-rate (10–20/min), high $V_T$ (8–12 mL/kg) (for pressure ventilation, the peak inspiratory pressure [PIP] needed to generate this Vt can be well greater than 25 $cmH_2O$), and prolonged Ti (0.5–0.8 seconds) ventilation in patients with sBPD, providing in association adequate positive end-expiratory pressure (PEEP), major than 8 to 10 $cmH_2O$ (may need PEEP >10–15 $cmH_2O$) and eventual adequate pressure support for spontaneous breaths (may be as high as the PIP needed on the mandatory vent breath) helping minute ventilation maintainment and achieving overall low respiratory rate.[7–9]

In association with this MV strategy in patients with sBPD we need to provide permissive hypercapnia and adjust $Fio_2$ to target higher $SpO_2$ values greater than 92% (92%–95%) or greater than or equal to 97% (97%–98%) in sBPD with PH.[6,9] Some important concepts could facilitate weaning from MV in sBPD infants: (1) the clinical variables of respiratory stability (ie, no retractions, no tachypnea, no recurrent cyanotic or bradycardic episodes), probably better reflect successful strategies than traditional metrics of $Paco_2$ or end-tidal $CO_2$[6]; (2) in patients with sBPD in whom MV provides adequate gas exchange and reduces work of breathing by promoting the growth and healing of the injured lungs with the others therapies, there is a slow but steady decrease in the amount of oxygen needed to provide stable saturation.[1,6] The focus should be to slowly and daily reduce the oxygen concentration (reducing no more than 10% respect to the previous $Fio_2$ a day) achieving $SpO_2$ targets.

When infants are stable for at least 24 hours in less than 40% $Fio_2$ to achieve $SpO_2$ targets with satisfactory gas exchange and without increase in work of breathing (Silverman score ≤3), extubation to noninvasive respiratory support should be attempted, even from relatively high $V_T$ (with corresponding high PIP values) and PEEP greater than or equal to 9 $cmH_2O$ (**Table 1**).

In our Unit, when mean arterial pressure (MAP) less than or equal to 14 $cmH_2O$ is reached with $Fio_2$ less than 40% to target higher $SpO_2$ values (≥92% [92%–95%] or ≥97% [97%–98%] in sBPD with PH) with satisfactory gas exchange and without increase in work of breathing for at least 24 hours, extubation to noninvasive respiratory support is attempted (see **Table 1**).

Reasonable tolerance limits during weaning and postextubation management could be (1) no more of 3 episodes of "spells" in 24 hours and/or 2 episodes in 2 consecutive hours; (2) reduction of the $SpO_2$ values at 85% to 90% for no more than 2 total hours per day; (3) reduction of the $SpO_2$ values at 80% to 85% for no more than 1 total hour per day; (4) no more than one brief episode of reduction in $SpO_2$ less than 80% over 24 hours that resolves without increasing more than 10% respect to the previous $Fio_2$ (see **Table 1**).

### Management of the Immediately Postextubation Period

After extubation, all infants should be adequately supported to provide adequate gas exchange, minimize V/Q mismatch, and promote growth rather than the sole purpose of avoiding reintubation. Different noninvasive ventilation (NIV) strategies are available:

1. Continuous positive airway pressure (CPAP): 10 to 14 $cmH_2O$. Maintaining a $Fio_2$ less than or equal to 0.40 to obtain $SpO_2$ values in the desired range (92%–95% and 97%–98% in sBPD with PH) will drive the slow reduction in the level of CPAP in the following days.

**Table 1**
**Suggested strategies to facilitate weaning from mechanical ventilation in infants with severe bronchopulmonary dysplasia**

| | |
|---|---|
| Weaning Strategies | Permissive hypercapnia<br>Slow and daily $Fio_2$ reduction (no more than 10%, respect to the previous a day) achieving $SpO_2$ targets (92%–95% or 95%–97% if sBPD and PH).<br>Tolerate relatively high $V_T$ and PEEP values |
| Attempt Extubation | MAP $\leq$ 14 cmH$_2$O for at least 24 h<br>$Fio_2$ < 40% achieving $SpO_2$ targets (92%–95% or 95%–97% if sBPD and PH) for at least 24 h<br>No increase of work of breathing |
| Tolerance Limits | No more of 3 episodes of "spells"in the 24 h and/or 2 in 2 consecutive hours;<br>Reduction of $SpO_2$ values 85%–90% for no more than 2 total hours per day;<br>Reduction of the $SpO_2$ values 80%–85% for no more than 1 total hour per day;<br>No more than one brief episode of reduction in $SpO_2$ <80% over 24 h that resolves without increasing more than 10% respect to the previous $Fio_2$ |
| Modify Noninvasive Respiratory Support and/or Consider Reintubation | Repeated episodes of apnea (>4 episodes of apnea per hour or >2 episodes of apnea per hour when ventilation with bag and mask was required)<br>Hypoxia (more than one prolonged episode of $SpO_2$ <80% over 24 h that resolves increasing more than 10% respect to the previous $Fio_{2)}$<br>Development of respiratory acidosis indicated by 2 consecutive blood gases ($Paco_2$ $\geq$65 mm Hg and pH <7.20)<br>Increased work of breathing |

2. Bilevel positive airway pressure or nasal intermittent positive pressure ventilation can be used as alternative to CPAP to improve oxygenation and/or ventilation.
3. Nasal high-frequency oscillatory ventilation (HFOV) as a rescue therapy to prevent the need for reintubation. We can start nasal HFOV if $Fio_2$ is greater than or equal to 0.50 and/or respiratory acidosis ($Pco_2$ >65 mm Hg [8.5 kPa] and pH <7.20) develops, despite optimal CPAP or noninvasive positive-pressure ventilation. The suggested starting parameters are as follows: MAP: 12 to 14 cmH$_2$O; I:E = 1:1; respiratory rate: 10 Hz; $\Delta$P: 25 to 30 cmH$_2$O.

The indications for modifying the parameters of NIV and/or considering reintubation should be (1) repeated episodes of apnea defined as greater than 4 episodes of apnea per hour or greater than 2 episodes of apnea per hour with bag and mask ventilation required; (2) hypoxia with more than 1 prolonged episode of reduction in $SpO_2$ less than 80% over 24 hours that resolves increasing more than 10% respect to the previous $Fio_2$; (3) development of respiratory acidosis indicated by 2 consecutive blood gases with $Paco_2$ greater than or equal to 65 mm Hg and pH <7.20; and (4) increased work of breathing (prolonged appareance and/or worsening of retractions [Silverman score >3] and/or tachypnea [respiratory rate >60 breaths/min]) (see **Table 1**).

### Weaning from Noninvasive Ventilation in Patients with Severe Bronchopulmonary Dysplasia

To the best of our knowledge, no studies have been conducted on weaning from NIV, particularly from CPAP and high-flow nasal cannula (HFNC) in the specific category of infants with established sBPD who require long-term NIV. In the literature, there are mainly generic indications for clinicians to use NIV in infants with sBPD. In these infants, an inadequate respiratory support can lead to many consequences such as poor somatic and pulmonary vascular bed growth and persistent V/Q mismatch that contributes to lung damage and subsequent development of PH.

Applying NIV with the aim of avoiding or limiting the duration of invasive respiratory support well beyond the immediate neonatal period cannot guarantee adequate respiratory support.

Indeed, infants diagnosed with evolving BPD, before the completion of the 36th week of PMA, can be well supported by NIV and undergo its progressive discontinuation. In these infants HFNC can be successfully used. The main perceived advantage of this technique is that the interface is simply to apply, less likely to cause skin trauma and better tolerated.

The NIV weaning strategy applicable to newborns with milder forms of BPD is more difficult to pursue in infants with established sBPD. In these infants, although there is no consensus on how to titrate the level of respiratory support, much attention is paid to suggest careful monitoring of the general health of the infant, his cardiorespiratory state, his tolerance to activities, and his growth.[7]

From a practical point of view, a scheme of weaning from NIV in infants with established sBPD has recently been proposed by Wright and colleagues.[10] To our knowledge these are the only investigators who address this topic by providing operational indications. They consider using NIV for long term only if the infant is able to maintain stability with no respiratory support or with only low oxygen flow when awake and requires NIV only during sleep (both night and naps) for a maximum of 16 hours/24 hours a day. Their approach is considered for both the infants on HFNC and the infants on CPAP. In infants on HFNC, in case of flow weaning failure, it is proposed to increase respiratory support by returning to the use of CPAP during sleep. If the conditions of the infant do not allow to gradually reduce the CPAP, the investigators suggest considering tracheostomy.

In our experience, HFNC represents a modality of respiratory support in infants with established sBPD, only after a period of CPAP and in which it has been possible to progressively reduce the pressure down to a value less than or equal to 6 $cmH_2O$ with a $Fio_2$ less than or equal to 0.25 (**Fig. 1**).

In this population of infants, a baseline CPAP greater than 8 $cmH_2O$ is generally required to counteract the increased pulmonary resistance and ensure adequate gas exchange.

We generally initiate the CPAP pressure reduction process in those infants who need a $Fio_2$ less than or equal to 0.25 to maintain the target SpO2 of 92% to 95%. In our experience, you need to proceed with caution before lowering your ongoing CPAP level: steps of CPAP reduction of 1 $cmH_2O$ every 48 to 72 hours are effective (see **Fig. 1**). An increase in $Fio_2$ greater than 30% for at least 6 hours, $Paco_2$ greater than 65 mm Hg, and pH <7.20 represent failure criteria. In this case, it is necessary to go back by setting the CPAP level of the previous step.

When the criteria for the transition to HFNC are reached and the need for noninvasive respiratory support persists, this modality of NIV is to be taken into consideration above all for the greater tolerance of the nasal aids that are more manageable for both the infant and the caregivers. HFNC allows a better interaction of the infant with the surrounding environment and is associated with a greater tolerance with a reduced nasal trauma. Generally, infants with established BPD need a starting flow rate greater than 6 L/min and sometimes up to 8 L/min.

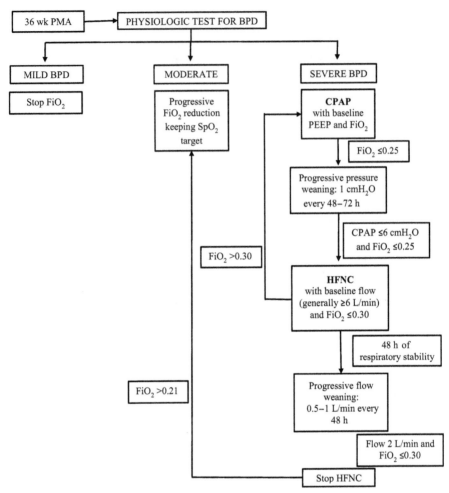

**Fig. 1.** Flow chart of the weaning from CPAP and HFNC in infants with established sBPD.

If after the transition from CPAP to HFNC there is an increase in $Fio_2$ greater than 0.30 and/or respiratory acidosis (pH <7.20 and $Paco_2 \geq 65$ mm Hg) and/or a Silvermann score greater than 3 and/or tachypnea (respiratory rate >60 breaths per minute) to maintain the target $SpO_2$ 92% to 95%, it is necessary to resume the previous CPAP setting.

If stability is maintained in HFNC for 48 hours, flow rate reduction can be performed subsequently. Based on our experience, it is necessary to wait at least 48 hours before being able to proceed with the reduction of 0.5 to 1 L/min until 2 L/min when discontinuation of HFNC is possible (see **Fig. 1**). Failure criteria include one of the following: increase in $Fio_2$ greater than 0.30 to maintain the target $SpO_2$ 92% to 95%; worsening blood gas with pH less than 7.20 and $Paco_2 \geq 65$ mm Hg; an increase in work of breathing with tachypnea (respiratory rate >60 breaths per minute) and/or Silverman score greater than 3; bradycardia or desaturation greater than 3 times within 1 hour or 1 episode of desaturation requiring positive pressure ventilation. In this case it is necessary to go back to the previous step that guaranteed respiratory stability and wait a further 48 to 72 hours before attempting a further reduction of the flow rate.

In conclusion, despite the widespread use of NIV also in the population of infants with established sBPD, no studies have been conducted on the best way of weaning CPAP or HFNC in this population. This certainly represents a research area to be developed in the near future.

SpO$_2$ target: 92% to 95%

For every step of CPAP or flow reduction, if the failure criteria are met, it is necessary to go back to the previous step that guaranteed respiratory stability.

## COMORBIDITES IMPAIRING WEANING

Various comorbidities, some not so rare, can coexist with BPD in preterm infants and affect the severity of lung disease, requiring interdisciplinary care. Beginning with treating the underlying disease can often allow the weaning of a baby apparently dependent on ventilation.

### Pulmonary Hypertension and Echocardiographic Investigation

The Pediatric Pulmonary Hypertension Network encouraged the use of standardized screening protocols for the evaluation of PH at 36 weeks PMA time for all infants with moderate or severe BPD.[11] It is known that PH contribute to the pathogenesis of BPD and can be diagnosed at later stages of disease.[12] It is strongly associated (up to 40%) with the severity of BPD, influencing the poor outcomes.[13] Performing echocardiogram at 36 weeks PMA should be a standardized screening protocol for all infants with any type of BPD to assess pulmonary pressure conditions. If echocardiogram screening demonstrates PH, recommendations suggest a follow-up initially frequent (1–2 weeks) to monitor response to interventions and then repeated less frequently (eg, monthly) related to clinical course.[11] A first approach is an adequate oxygen supplementation to avoid intermittent or chronic hypoxemia. The European network recommends maintaining systemic arterial O$_2$ saturation (SaO$_2$) of greater than 95% for proven BPD-associated pulmonary hypertension.[14] For specific argumentation on PH-targeted therapy in BPD we remand to recent updates.[11,15] Weaning from drugs can be considered after various echocardiograms showing resolution of PH.

### Other Investigations

Additional studies often include bronchoscopy for anatomic and dynamic airway lesions or gastrointestinal series, pH or impedance probe, and swallow studies. Atypical clinical features such as coughing, desaturation during feeds, cyanotic episodes, stridor, and abnormal cry warrant further investigations. This approach generally includes an extensive evaluation for structural airway abnormal anatomic and dynamic airway lesions (vocal cord paralysis, airway stenosis, tracheomalacia, and granulomas), assessment of bronchial hyperreactivity, chronic reflux, aspiration, and incoordinate swallow. Infants who have sBPD, inconsistent with their degree of prematurity, (eg, $\geq$ 29 weeks gestational age) should have lung computed tonography scan, genetic studies, and possible lung biopsy to evaluate the potential diagnosis of developmental lung diseases (alveolar capillary dysplasia, surfactant protein deficiencies, pulmonary lymphangiectasia)[16] (**Fig. 2**).

## TRACHEOSTOMY

Even using the best strategy, some infants with BPD cannot be weaned from invasive or NIV. For this reason, the tracheostomy has been increasingly performed in infants

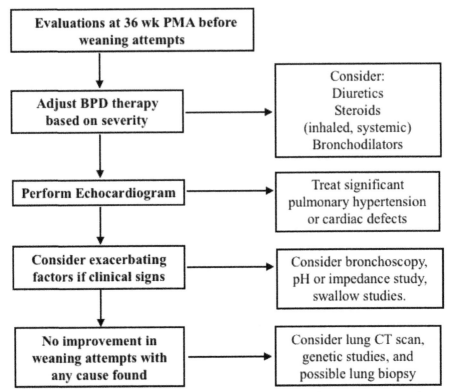

**Fig. 2.** Schematic approach for management of major comorbidities impairing weaning.

with BPD in the last decade.[17] In neonatal intensive care unit some infants remain intubated for months until the decision to perform a tracheostomy is taken. On one hand, this is due to the lack of randomized trials and strong evidence of benefits; on the other hand this decision is challenging because of the concern about the several complications of the procedure that could even be life threatening.[18–22] In a cohort of 304 infants born before the 30 week of gestation, DeMauro and colleagues showed that tracheostomy was associated with a significantly increased risk for the composite primary outcome of death or neurodevelopmental impairment (NDI).[20] Nevertheless, infants affected by severe BPD, who have been ventilated for long times, are at high risk for death or NDI, and tracheostomy may just be a marker for this risk.[20] Moreover, DeMauro and colleagues showed that the risk of death or developmental impairment at 18 to 22 months was significantly lower among infants who underwent tracheostomy before 120 days of life as compared with those who underwent tracheostomy after 120 days.[21] Earlier infant tracheostomy may facilitate long-term ventilation that may reduce work of breathing and promote growth. Tracheostomy decreases the need for pharmacologic sedation, allowing the infant to engage in developmentally appropriate activities such as physiotherapy sessions. Eventually, this could improve cognitive and motor outcomes for preterm infants.[19,23]

The decision to put a tracheostomy is even more complex in infants on NIV, who seems to be close to weaning, but sometimes remain on NIV for months. Clinicians should not forget that facial deformity, oromotor retardation, gastric distension, as well as substantial interference with daily activities and parental interactions are not insignificant risks of NIV.[24] Nevertheless, there is no published consensus opinion for optimal timing of tracheostomy in BPD infants. Based on literature data, tracheostomy in infants with BPD is usually performed between 40 and 50 weeks of PMA.[22,25] It is reasonable to begin considering tracheostomy as the infant approaches term gestation and still requires high-level respiratory support (either invasive mechanical ventilation or high-level noninvasive support).[26]

We suggest to verify eligibility of the baby assessing his respiratory state at term-equivalent age. This evaluation should take into account several parameters. An infant is likely to be soon weaned if he does not need an "aggressive" respiratory support in order to achieve and maintain all of these: (1) absence of severe respiratory distress (including retractions, head-bobbing, dyspnoea, and "spells"), (2) good growth (both weight gain and linear growth), (3) ability to participate in developmentally appropriate activities, (4) stability of BPD-associated pulmonary hypertension, if present, and (5) ability of feeding. We define respiratory support as "aggressive" if invasive mechanical ventilation is needed or when the baby is on NIV and he needs more than 40% oxygen or an MAP higher than 10 cmH$_2$O to maintain a stable SpO$_2$ values greater than or equal to 92% (92%–95%) or greater than or equal to 97% (97%–98%) in sBPD with PH. In a secondary analysis of data from a randomized trial about late surfactant in extremely preterm newborns, Wai and colleagues showed that differences in MAP over time between the tracheotomy and no tracheotomy groups diverged well before tracheotomy was performed.[25] They suggest that trends in MAP, as well as absolute MAP levels at 90 days of age, can be used to help guide clinical decisions regarding the timing of tracheotomy.[25] In case of doubt, a trend in increasing MAP between 36 and 40 weeks of PMA indicates the need to place a tracheostomy. After the decision is made and a tracheostomy is performed, a multidisciplinary team of specialists (including physicians, surgeons, nursing, respiratory therapists, physical therapists, speech therapists, audiologists, nutrition specialists) is needed to care for the patient.[21] This team is essential to ensure the good outcome of the procedure and avoid life-threatening complications as well.[21]

## DISCHARGE AT HOME OF INFANTS WITH SEVERE BRONCHOPULMONARY DISPLASIA

The 3 physiologic competencies that are generally recognized as essential before hospital discharge of the preterm infant are oral feeding sufficient to support appropriate growth, the ability to maintain normal body temperature in a home environment, and sufficiently mature respiratory control. Home oxygen therapy is, anyway, an option to facilitate discharge of infants with sBPD as an alternative to prolonged hospitalization. Determining the appropriate timing to safely discharge an oxygen-dependent infant from the hospital, after a stay in the neonatal intensive care unit, can be complicated. This decision is made based on the infant's medical stability and the availability of care providers. Clinically stable means stable oxygen requirement less than or equal to 30% for at least 2 weeks and less than or equal to 40% in babies mechanically ventilated with tracheostomy to maintain saturations greater than 92%. In addition, the infant needs to be able to tolerate a nutritional regimen that allows adequate growth.[27]

Discharge of the ventilator-/oxygen-dependent child requires a multidisciplinary approach. Greater than 30% of infants with BPD require supplemental oxygen at the time of discharge. Despite this there are no evidence-based guidelines or consensus statements regarding oxygen weaning in patients with BPD.[28]

In our unit in the last 2 years only 3 out of 51 (5.8%) patients with BPD have been discharged with home oxygen therapy. After discharge of patients with BPD, we first decrease flow rates and then the duration of time that the patient receives oxygen supplementation. Although there are no guidelines regarding oxygen weaning, experts recommend weaning oxygen during the day time first, followed by weaning oxygen at night time.[29] Some investigators recommend obtaining a polysomnogram to rule out nocturnal hypoxemia before oxygen weaning.[30] Clinical criteria including growth and clinical examination have to guide weaning oxygen supplementation in addition to monitoring oxygen saturations. It is important to note that in addition to oxygen saturation, achieving adequate somatic growth and prevention or resolution of the signs of PH are important outcomes to consider before discontinuing supplemental oxygen therapy. When growth is poor, the use of nocturnal oxygen may need to be extended.[6] In our experience all the babies have been weaned within 12 months of PMA.

## BEST PRACTICES BOX

What is the current practice for the ventilator management of patients affected by severe bronchopulmonary dysplasia
*To adopt the similar ventilator strategies used during the acute phase of neonatal lung disease.*

What changes in current practice are likely to improve outcomes?
*The goals of mechanical ventilation in the infants with severe bronchopulmonary dysplasia (sBPD) are to reach adequate gas exchange, to minimize ventilation/perfusion mismatch, to provide relatively stable respiratory support reducing the work of breathing and respiratory distress (no retractions, no tachypnea, no recurrent cyanotic or bradycardic episodes), reducing the need for chronic sedation, preventing the development or progression of pulmonary hypertension and promoting optimal growth (both somatic and alveolar/vascular growth);*

Is there a Clinical Algorithm? If so, please include
*Table 1: Algorithm to facilitate weaning from invasive mechanical ventilation in infants with with severe bronchopulmonary dysplasia (sBPD).*
*Figure 1: Flow chart to facilitate weaning from non invasive mechanical ventilation (CPAP, HFNC) in infants with with severe bronchopulmonary dysplasia (sBPD).*
Figure 2: Flow chart for the approach for management of major comorbidities impairing weaning.

## CLINICAL CARE POINTS

- Identifying phenotypical presentation of severe bronchopulmonary dysplasia (sBPD) and its underlying lung pathology represents the first important step in determining the appropriate individual management strategy in each patient;

- The invasive ventilation strategy for patients affected by sBPD includes slow-rate (10-20/min), high tidal volume ($V_T$) (8-12 ml/kg with peak inspiratory pressure to generate this $V_T$ often well above 25 cm $H_2O$) and prolonged inspiratory time (Ti) (0.5-0.8 seconds), providing in association adequate positive end-expiratory pressure, major than 8-10 cm $H_2O$ and eventual adequate pressure support (PS) for spontaneous breaths, helping minute ventilation maintenance and achieving overall low respiratory rate.

- The focus is to slowly and daily reduce the oxygen concentration (no more than 10%, respect to the previous $FiO_2$ a day) achieving $SpO_2$targets. When infants are stable for at least 24 hours in less than 40% $FiO_2$with satisfactory gas exchange and without increase in work of breathing (Silverman score $\leq$ 3), extubation to non-invasive respiratory support should be attempted, even from relatively high $V_T$, high PEEP values ($\geq$ 9 cm $H_2O$) and high MAP values ($\leq$ 14 cm$H_2O$).

## DISCLOSURE

The authors have nothing to disclose.

## REFERENCES

1. Thébaud B, Goss KN, Laughon M, et al. Bronchopulmonary dysplasia. Nat Rev Dis Primers 2019;5(1):78.
2. Jobe AH, Bancalari E. Bronchopulmonary dysplasia. Am J Respir Crit Care Med 2001;163(7):1723–9.
3. Walsh MC, Wilson-Costello D, Zadell A, et al. Safety, reliability, and validity of a physiologic definition of bronchopulmonary dysplasia. J Perinatol 2003;23(6): 451–6.
4. Higgins RD, Jobe AH, Koso-Thomas M, et al. Bronchopulmonary dysplasia: executive summary of a workshop. J Pediatr 2018;197:300–8.
5. Vento G, Vendettuoli V, Aurilia C, et al. A modified physiologic test for bronchopulmonary dysplasia: a clinical tool for weaning from CPAP and/or oxygen-therapy the premature babies? Ital J Pediatr 2019;45(1):2.
6. Abman SH, Collaco JM, Shepherd EG, et al. Bronchopulmonary dysplasia collaborative. Interdisciplinary care of children with severe bronchopulmonary dysplasia. J Pediatr 2017;181:12–28.e1.
7. Jensen EA, Dysart K, Gantz MG, et al. The diagnosis of bronchopulmonary dysplasia in very preterm infants: an evidence- based approach. Am J Respir Crit Care Med 2019;200(6):751–9.
8. Zhang H, Fox WW. Management of the infant with bronchopulmonary dysplasia. In: Goldsmith JP, Karotkin EH, Keszler M, et al. Assisted ventilation of the neonate: an evidence-based approach to newborn respiratory care. Sixth edition. USA: Elsevier; 2016. 380-390.
9. Abman SH, Nelin LD. Management of the infant with severe bronchopulmonary dysplasia. In: Bancalari E, editor. The newborn lung: neonatology questions and controversies. Philadelphia (PA): Elsevier Saunders; 2012. p. 407–25.
10. Wright MFA, Wallis C. Investigation and management of the long-term ventilated premature infant. Early Hum Dev 2018;126:10–7.
11. Krishnan U, Feinstein JA, Adatia I, et al. Evaluation and management of pulmonary hypertension in children with bronchopulmonary dysplasia. J Pediatr 2017;188:24–34.e1.
12. Kinsella JP, Greenough A, Abman SH. Bronchopulmonary dysplasia. Lancet 2006;367(9520):1421–31.
13. Venkataraman R, Kamaluddeen M, Hasan SU, et al. Intratracheal Administration of budesonide-surfactant in prevention of bronchopulmonary dysplasia in very low birth weight infants: a systematic review and meta-analysis. Pediatr Pulmonol 2017;52(7):968–75.
14. Hilgendorff A, Apitz C, Bonnet D, et al. Pulmonary hypertension associated with acute or chronic lung diseases in the preterm and term neonate and infant. The

European Paediatric Pulmonary Vascular Disease Network, endorsed by ISHLT and DGPK. Heart 2016;102(Suppl 2):ii49–56.

15. Berkelhamer S, Mestan KK, Steinhorn R. An update on the diagnosis and management of bronchopulmonary dysplasia (BPD)-associated pulmonary hypertension. Semin Perinatol 2018;42(7):432–43.

16. Kurland G, Deterding RR, Hagood JS, et al. An official American Thoracic Society clinical practice guideline: classification, evaluation, and management of childhood interstitial lung disease in infancy. Am J Respir Crit Care Med 2013; 188(3):376–94.

17. Wang CS, Kou Y, Shah GB, et al. Tracheostomy in extremely preterm neonates in the United States: a cross-sectional analysis. Laryngoscope 2019;130(8): 2056–62.

18. Walsh J, Rastatter J. Neonatal tracheostomy. Clin Perinatol 2018;45:805–16.

19. Akangire G, Taylor GB, McAnany S, et al. Respiratory, growth, and survival outcomes of infants with tracheostomy and ventilator dependence. Pediatr Res 2020;1–9.

20. DeMauro SB, D'Agostino JA, Bann C, et al. Developmental outcomes of very preterm infants with Tracheostomies. J Pediatr 2014;164(6):1303–10.

21. DeMauro SB, Wei JL, Lin RJ. Perspectives on neonatal and infant tracheostomy. Semin Fetal Neonatal Med 2016;21:285–91.

22. Upadhyay K, Vallarino DA, Talati AJ. Outcomes of neonates with tracheostomy secondary to bronchopulmonary dysplasia. BMC Pediatr 2020;20(1):414.

23. Luo J, Shepard S, Nilan K, et al. Improved growth and developmental activity post tracheostomy in preterm infants with severe BPD. Pediatr Pulmonol 2018; 53(9):1237–44.

24. Rabatin JT, Gay PC. Noninvasive ventilation. Mayo Clin Proc 1999;74: 817–20, 40.

25. Wai KC, Keller RL, Lusk LA, et al. Characteristics of extremely low gestational age newborns undergoing tracheotomy: a secondary analysis of the trial of late surfactant randomized clinical trial. JAMA Otolaryngol Head Neck Surg 2017; 143(1):13–9.

26. Koltsida G, Konstantinopoulou S. Long term outcomes in chronic lung disease requiring tracheostomy and chronic mechanical ventilation. Semin Fetal Neonatal Med 2019;24(5):101044.

27. American Academy of Pediatrics Committee on Fetus and Newborn. Hospital discharge of the high-risk neonate. Pediatr Actions 2008;122(5):1119–26.

28. Palm K, Simoneau T, Sawicki G, et al. Assessment of current strategies for weaning premature infants from supplemental oxygen in the outpatient setting. Adv Neonatal Care 2011;11:349–56.

29. Bancalari E, Wilson Costello D, Iben SC. Management of infants with bronchopulmonarydysplasia in North America. EarlyHumDev 2005;81:171–9.

30. Khetan R, Hurley M, Spencer S, et al. Bronchopulmonary dysplasia within and beyond the neonatal unit. Adv Neonatal Care 2016;16:17–25.

# UNITED STATES POSTAL SERVICE® Statement of Ownership, Management, and Circulation (All Periodicals Publications Except Requester Publications)

| 1. Publication Title | 2. Publication Number | | 3. Filing Date |
|---|---|---|---|
| CLINICS IN PERINATOLOGY | 001 – 744 | | 9/18/2021 |

| 4. Issue Frequency | 5. Number of Issues Published Annually | 6. Annual Subscription Price |
|---|---|---|
| MAR, JUN, SEP, DEC | 4 | $321.00 |

7. Complete Mailing Address of Known Office of Publication (Not printer) (Street, city, county, state, and ZIP+4®)

ELSEVIER INC.
230 Park Avenue, Suite 800
New York, NY 10169

Contact Person
Malathi Samayan
Telephone (Include area code)
91-44-4299-4507

8. Complete Mailing Address of Headquarters or General Business Office of Publisher (Not printer)

ELSEVIER INC.
230 Park Avenue, Suite 800
New York, NY 10169

9. Full Names and Complete Mailing Addresses of Publisher, Editor, and Managing Editor (Do not leave blank)

Publisher (Name and complete mailing address)

DOLORES MELONI, ELSEVIER INC.
1600 JOHN F KENNEDY BLVD. SUITE 1800
PHILADELPHIA, PA 19103-2899

Editor (Name and complete mailing address)

KERRY HOLLAND, ELSEVIER INC.
1600 JOHN F KENNEDY BLVD. SUITE 1800
PHILADELPHIA, PA 19103-2899

Managing Editor (Name and complete mailing address)

PATRICK MANLEY, ELSEVIER INC.
1600 JOHN F KENNEDY BLVD. SUITE 1800
PHILADELPHIA, PA 19103-2899

10. Owner (Do not leave blank. If the publication is owned by a corporation, give the name and address of the corporation immediately followed by the names and addresses of all stockholders owning or holding 1 percent or more of the total amount of stock. If not owned by a corporation, give the names and addresses of the individual owners. If owned by a partnership or other unincorporated firm, give its name and address as well as those of each individual owner. If the publication is published by a nonprofit organization, give its name and address.)

| Full Name | Complete Mailing Address |
|---|---|
| WHOLLY OWNED SUBSIDIARY OF REED/ELSEVIER, US HOLDINGS | 1600 JOHN F KENNEDY BLVD. SUITE 1800 PHILADELPHIA, PA 19103-2899 |

11. Known Bondholders, Mortgagees, and Other Security Holders Owning or Holding 1 Percent or More of Total Amount of Bonds, Mortgages, or Other Securities. If none, check box ▶ ☐ None

| Full Name | Complete Mailing Address |
|---|---|
| N/A | |

12. Tax Status (For completion by nonprofit organizations authorized to mail at nonprofit rates) (Check one)
The purpose, function, and nonprofit status of this organization and the exempt status for federal income tax purposes:
☒ Has Not Changed During Preceding 12 Months
☐ Has Changed During Preceding 12 Months (Publisher must submit explanation of change with this statement)

PS Form 3526, July 2014 [Page 1 of 4 (see instructions page 4)]   PSN: 7530-01-000-9931   PRIVACY NOTICE: See our privacy policy on www.usps.com.

---

| 13. Publication Title | | 14. Issue Date for Circulation Data Below |
|---|---|---|
| CLINICS IN PERINATOLOGY | | JUNE 2021 |

| 15. Extent and Nature of Circulation | | | Average No. Copies Each Issue During Preceding 12 Months | No. Copies of Single Issue Published Nearest to Filing Date |
|---|---|---|---|---|
| a. Total Number of Copies (Net press run) | | | 564 | 492 |
| b. Paid Circulation (By Mail and Outside the Mail) | (1) | Mailed Outside-County Paid Subscriptions Stated on PS Form 3541 (Include paid distribution above nominal rate, advertiser's proof copies, and exchange copies) | 427 | 378 |
| | (2) | Mailed In-County Paid Subscriptions Stated on PS Form 3541 (Include paid distribution above nominal rate, advertiser's proof copies, and exchange copies) | 0 | 0 |
| | (3) | Paid Distribution Outside the Mails Including Sales Through Dealers and Carriers, Street Vendors, Counter Sales, and Other Paid Distribution Outside USPS® | 103 | 77 |
| | (4) | Paid Distribution by Other Classes of Mail Through the USPS (e.g. First-Class Mail®) | 0 | 0 |
| c. Total Paid Distribution (Sum of 15b (1), (2), (3), and (4)) | | ▶ | 530 | 455 |
| d. Free or Nominal Rate Distribution (By Mail and Outside the Mail) | (1) | Free or Nominal Rate Outside-County Copies Included on PS Form 3541 | 16 | 19 |
| | (2) | Free or Nominal Rate In-County Copies Included on PS Form 3541 | 0 | 0 |
| | (3) | Free or Nominal Rate Copies Mailed at Other Classes Through the USPS (e.g. First-Class Mail) | 0 | 0 |
| | (4) | Free or Nominal Rate Distribution Outside the Mail (Carriers or other means) | 0 | 0 |
| e. Total Free or Nominal Rate Distribution (Sum of 15d (1), (2), (3) and (4)) | | ▶ | 16 | 19 |
| f. Total Distribution (Sum of 15c and 15e) | | ▶ | 546 | 474 |
| g. Copies not Distributed (See Instructions to Publishers #4 (page #3)) | | ▶ | 18 | 18 |
| h. Total (Sum of 15f and g) | | ▶ | 564 | 492 |
| i. Percent Paid (15c divided by 15f times 100) | | ▶ | 97.06% | 95.99% |

* If you are claiming electronic copies, go to line 16 on page 3. If you are not claiming electronic copies, skip to line 17 on page 3.

| 16. Electronic Copy Circulation | | Average No. Copies Each Issue During Preceding 12 Months | No. Copies of Single Issue Published Nearest to Filing Date |
|---|---|---|---|
| a. Paid Electronic Copies | ▶ | | |
| b. Total Paid Print Copies (Line 15c) + Paid Electronic Copies (Line 16a) | ▶ | | |
| c. Total Print Distribution (Line 15f) + Paid Electronic Copies (Line 16a) | ▶ | | |
| d. Percent Paid (Both Print & Electronic Copies) (16b divided by 16c × 100) | ▶ | | |

☒ I certify that 50% of all my distributed copies (electronic and print) are paid above a nominal price.

17. Publication of Statement of Ownership

☒ If the publication is a general publication, publication of this statement is required. Will be printed in the DECEMBER 2021 issue of this publication.   ☐ Publication not required.

18. Signature and Title of Editor, Publisher, Business Manager, or Owner

Malathi Samayan   Malathi Samayan - Distribution Controller   Date 9/18/2021

I certify that all information furnished on this form is true and complete. I understand that anyone who furnishes false or misleading information on this form or who omits material or information requested on the form may be subject to criminal sanctions (including fines and imprisonment) and/or civil sanctions (including civil penalties).

PS Form 3526, July 2014 (Page 3 of 4)   PRIVACY NOTICE: See our privacy policy on www.usps.com

Printed and bound by CPI Group (UK) Ltd, Croydon, CR0 4YY

03/10/2024

01040467-0005